ANNUAL EDITIONS

Aging 10/11

Twenty-Third Edition

P9-CAL-524

EDITOR

Harold Cox
Indiana State University

Harold Cox, professor of sociology at Indiana State University, has published several articles in the field of gerontology. He is the author of *Later Life: The Realities of Aging* (Prentice Hall, 2006). He is a member of the Gerontological Society of America and the American Sociological Association's Occupation and Professions Section and Youth Aging Section.

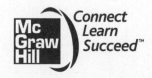

McGraw Hill

Connect
Learn
Succeed™

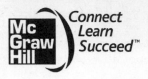

The McGraw-Hill Companies

Mc Graw Hill

Connect
Learn
Succeed™

ANNUAL EDITIONS: AGING, TWENTY-THIRD EDITION

Published by McGraw-Hill, a business unit of The McGraw-Hill Companies, Inc., 1221 Avenue of the Americas, New York, NY 10020. Copyright © 2011 by The McGraw-Hill Companies, Inc. All rights reserved. Previous edition(s) 2008, 2009, 2010. No part of this publication may be reproduced or distributed in any form or by any means, or stored in a database or retrieval system, without the prior written consent of The McGraw-Hill Companies, Inc., including, but not limited to, in any network or other electronic storage or transmission, or broadcast for distance learning.

Some ancillaries, including electronic and print components, may not be available to customers outside the United States.

Annual Editions® is a registered trademark of The McGraw-Hill Companies, Inc.

Annual Editions is published by the **Contemporary Learning Series** group within the McGraw-Hill Higher Education division.

1 2 3 4 5 6 7 8 9 0 WDQ/WDQ 1 0 9 8 7 6 5 4 3 2 1 0

ISBN 978–0–07–805059–6
MHID 0–07–805059–6
ISSN 0272–3808

Managing Editor: *Larry Loeppke*
Developmental Editor: *Debra Henricks*
Editorial Coordinator: *Mary Foust*
Editorial Assistant: *Cindy Hedley*
Production Service Assistant: *Rita Hingtgen*
Permissions Coordinator: *DeAnna Dausner*
Senior Marketing Manager: *Julie Keck*
Senior Marketing Communications Specialist: *Mary Klein*
Marketing Coordinator: *Alice Link*
Director Specialized Production: *Faye Schilling*
Senior Project Manager: *Joyce Watters*
Design Coordinator: *Margarite Reynolds*
Production Supervisor: *Sue Culbertson*
Cover Graphics: *Kristine Jubeck*

Compositor: Laserwords Private Limited
Cover Images: © Digital Vision/Getty Images (inset); © Corbis/RF (background)

Library in Congress Cataloging-in-Publication Data
Main entry under title: Annual Editions: Aging. 2010/2011.
   1. Aging—Periodicals. I. Cox, Harold, *comp*. II. Title: Aging.
658'.05

www.mhhe.com

Editors/Academic Advisory Board

Members of the Academic Advisory Board are instrumental in the final selection of articles for each edition of ANNUAL EDITIONS. Their review of articles for content, level, and appropriateness provides critical direction to the editors and staff. We think that you will find their careful consideration well reflected in this volume.

ANNUAL EDITIONS: Aging 10/11
23rd Edition

EDITOR

Harold Cox
Indiana State University

ACADEMIC ADVISORY BOARD MEMBERS

Preface

In publishing ANNUAL EDITIONS we recognize the enormous role played by the magazines, newspapers, and journals of the public press in providing current, first-rate educational information in a broad spectrum of interest areas. Many of these articles are appropriate for students, researchers, and professionals seeking accurate, current material to help bridge the gap between principles and theories and the real world. These articles, however, become more useful for study when those of lasting value are carefully collected, organized, indexed, and reproduced in a low-cost format, which provides easy and permanent access when the material is needed. That is the role played by ANNUAL EDITIONS.

The decline of the crude birth rate in the United States and other industrialized nations combined with improving food supplies, sanitation, and medical technology has resulted in an ever-increasing number and percentage of people remaining alive and healthy well into their retirement years. The result is a shifting age composition of the populations in these nations—a population composed of fewer people under age 20 and more people 65 and older. In 1900, in the United States, approximately 3 million Americans were 65 years old and above, and they comprised 4 percent of the population. In 2000, there were 36 million persons 65 years old and above, and they represented 13 percent of the total population. The most rapid increase in the number of older persons is expected between 2010 and 2030, when the "baby boom" generation reaches the age of 65. Demographers predict that by 2030 there will be 66 million older persons representing approximately 22 percent of the total population. The growing number of older people has made many of the problems of aging immediately visible to the average American. These problems have become widespread topics of concern for political leaders, government planners, and average citizens. Moreover, the aging of the population has become perceived as a phenomenon of the United States and the industrialized countries of Western Europe—it is also occurring in the underdeveloped countries of the world as well. An increasing percentage of the world's population is now defined as aged.

Today, almost all middle-aged people expect to live to retirement age and beyond. Both the middle-aged and the elderly have pushed for solutions to the problems confronting older Americans. Everyone seems to agree that granting the elderly a secure and comfortable status is desirable. Voluntary associations, communities, and state and federal governments have committed themselves to improving the lives of older persons. Many programs for senior citizens, both public and private, have emerged in the last 50 years.

The change in the age composition of the population has not gone unnoticed by the media or the academic community. The number of articles appearing in the popular press and professional journals has increased dramatically over the last several years. While scientists have been concerned with the aging process for some time, in the last three decades there has been an expanding volume of research and writing on this subject. This growing interest has resulted in this twenty-third edition of *Annual Editions: Aging 10/11.*

This volume is representative of the field of gerontology in that it is interdisciplinary in its approach, including articles from the biological sciences, medicine, nursing, psychology, sociology, and social work. The articles are taken from the popular press, government publications, and scientific journals. They represent a wide cross-section of authors, perspectives, and issues related to the aging process. They were chosen because they address the most relevant and current problems in the field of aging and present a variety of divergent views on the appropriate solutions to these problems. The topics covered include demographic trends, the aging process, longevity, social attitudes toward old age, problems and potentials of aging, retirement, death, living environments in later life, and social policies, programs, and services for older Americans. The articles are organized into an anthology that is useful for both the student and the teacher.

The goal of *Annual Editions: Aging 10/11* is to choose articles that are pertinent, well written, and helpful to those concerned with the field of gerontology. Comments, suggestions, or constructive criticism are welcomed to help improve future editions of this book. Please complete and return the postage-paid article rating form on the last page of this volume. Any anthology can be improved. This one will continue to be improved—annually.

Harold Cox

Harold Cox
Editor

Contents

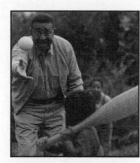

UNIT 1
The Phenomenon of Aging

The concepts in bold italics are developed in the article. For further expansion, please refer to the Topic Guide.

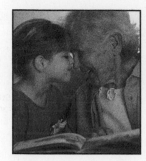

UNIT 2
The Quality of Later Life

UNIT 3
Societal Attitudes toward Old Age

The concepts in bold italics are developed in the article. For further expansion, please refer to the Topic Guide.

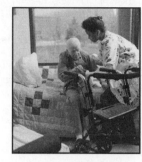

UNIT 4
Problems and Potentials of Aging

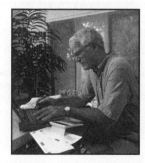

UNIT 5
Retirement: American Dream or Dilemma?

The concepts in bold italics are developed in the article. For further expansion, please refer to the Topic Guide.

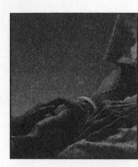

UNIT 6
The Experience of Dying

The concepts in bold italics are developed in the article. For further expansion, please refer to the Topic Guide.

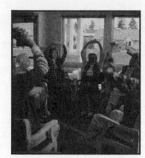

UNIT 7
Living Environment in Later Life

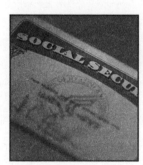

UNIT 8
Social Policies, Programs, and Services
for Older Americans

The concepts in bold italics are developed in the article. For further expansion, please refer to the Topic Guide.

The concepts in bold italics are developed in the article. For further expansion, please refer to the Topic Guide.

Correlation Guide

The *Annual Editions* series provides students with convenient, inexpensive access to current, carefully selected articles from the public press. **Annual Editions: Aging 10/11** is an easy-to-use reader that presents articles on important topics such as *living longer, retirement, health care, dying,* and many more. For more information on *Annual Editions* and other *McGraw-Hill Contemporary Learning Series* titles, visit www.mhhe.com/cls.

This convenient guide matches the units in **Annual Editions: Aging 10/11** with the corresponding chapters in two of our best-selling McGraw-Hill Aging textbooks by Quadagno and Hoyer/Roodin.

Annual Editions: Aging 10/11	Aging and The Life Course: An Introduction to Social Gerontology, 5/e by Quadagno	Adult Development and Aging, 6/e by Hoyer/Roodin
Unit 1: The Phenomenon of Aging	**Chapter 1:** The Field of Social Gerontology **Chapter 2:** Life Course Transitions **Chapter 3:** Theories of Aging	**Chapter 1:** Adult Development and Aging: An Introduction **Chapter 3:** Physiological and Sensory Processes
Unit 2: The Quality of Later Life	**Chapter 6:** Biological Perspectives on Aging	**Chapter 2:** Cultural and Ethnic Diversity **Chapter 3:** Physiological and Sensory Processes
Unit 3: Societal Attitudes toward Old Age	**Chapter 7:** Psychological Perspectives on Aging	**Chapter 2:** Cultural and Ethnic Diversity **Chapter 3:** Physiological and Sensory Processes **Chapter 5:** Mental Health
Unit 4: Problems and Potentials of Aging	**Chapter 6:** Biological Perspectives on Aging **Chapter 7:** Psychological Perspectives on Aging **Chapter 8:** Family Relationships and Social Support Systems **Chapter 11:** Health and Health Care **Chapter 12:** Caring for the Frail Elderly	**Chapter 4:** Coping and Adaptation **Chapter 5:** Mental Health **Chapter 6:** Physical Health **Chapter 7:** Memory, Attention, and Learning **Chapter 11:** Relationships
Unit 5: Retirement: American Dream or Dilemma?	**Chapter 10:** Work and Retirement **Chapter 14:** The Economics of Aging	**Chapter 12:** Work, Leisure, and Retirement
Unit 6: The Experience of Dying	**Chapter 13:** Death, Dying and Bereavement	**Chapter 13:** Approaching Death
Unit 7: Living Environment in Later Life	**Chapter 8:** Family Relationships and Social Support Systems **Chapter 9:** Living Arrangements **Chapter 12:** Caring for the Frail Elderly **Chapter 15:** Poverty and Inequality	**Chapter 11:** Relationships **Chapter 13:** Approaching Death
Unit 8: Social Policies, Programs, and Services for Older Americans	**Chapter 4:** Demography of Aging **Chapter 5:** Old Age and the Welfare State **Chapter 11:** Health and Health Care **Chapter 14:** The Economics of Aging **Chapter 15:** Poverty and Inequality **Chapter 16:** The Politics of Aging	**Chapter 12:** Work, Leisure, and Retirement **Chapter 13:** Approaching Death

Topic Guide

This topic guide suggests how the selections in this book relate to the subjects covered in your course. You may want to use the topics listed on these pages to search the Web more easily.

On the following pages a number of websites have been gathered specifically for this book. They are arranged to reflect the units of this Annual Editions reader. You can link to these sites by going to *http://www.mhhe.com/cls.*

All the articles that relate to each topic are listed below the bold-faced term.

Internet References

The following Internet sites have been selected to support the articles found in this reader. These sites were available at the time of publication. However, because websites often change their structure and content, the information listed may no longer be available. We invite you to visit http://www.mhhe.com/cls for easy access to these sites.

Annual Editions: Aging 10/11

General Sources

Alliance for Aging Research
http://www.agingresearch.org

The nation's leading nonprofit organization dedicated to improving the health and independence of Americans as they age through public and private funding of medical research and geriatric education.

ElderCare Online
http://www.ec-online.net

This site provides numerous links to eldercare resources. Information on health, living, aging, finance, and social issues can be found here.

FirstGov
http://www.firstgov.gov

Whatever you want or need from the U.S. government, it's here on FirstGov.gov. You'll find a rich treasure of online information, services, and resources.

UNIT 1: The Phenomenon of Aging

The Aging Research Centre
http://www.arclab.org

The Aging Research Centre is dedicated to providing a service that allows researchers to find information that is related to the study of the aging process.

Centenarians
http://www.hcoa.org/centenarians/centenarians.htm

There are approximately 70,000 centenarians in the United States. This site provides resources and information for and about centenarians.

National Center for Health Statistics
http://www.cdc.gov/nchs/agingact.htm

NCHS is the federal government's principal vital and health statistics agency. NCHS is a part of the Centers for Disease Control and Prevention, U.S. Department of Health and Human Services.

UNIT 2: The Quality of Later Life

Aging with Dignity
http://www.agingwithdignity.org

The nonprofit Aging with Dignity was established to provide people with the practical information, advice, and legal tools needed to help their loved ones get proper care.

The Gerontological Society of America
http://www.geron.org

The Gerontological Society of America promotes the scientific study of aging, and it fosters growth and diffusion of knowledge relating to problems of aging and of the sciences contributing to their understanding.

The National Council on the Aging
http://www.ncoa.org

The National Council on the Aging, Inc., is a center of leadership and nationwide expertise in the issues of aging. This private, nonprofit association is committed to enhancing the field of aging through leadership, service, education, and advocacy.

UNIT 3: Societal Attitudes toward Old Age

Adult Development and Aging: Division 20 of the American Psychological Association
http://www.iog.wayne.edu/APADIV20/APADIV20.HTM

This group is dedicated to studying the psychology of adult development and aging.

American Society on Aging
http://www.asaging.org/index.cfm

The American Society on Aging is the largest and most dynamic network of professionals in the field of aging.

Canadian Psychological Association
http://www.cpa.ca

This is the contents page of the Canadian Psychological Association. Material on aging and human development can be found at this site.

UNIT 4: Problems and Potentials of Aging

Alzheimer's Association
http://www.alz.org

The Alzheimer's Association is dedicated to researching the prevention, cures, and treatments of Alzheimer's disease and related disorders and providing support and assistance to afflicted patients and their families.

A.P.T.A. Section on Geriatrics
http://geriatricspt.org

This is a component of the American Physical Therapy Association. At this site, information regarding consumer and health information for older adults can be found.

Caregiver's Handbook
http://www.acsu.buffalo.edu/~drstall/hndbk0.html

This site is an online handbook for caregivers. Topics include nutrition, medical aspects of caregiving, and liabilities of caregiving.

Caregiver Survival Resources
http://www.caregiver.com

Information on books, and seminars and information for caregivers can be found at this site.

AARP Health Information
http://www.aarp.org/bulletin

Information on a BMI calculator, the USDA food pyramid, healthy recipes, and health-related articles can be found at this site.

Internet References

International Food Information Council
http://www.ific.org

At this site, you can find information regarding nutritional needs for aging adults. The site focuses on information for educators and students, publications, and nutritional information.

University of California at Irvine: Institute for Brain Aging and Dementia
http://www.alz.uci.edu

The Institute for Brain Aging and Dementia is dedicated to the study of Alzheimer's and the causes of mental disabilities for the elderly.

UNIT 5: Retirement: American Dream or Dilemma?

American Association of Retired People
http://www.aarp.org

The AARP is the nation's leading organization for people 50 and older. AARP serves their needs through information, education, advocacy, and community service.

Health and Retirement Study (HRS)
http://www.umich.edu/~hrswww

The University of Michigan Health and Retirement Study surveys more than 22,000 Americans over the age of 50 every two years. Supported by the National Institute on Aging, the study paints an emerging portrait of an aging America: physical and mental health, insurance coverage, financial status, family support systems, labor market status, and retirement planning.

UNIT 6: The Experience of Dying

Agency for Health Care Policy and Research
http://www.ahcpr.gov

Information on the dying process in the context of U.S. health policy is provided here, along with a search mechanism. The agency is part of the Department of Health and Human Services.

Growth House, Inc.
http://www.growthhouse.org

This award-winning website is an international gateway to resources for life-threatening illness and end-of-life care.

Hospice Foundation of America
http://www.HospiceFoundation.org

On this page, you can learn about hospice care, how to select a hospice, and how to find a hospice near you.

UNIT 7: Living Environment in Later Life

American Association of Homes and Services for the Aging
http://www.aahsa.org

The American Association of Homes and Services for the Aging represents a not-for-profit organization dedicated to providing high-quality health care, housing, and services to the nation's elderly.

Center for Demographic Studies
http://cds.duke.edu

The Center for Demographic Studies is located in the heart of the Duke campus. The primary focus of its research is long-term care for elderly populations, specifically those 65 years of age and older.

Guide to Retirement Living Online
http://www.retirement-living.com

An online version of a free publication, this site provides information about nursing homes, continuous care communities, independent living, home health care, and adult day care centers.

The United States Department of Housing and Urban Development
http://www.hud.gov

News regarding housing for aging adults can be found at this site sponsored by the U.S. federal government.

UNIT 8: Social Policies, Programs, and Services for Older Americans

Administration on Aging
http://www.aoa.dhhs.gov

This site, housed on the Department of Health and Human Services website, provides information for older persons and their families. There is also information for educators and students regarding the elderly.

American Federation for Aging Research
http://www.afar.org

Since 1981, the American Federation for Aging Research (AFAR) has helped scientists begin and further careers in aging research and geriatric medicine.

American Geriatrics Society
http://www.americangeriatrics.org

This organization addresses the needs of our rapidly aging population. At this site, you can find information on health care and other social issues facing the elderly.

Community Transportation Association of America
http://www.ctaa.org

C.T.A.A. is a nonprofit organization dedicated to mobility for all people, regardless of wealth, disability, age, or accessibility.

Consumer Reports State Inspection Surveys
http://www.ConsumerReports.org

To learn how to get state inspection surveys and to contact the ombudsman's office, click on "Personal Finance," then select "Assisted Living."

Medicare Consumer Information from the Health Care Finance Association
http://cms.hhs.gov/default.asp?fromhcfadotgov=true

This site is devoted to explaining Medicare and Medicaid costs to consumers.

National Institutes of Health
http://www.nih.gov

Information on health issues can be found at this government site. There is quite a bit of information relating to health issues and the aging population in the United States.

The United States Senate: Special Committee on Aging
http://www.senate.gov/~aging

This committee, chaired by Senator Gordon Smith of Oregon, deals with the issues surrounding the elderly in America. At this site, you can download committee hearing information, news, and committee publications.

UNIT 1

The Phenomenon of Aging

Unit Selections

1. **Elderly Americans,** Christine L. Himes
2. **You Can Stop "Normal" Aging,** Dr. Henry S. Lodge
3. **Living Longer: Diet and Exercise,** Donna Jackson Nakazawa and Susan Crandell
4. **Secrets to Longevity,** Cathy Gulli
5. **Will You Live to Be 100?,** Thomas Perls and Margery Hutter Silver
6. **Faulty Fountains of Youth,** Patrick Barry

Key Points to Consider

- What factors contribute to the increasing life expectancy of the American people? What challenges do aging Americans face?

- Why are older Americans healthier than ever before?

- Will it ever be possible to slow down the aging process? Would this be desirable? Why or why not?

- What do centenarians living in *blue zones* believe are the factors that contribute to their long and healthy lives?

- In "Living Longer: Science," what changes are recommended in the areas of diet, environment, exercise, and stress to increase the individual's health and longevity?

Student Website
www.mhhe.com/cls

Internet References

The Aging Research Centre
http://www.arclab.org

Centenarians
http://www.hcoa.org/centenarians/centenarians.htm

National Center for Health Statistics
http://www.cdc.gov/nchs/agingact.htm

The process of aging is complex and includes biological, psychological, sociological, and behavioral changes. Biologically, the body gradually loses the ability to renew itself. Various body functions begin to slow down, and the vital senses become less acute. Psychologically, aging persons experience changing sensory processes; perception, motor skills, problem-solving ability, and drives and emotions are frequently altered. Sociologically, they must cope with the changing roles and definitions of self that society imposes on the individual. For instance, the role expectations and the status of grandparents is different from those of parents, and the roles of the retired are quite different from those of the employed. Being defined as "old" may be desirable or undesirable, depending on the particular culture and its values. Behaviorally, aging individuals may move slower and with less dexterity. Because they are assuming new roles and are viewed differently by others, their attitudes about themselves, their emotions, and, ultimately, their behavior can be expected to change.

Those studying the process of aging often use developmental theories of the life cycle—a sequence of predictable phases that begins with birth and ends with death—to explain individuals' behavior at various stages of their lives. An individual's age, therefore, is important because it provides clues about his or her behavior at a particular phase of the life cycle—be it childhood, adolescence, adulthood, middle age, or old age. There is, however, the greatest variation in terms of health and human development among older people than among any other age group.

While every 3-year-old child can be predicted to have certain developmental experiences, there is a wide variation in the behavior of 65-year-old people. By age 65, we find that some people are in good health, employed, and performing important work tasks. Others of this cohort are retired but in good health or are retired and in poor health. Still others have died prior to the age of 65. The articles in this section are written from biological, psychological, and sociological perspectives. These disciplines attempt to explain the effects of aging and the resulting choices in lifestyle, as well as the wider, cultural implications of an older population.

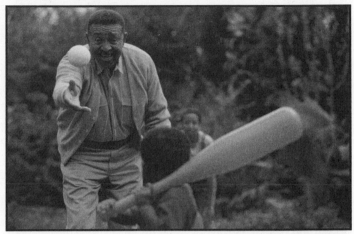

© Steve Mason/Getty Images

In the article "Elderly Americans," Christine L. Himes delineates the increases in life expectancy and the aging of the American population that has occurred during the last century. In "You Can Stop 'Normal' Aging," Henry Lodge gives a number of suggestions on what could be done to slow the aging process. In "Living Longer: Diet and Exercise," the authors discuss how the research findings in the areas of diet and exercise, if followed, could increase the individual's life expectancy by a number of years. In "Secrets to Longevity," Cathy Gulli points out why people live longer in the blue zones and what we could do to emulate the lifestyle.

Thomas Perls and Margery Hutter Silver conducted a study at Harvard Medical School of long-living individuals. Following their research, they came up with a quiz that included dietary and lifestyle choices, as well as family histories to help an individual determine what his or her probabilities are of living to a very old age. In "Faulty Fountains of Youth," Patrick Barry explains how scientists, by carefully looking at the changes in the human bodies' stem cells, see how these cells may contribute to those physical characteristics that we consider to be signs of aging.

Elderly Americans

CHRISTINE L. HIMES

The United States is in the midst of a profound demographic change: the rapid aging of its population. The 2000 Census counted nearly 35 million people in the United States 65 years of age or older, about one of every eight Americans. By 2030, demographers estimate that one in five Americans will be age 65 or older, which is nearly four times the proportion of elderly 100 years earlier, in 1930. The effects of this older age profile will reverberate throughout the American economy and society in the next 50 years. Preparing for these changes involves more than the study of demographic trends; it also requires an understanding of the growing diversity within the older population.

The lives and well-being of older Americans attract increasing attention as the elderly share of the U.S. population rises: One-fifth will be 65 or older in 2030.

The aging of the U.S. population in the next 20 years is being propelled by one of the most powerful demographic forces in the United States in the last century: the "baby boom" cohort, born between 1946 and 1964. This group of 76 million children grabbed media attention as it moved toward adulthood—changing school systems, colleges, and the workplace. And, this same group of people will change the profile and expectations of old age in the United States over the next 30 years as it moves past age 65. The potential effects of the baby boom on the systems of old-age assistance already are being evaluated. This cohort's consumption patterns, demand for leisure, and use of health care, for example, will leave an indelible mark on U.S. society in the 21st century. Understanding their characteristics as they near older ages will help us anticipate baby-boomers' future needs and their effects on the population.

Until the last 50 years, most gains in life expectancy came as the result of improved child mortality. The survival of larger proportions of infants and children to adulthood radically increased average life expectancy in the United States and many other countries over the past century. Now, gains are coming at the end of life as greater proportions of 65-year-olds are living until age 85, and more 85-year-olds are living into their 90s. These

changes raise a multitude of questions: How will these years of added life be spent? Will increased longevity lead to a greater role for the elderly in our society? What are the limits of life expectancy?

Increasing life expectancy, especially accompanied by low fertility, changes the structure of families. Families are becoming more "vertical," with fewer members in each generation, but more generations alive at any one time. Historically, families have played a prominent role in the lives of elderly people. Is this likely to change?

As much as any stage of the life course, old age is a time of growth, diversity, and change. Elderly Americans are among the wealthiest and among the poorest in our nation. They come from a variety of racial and ethnic backgrounds. Some are employed full-time, while others require full-time care. While general health has improved, many elderly suffer from poor health.

The older population in the 21st century will come to later life with different experiences than did older Americans in the last century—more women will have been divorced, more will have worked in the labor force, more will be childless. How will these experiences shape their later years?

The answers to these questions are complex. In some cases, we are confident in our predictions of the future. But for many aspects of life for the elderly, we are entering new territory. This report explores the characteristics of the current older population and speculates how older Americans may differ in the future. It also looks at the impact of aging on the U.S. society and economy.

Increasing Numbers

The United States has seen its elderly population—defined as those age 65 or older—grow more than tenfold during the 20th century. There were just over 3 million Americans age 65 or older in 1900, and nearly 35 million in 2000.

At the dawn of the 20th century, three demographic trends—high fertility, declining infant and child mortality, and high rates of international immigration—were acting in concert in the United States and were keeping the population young. The age distribution of the U.S. population was heavily skewed toward younger ages in 1900, as illustrated by the broad base of the population age-sex pyramid for that year in Figure 1. The pyramid, which shows the proportion of each age and sex group in the population, also reveals that the elderly made up a tiny share

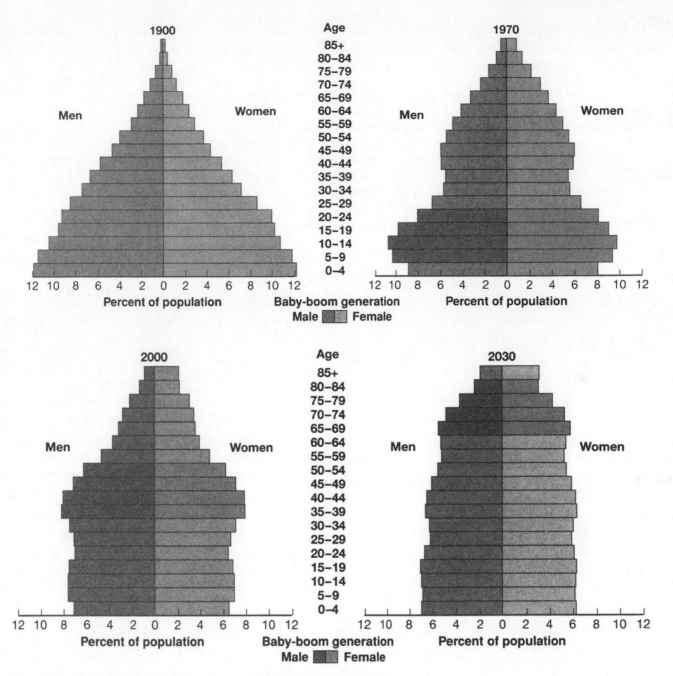

Figure 1 U.S. Population by Age and Sex, 1900, 1970, 2000, and 2030.

Sources: U.S. Census Bureau Publications: *Historical Statistics of the United States: Colonial Times to 1970* (1975); *Census 2000 Summary File* (SFI) (http://factfinder.census.gov, accessed Sept. 5, 2001); and "Population Projections of the United States by Age, Sex, Race, Hispanic Origin, and Nativity: 1999 to 2100" (www.census.gov/population/projections/nation/summary/np-t4-a.txt, accessed Sept. 25, 2001).

Note. U.S. population in 1900 does not include Alaska or Hawaii. The baby-boom generation includes persons born between 1946 and 1964.

of the U.S. population in 1900. Only 4 percent of Americans were age 65 of older, while more than one-half (54 percent) were under age 25.

But adult health improved and fertility fell during the first half of the century. The inflow of international immigrants slowed considerably after 1920. These trends caused an aging of the U.S. population, but they were interrupted after World War II by the baby boom. In the post-war years, Americans were marrying and starting families at younger ages and in

greater percentages than they had during the Great Depression. The surge in births between 1946 and 1964 resulted from a decline in childlessness (more women had at least one child) combined with larger family sizes (more women had three or more children). The sustained increase in birth rates during their 19-year period fueled a rapid increase in the child population. By 1970, these baby boomers had moved into their teen and young adult years, creating a bulge in that year's age-sex pyramid shown in Figure 1.

The baby boom was followed by a precipitous decline in fertility: the "baby bust." Young American women reaching adulthood in the late 1960s and 1970s were slower to marry and start families than their older counterparts, and they had fewer children when they did start families. U.S. fertility sank to an all-time low. The average age of the population started to climb as the large baby boom generation moved into adulthood, and was replaced by the much smaller baby-bust cohort. By 2000, the baby-boom bulge had moved up to the middle adult ages. The population's age structure at younger and older ages became more evenly distributed as fluctuations in fertility diminished and survival at the oldest ages increased. By 2030, the large baby-boom cohorts will be age 65 and older, and U.S. Census Bureau projections show that the American population will be relatively evenly distributed across age groups, as Figure 1 shows.

The radical shift in the U.S. population age structure over the last 100 years provides only one part of the story of the U.S. elderly population. Another remarkable aspect is the rapid growth in the number of elderly, and the increasing numbers of Americans at the oldest ages, above ages 85 or 90. The most rapid growth in the 65-or-older age group occurred between the 1920s and the 1950s (see Table 1). During each of these decades, the older population increased by at least 34 percent, reaching 16.6 million in 1960. The percentage increase slowed after 1960, and between 1990 and 2000, the population age 65 or older increased by just 12 percent. Since the growth of the

older population largely reflects past patterns of fertility, and U.S. fertility rates plummeted in the 1930s, the first decade of the 21st century will also see relatively slow growth of the elderly population. Fewer people will be turning 65 and entering the ranks of "the elderly." Not until the first of the baby-boom generation reaches age 65 between 2010 and 2020 will we see the same rates of increase as those experienced in the mid-20th century.

In the 1940s and 1950s, the rapid growth at the top of the pyramid was matched by growth in the younger ages—the total U.S. population was growing rapidly, and the general profile was still fairly young. That was not the case in the second half of the 20th century, as the share of the population age 65 or older increased to around 12 percent. The elderly share will increase much faster in the first half of the 21st century. This growth in the percentage age 65 or older constitutes population aging.

Many policymakers and health care providers are more concerned about the sheer size of the aging baby-boom generation than the baby boom's share of the total population. The oldest members of this group will reach age 65 in 2011, and by 2029, the youngest baby boomers will have reached age 65. This large group will continue to move into old age at a time of slow growth among younger age groups. The Census Bureau projects that 54 million Americans will be age 65 or older in 2020; by 2060, the number is projected to approach

Table 1 U.S. Total Population and Population Age 65 or Older, 1900–2060

| Year | Population (in thousands) | | Percent 65+ | Percent Increase from Preceding Decade | |
	Total	Age 65+		Total	Age 65+
Actual					
1900	75,995	3,080	4.1		
1910	91,972	3,950	4.3	21.0	28.2
1920	105,711	4,933	4.7	14.9	24.9
1930	122,755	6,634	5.4	16.1	34.5
1940	131,669	9,019	6.8	7.2	36.0
1950	150,697	12,270	8.1	14.5	36.0
1960	179,323	16,560	9.2	19.0	35.0
1970	203,212	20,066	9.9	13.4	21.2
1980	226,546	25,549	11.3	11.5	27.3
1990	248,710	31,242	12.6	9.8	22.3
2000	281,422	34,992	12.4	13.2	12.0
Projections					
2020	324,927	53,733	16.5	8.4	35.3
2040	377,350	77,177	20.5	7.5	9.8
2060	432,011	89,840	20.8	7.0	9.6

Sources: U.S. Census Bureau publications: *Historical Statistics of the United States: Colonial Times to 1970* (1975); *1980 Census of Population: General Population Characteristics* (PC80-1-B1); *1990 Census of Populations: General Population Characteristics* (1990-CP1); *Census 2000 Demographic Profile,* (www.census.gov/Press-Release/www/2001/tables/dp_us_2000.xls, accessed Sept. 19, 2001); and *Population Projections of the United States by Age, Sex, Race, Hispanic Origin, and Nativity: 1999 to 2100* (www.census.gov/population/projections/nation/summary/np-t4-a.txt, accessed Sept. 25, 2001).

Note. Data from 1900 to 1950 exclude Alaska and Hawaii. All data refer to the resident U.S. population.

90 million. The size of this group, and the general aging of the population, are important in planning for the future. Older Americans increasingly are healthy and active and able to take on new roles. At the same time, increasing numbers of older people will need assistance with housing, health care, and other services.

The Oldest-Old

The older population is also aging as more people are surviving into their 80s and 90s. In the 2000 Census, nearly one-half of Americans age 65 or older were above age 74, compared with less than one-third in 1950; one in eight were age 85 or older in 2000, compared with one in 20 in 1950 (see Figure 2).

As the baby boomers enter their late 60s and early 70s around 2020, the U.S. elderly population will be younger: The percentage ages 65 to 74 will rise to 58 percent, as shown in Figure 2. By 2040, however, just 44 percent will be 65 to 74, and 56 percent of all elderly will be age 75 or older.

Those age 85 or older, the "oldest-old," are the fastest growing segment of the elderly population. While those 85 or older made up only about 1.5 percent of the total U.S. population in 2000, they constituted about 12 percent of all elderly. More than 4 million people in the United States were 85 or older in the 2000 Census, and by 2050, a projected 19 million will be age 85 or older. These oldest-old will make up nearly 5 percent of the total population, and more than 20 percent of all elderly Americans. This group is of special interest to planners because those 85 or older are more likely to require health services.

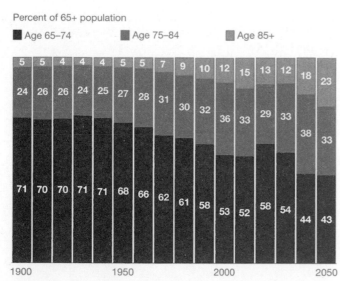

Figure 2   Age Distribution of Older Americans, 1900–2000, and Projection to 2050.

Sources: U.S. Census Bureau publications: *Historical Statistics of the United States: Colonial Times to 1970* (1975); *1980 Census of Population: General Population Characteristics* (PC80-1-B1); *1990 Census of Populations: General Population Characteristics* (1990-CP1); *Census 2000 Demographic Profile,* (www.census.gov/2001/tables/dp_us_2000.xls, accessed Sept. 19, 2001); and "Projections of the Resident Population by Age, Sex, Race, Hispanic Origin, 1990 to 2100" (www.census. gov/population/www/projections/natdet-D1A.html, accessed July 6, 2001).

Gender Gap

Women outnumber men at every age among the elderly. In 2000, there were an estimated three women for every two men age 65 or older, and the sex ratio is even more skewed among the oldest-old.

The preponderance of women among the elderly reflects the higher death rates for men than women at every age. There are approximately 105 male babies born for every 100 female babies, but higher male death rates cause the sex ratio to decline as age increases, and around age 35, females outnumber males in the United States. At age 85 and older, the ratio is 41 men per 100 women.[1]

Changes in the leading causes and average ages of death affect a population's sex ratio. In 1900, the average sex ratio for the U.S. total population was 104 men for every 100 women. But during the early 1900s, improvements in health care during and after pregnancy lowered maternal mortality, and a greater proportion of women survived to older ages. Adult male mortality improved much more slowly; death rates for adult men plateaued during the 1960s.

In recent years, however, male mortality improved faster than female mortality, primarily because of a marked decline in deaths from heart disease. The gender gap at the older ages has narrowed, and it is expected to narrow further. The U.S. Census Bureau projects the sex ratio for those age 65 or older to rise to 79 men for every 100 women by 2050. A sex ratio of 62 is anticipated for those age 85 or older.

Most elderly women today will outlive their spouses and face the challenges of later life alone: Older women who are widowed or divorced are less likely than older men to remarry. Older women are more likely than older men to be poor, to live alone, to enter nursing homes, and to depend on people other than their spouses for care. Many of the difficulties of growing older are compounded by past discrimination that disadvantaged women in the workplace and now threatens their economic security.

As the sex differential in mortality diminishes, these differences may lessen, but changes in marriage and work patterns, family structures, and fertility may mean that a greater proportion of older women will not have children or a living spouse. High divorce rates and declining rates of marriage, for instance, mean that many older women will not have spousal benefits available to them through pensions or Social Security.

Ethnic Diversity

The U.S. elderly population is becoming more racially and ethnically diverse, although not as rapidly as is the total U.S. population. In 2000, about 84 percent of the elderly population were non-Hispanic white, compared with 69 percent of the total U.S. population. By 2050, the proportion of elderly who are non-Hispanic white is projected to drop to 64 percent as the growing minority populations move into old age (see Figure 3). Although Hispanics made up only about 5 percent of the elderly population in 2000, 16 percent of the elderly population of 2050 is likely to be Hispanic. Similarly, blacks accounted

Percent of population age 65+

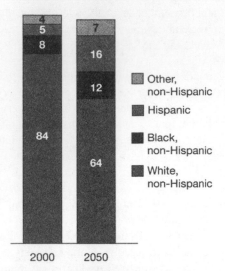

Figure 3 Elderly Americans by Race and Ethnicity, 2000 and 2050.

Sources: U.S. Census Bureau, *Census 2000 Demographic Profile* (2001); and U.S. Census Bureau, "Projections of the Resident Population by Age, Sex, Race and Hispanic Origin, 1999–2100" (www.census.gov/population/www/projections/natdet-D1A.html, accessed Sept. 19, 2001).

Note. The 2000 figures refer to residents who identified with one race. About 2% of Americans identified with more than one race in the 2000 census.

for 8 percent of the elderly population in 2000, but are expected to make up 12 percent of elderly Americans in 2050.

The major racial and ethnic groups are aging at different rates, depending upon fertility, mortality, and immigration among these groups. Immigration has a growing influence on the age structure of racial and ethnic minority groups. Although most immigrants tend to be in their young adult ages, when people are most likely and willing to assume the risks of moving to a new country, U.S. immigration policy also favors the entry of parents and other family members of these young immigrants. The number of immigrants age 65 or older is rapidly increasing as more foreign-born elderly move to the United States from Latin America, Asia, or Africa to join their children.[2] These older immigrants, plus the aging of immigrants who entered as young adults, are altering the ethnic makeup of elderly Americans.

Notes

1. U.S. Census Bureau, *Population Projections of the United States by Age, Sex, Race, Hispanic Origin, and Nativity: 1999 to 2100* (2000), accessed online at: www.census.gov/population/projections/nation/summary/np-t3-a.txt, on Sept. 19, 2001.

2. Janet M. Wilmoth, Gordon F. DeJong, and Christine L. Himes, "Immigrant and Non-Immigrant Living Arrangements in Later Life," *International Journal of Sociology and Social Policy* 17 (1997): 57–82.

You Can Stop "Normal" Aging

New research reveals surprising facts about our changing bodies.

DR. HENRY S. LODGE

From your body's point of view, "normal" aging isn't normal at all. It's a choice you make by the way you live your life. The other choice is to tell your cells to grow—to build a strong, vibrant body and mind.

Let's have a look at standard American aging. Barbara D. had a baby when she was 34, gave up exercise and gained 50 pounds. Exhausted and depressed, Barbara thought youth, energy and optimism were all in her rearview mirror. Jon M., 55, had fallen even farther down the slippery slope. He was stuck in the corporate world of stress, long hours and doughnuts. At 255 pounds, he had knees that hurt and a back that ached. He developed high blood pressure and eventually diabetes. Life was looking grim.

Most aging is just the dry rot we program into our cells by sedentary living, junk food and stress.

Jon and Barbara weren't getting old; they had let their bodies decay. Most aging is just the dry rot we program into our cells by sedentary living, junk food and stress. Yes, we do have to get old, and ultimately we do have to die. But our bodies are designed to age slowly and remarkably well. Most of what we see and fear is decay, and decay is only one choice. Growth is the other.

After two years of misery, Barbara started exercising and is now in the best shape of her life. She just finished a sprint triathlon and, at 37, feels like she is 20. Jon started eating better and exercising too—slowly at first, but he stuck with it. He has since lost 50 pounds, the pain in his knees and back has disappeared, and his diabetes is gone. Today, Jon is 60 and living his life in the body of a healthy 30-year-old. He will die one day, but he is likely to live like a young man until he gets there.

The hard reality of our biology is that we are built to move. Exercise is the master signaling system that tells our cells to grow instead of fade. When we exercise, that process of growth spreads throughout every cell in our bodies, making us functionally younger. Not a little bit younger—a lot younger. True biological aging is a surprisingly slow and graceful process. You can live out your life in a powerful, healthy body if you are willing to put in the work.

Let's take a step back to see how exercise works at the cellular level. Your body is made up of trillions of cells that live mostly for a few weeks or months, die and are replaced by new cells in an endless cycle. For example, your taste buds live only a few hours, white blood cells live 10 days, and your muscle cells live about three months. Even your bones dissolve and are replaced, over and over again. A few key stem cells in each organ and your brain cells are the only ones that stick around for the duration. All of your other cells are in a constant state of renewal.

You replace about 1% of your cells every day. That means 1% of your body is brand-new today, and you will get another 1% tomorrow. Think of it as getting a whole new body every three months. It's not entirely accurate, but it's pretty close. Viewed that way, you are walking around in a body that is brand-new since Christmas—new lungs, new liver, new muscles, new skin. Look down at your legs and realize that you are going to have new ones by the Fourth of July. Whether that body is functionally younger or older is a choice you make by how you live.

You choose whether those new cells come in stronger or weaker. You choose whether they grow or decay each day from then on. Your cells don't care which choice you make. They just follow the directions you send. Exercise, and your cells get stronger; sit down, and they decay.

This whole system evolved over billions of years out in nature, where all animals face two great cellular challenges: The first is to grow strong, fast and fit in the spring, when food abounds and there are calories to fuel hungry muscles, bones and brains. The second is to decay as fast as possible in the winter, when calories disappear and surviving starvation is the key to life. You would think that food is the controlling signal for this, but it's not. Motion controls your system.

When you don't exercise, your muscles let out a steady trickle of chemicals that tell every cell to decay, day after day after day.

Though we've moved indoors and left that life behind, our cells still think we're living out on the savannah, struggling to stay alive each day. There are no microwaves or supermarkets in nature. If you want to eat, you have to hunt or forage every single day. That movement is a signal that it's time to grow. So, when you exercise, your muscles release specific substances that travel throughout your bloodstream, telling your cells to grow. Sedentary muscles, on the other hand, let out a steady trickle of chemicals that whisper to every cell to decay, day after day after day.

Men like Jon, who go from sedentary to fit, cut their risk of dying from a heart attack by 75% over five years. Women cut their risk by 80%—and heart attacks are the largest single killer of women. Both men and women can double their leg strength with three months of exercise, and most of us can double it again in another three months. This is true whether you're in your 30s or your 90s. It's not a miracle or a mystery. It's your biology, and you're in charge.

The other master signal to our cells—equal and, in some respects, even more important than exercise—is emotion. One of the most fascinating revelations of the last decade is that emotions change our cells through the same molecular pathways as exercise. Anger, stress and loneliness are signals for "starvation" and chronic danger. They "melt" our bodies as surely as sedentary living. Optimism, love and community trigger the process of growth, building our bodies, hearts and minds.

Men who have a heart attack and come home to a family are four times less likely to die of a second heart attack. Women battling heart disease or cancer do better in direct proportion to the number of close friends and relatives they have. Babies in the ICU who are touched more often are more likely to survive. Everywhere you look, you see the role of emotion in our biology. Like exercise, it's a choice.

It's hard to exercise every day. And with our busy lives, it's even harder to find the time and energy to maintain relationships and build communities. But it's worth it when you consider the alternative. Go for a walk or a run, and think about it. Deep in our cells, down at the level of molecular genetics, we are wired to exercise and to care. We're beginning to wake up to that as a nation, but you might not want to wait. You might want to join Barbara, Jon and millions of others and change your life. Start today. Your cells are listening.

DR. HENRY S. LODGE is on the faculty of Columbia Medical School and is co-author of "Younger Next Year" (Workman).

Living Longer: Diet and Exercise
Diet

In the search for the fountain of youth, researchers keep coming back to one fact: what you eat has a tremendous impact not only on your health but on your longevity. Here's why every bite you take counts.

DONNA JACKSON NAKAZAWA

It's hard to get through your first cup of morning coffee without reading a headline about food. Eat blueberries! Inhale kale! Such antioxidant-rich foods will clear your arteries and help prevent the buildup of Alzheimer's plaque in your brain. Add in a cup of green tea in the morning and swish down an ounce or two of dark chocolate with a glass of red wine in the evening and you will be nicely tanked up on healthy fuel for the day.

Or will you? Almost every day, it seems, new studies emerge on the antiaging properties of various foods. One day, soy is good; the next, we find out soy's health benefits may have been oversold. To add to the confusion, this year *The Journal of the American Medical Association (JAMA)* published a study that found caloric restriction—eating about 25 percent less than normal—could extend your life.

So which headlines should we believe? And why should we believe them? The answers lie in research that shows exactly how various foods work at the cellular level. In particular, antioxidant-rich fruits and vegetables are emerging as powerful medicine in the fight against cellular aging.

Here's how it works. In the normal process of metabolism, cells produce unstable oxygen molecules—called free radicals—that damage cells. Worse still, the older we get, the more free radicals we produce. Recent studies suggest that the havoc free radicals wreak "plays a central role in virtually every age-related disease, including cardiovascular diseases such as stroke and atherosclerosis, Parkinson's disease, Alzheimer's, and type 2 diabetes," says Mark Mattson, Ph.D., chief of the Laboratory of Neurosciences at the National Institute on Aging at the National Institutes of Health.

It sounds pretty grim, but in this battle there are, thankfully, superheroes. Enter the vibrant world of antioxidants—substances that bind with free radicals and inhibit them from damaging cells. They are abundant in the most colorful fruits and vegetables, including spinach, broccoli, spirulina (blue-green algae), red apples, cranberries, blueberries, cherries, and grapes, as well as in chocolate and red wine. When you hear doctors say that eating five helpings of fruits and vegetables a day is good for you, antioxidants are the main reason. In the past five years an impressive body of research has emerged showing how antioxidants may protect the body and brain against the ravages of aging.

Paula Bickford, Ph.D., a researcher at the University of South Florida Center of Excellence for Aging and Brain Repair, is particularly interested in the role of antioxidants in brain health. The brain is a good place to study the benefits of antioxidants, says Bickford, because it has one of the highest percentages of fats of any organ in the body, and it is in our fats that free radicals inflict much of their damage. As we age, "communications between neurons become damaged, kind of like what happened to the Tin Man in *The Wizard of Oz*," she explains. "Oxidative damage caused the Tin Man to grow rusty—until Dorothy came along and oiled him." Similarly, antioxidants help to "regrease the lines of communication" in the cells in our brain, says Bickford.

To measure how the communication between cells was affected when groups of rats ate different diets, Bickford and her colleagues placed electrodes in the brains of 20-month-old rats—the equivalent of 60-year-old humans. She then fed one group of rats a diet supplemented with spirulina, another with apples, and a third with cucumbers, which lack the antioxidant qualities of spirulina and apples. Bickford and her colleagues were surprised by the robustness with which "both the spirulina and apple groups demonstrated improved neuron function in the brain, a suppression of inflammatory substances in the brain, and a decrease in oxidative damage." By contrast, there was no improvement in rats fed a diet containing cucumbers. Bickford, who calls the findings "dramatic," reproduced her results in another study, in which rats fed a spinach-rich diet had a reversal in the loss of learning ability that occurs with age.

Most recently, Bickford examined whether eating a diet high in antioxidant-rich spinach and blueberries makes a difference in lab animals suffering from stroke and Parkinson's. "We've seen very positive effects with both of these diseases, as well," she says. "We believe that antioxidants can help people either to delay the onset or to slow the progression of a range of diseases that we tend to get as we age."

Tempting though it may be now to go out and gorge on antioxidant-rich dark chocolate, resist the urge. The hottest discovery in the search to find the fountain of youth through the foods we eat is to—gulp!—eat a lot less of them. A 2006 article in *JAMA* caused a stir by announcing that in both men and women, caloric restriction—as spartan as 890 calories a day—resulted in a decrease in fasting insulin levels and body temperature, two biomarkers of longevity. Why? Because restricting calories also helps to eliminate those nefarious free radicals. Mattson explains: "When you overeat and more energy comes into the cells than you burn off by being active, you are going to have more excess free radicals roaming around." Still, he advises, don't panic over the idea of having to subsist on 890 calories a day. Mattson, who calls such a diet "starvation," believes we can all gain the benefits of healthy eating with a lot less pain.

Richard Miller, M.D., Ph.D., professor of pathology and geriatric medicine at the University of Michigan, agrees. He has spent the last 20 years studying the ways in which dietary and genetic changes can slow the aging process. The research has shown that mice, rats, and monkeys that have undergone severe caloric restriction demonstrate all kinds of mental and physical benefits such as better mental function, less joint disease, and even fewer cases of cataracts. But it's unrealistic to try to replicate that in humans. "To copy what's happening in the lab, a man weighing 200 pounds would have to decrease his caloric intake by 40 percent for life, which would put him at about 120 pounds," Miller explains. "That's just not tenable."

Instead, Mattson and Miller advocate a more moderate approach. According to the Centers for Disease Control and Prevention, the average man in the United States consumes about 2,475 calories a day. That's roughly 500 more, on average, than he really needs. Likewise, the average American woman consumes 1,833 calories, yet probably needs only about 1,600. One way to ratchet down your caloric consumption would be to follow this simple equation: men should aim for about 500 calories at both breakfast and lunch, while women should strive for about 300 at each meal. Both sexes can then shoot for 1,000 calories at dinner.

Bickford, who prefers to think of caloric restriction as caloric selection, underscores the importance of getting as much of your caloric intake as you can not only from antioxidant-rich fruits and vegetables but also from nuts and flaxseed, which are loaded with vitamin E and omega-3 and omega-6 fatty acids. In fact, Bickford takes a page out of her own lab studies and starts

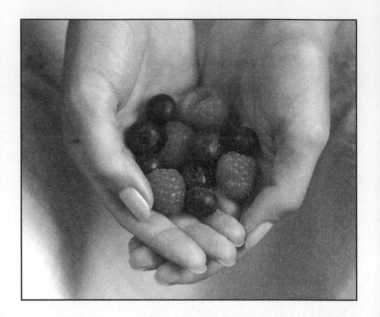

her day with an antioxidant smoothie. You can try it at home by blending together one cup of frozen blueberries with half a tablespoon of spirulina (available in any health food store), half a cup of nonfat plain yogurt, one teaspoon of ground flaxseed, one tablespoon of almond butter or a half-handful of almonds, and a dash of soy milk. Consider what's in that blender as a gas tank full of high-antioxidant fuel for the day.

Of course, one can't help but ask: what's the fun of living to 102 if you're subsisting on spirulina shakes? Not to worry. If you splurge on a stack of pancakes with eggs, bacon, and sausage—packing in 2,000 calories before 10 A.M.—you can always take heart in new data about to emerge from Mattson's lab, which show that periodic fasting—skipping a meal here and there—can also help to eliminate free radicals quite beautifully. "From an evolutionary standpoint we just aren't used to constant access to food," he explains. "Our bodies are used to going days without eating anything. Yet all of a sudden, we are taking in calories all day long."

In other words, we have gone from thousands of years of intermittently restricting our calories and eating a high-antioxidant diet to, in the past century, constantly eating a low-antioxidant diet. And that means more free radicals and more disease. So indulge in the pancakes or the cheese steak, but not both. Then skip a couple of meals and make your next one an all-out antioxidant feast. It may be counter to the don't-skip-meals philosophy our mothers all taught us; yet as it turns out, Mother Nature just might know better.

DONNA JACKSON NAKAZAWA is a health writer whose next book, a medical mystery about what's behind rising rates of autoimmune disease, will be published by Touchstone/Simon & Schuster in 2007.

Exercise

Regular physical activity has been shown to reduce your risk of heart attack, stroke, Alzheimer's, and some cancers. Now we're finding it also may add years to your life. That's powerful medicine indeed.

SUSAN CRANDELL

There are no guarantees in life and even fewer in death. But if you wish to prolong the former and delay the latter, scientists can now pretty much promise that regular exercise will help. "So many of what we thought were symptoms of aging are actually symptoms of disuse," says Pamela Peeke, M.D., a University of Maryland researcher and author of *Body for Life for Women* (Rodale, 2005). "This is a monster statement." It means that your health is not just a throw of the genetic dice but a factor that is largely under your control. "Our bodies are built for obsolescence after 50," Peeke says. "Up to 50 you can get away with not exercising; after that, you start paying the price."

The most dramatic declines due to aging are in muscle strength. "Unless you do resistance exercise—strength training with weights or elastic bands—you lose six pounds of muscle a decade," says Wayne Westcott, Ph.D., the highly respected fitness research director at the South Shore YMCA in Quincy, Massachusetts. That change in body composition not only saps our strength; it also lowers our metabolism and exposes us to greater risk of age-related disease. In fact, the loss of muscle (and accompanying increase in body fat) puts extra strain on the heart, alters sugar metabolism (increasing the risk for diabetes), and can tip the balance of healthy lipids in the blood, leading to heart attack and stroke.

Building muscle is much easier than you might think. Strength training just 20 minutes a day, two or three times a week, for 10 to 12 weeks can rebuild three pounds of muscle and increase your metabolism by 7 percent. Do you really need a boost in metabolism? Yes, if you want to feel more energetic, more alert, more vital and alive. Plus, the added muscle has a halo effect on many systems of the body, reducing blood pressure, improving your ability to use glucose from the blood by 25 percent, increasing bone mass by 1 to 3 percent, and improving gastrointestinal efficiency by 55 percent. "It's like going from a four-cylinder engine to a six," Westcott says.

If that's not enough to get your attention, consider this: a regular exercise program (30 minutes of physical activity at least three days a week) can reduce your risk of dying in the next eight years by 40 percent, improve brain function, cut your risk of Alzheimer's disease by up to 60 percent, and blunt the symptoms of depression. This is powerful medicine, given that 80 percent of the population over 65 suffers from at least one chronic condition, and half have two or more, according to a report from the Census Bureau and the National Institute on Aging.

What is it about physical activity that makes it such a panacea? As scientists learn more about how the aging process works, they're finding that exercise—both aerobic exercise and strength training—has a tremendous impact on every cell in the body, reducing inflammation, increasing blood flow, and even reversing the natural declines in oxygen efficiency and muscle mass that come with aging.

Westcott points to a study his organization conducted at a nursing home in Orange City, Florida. Nineteen men and women with an average age of 89, most of whom used wheelchairs, did just ten minutes of strength training a week. "After 14 weeks almost everybody was out of their wheelchairs," Westcott says. "One woman moved back into independent living." The results were published in *Mature Fitness*.

Another inspiring study, published last spring in the *Journal of the American College of Cardiology,* reported that people in their 60s and 70s who walked or jogged, biked, and stretched for 90 minutes three times a week for six months increased their exercise efficiency—their ability to exercise harder without expending more energy—by a whopping 30 percent. But here's the shocker: a comparison group of people in their 20s and 30s showed an efficiency increase of just 2 percent. The results caught even study author Wayne C. Levy, M.D., an associate professor of cardiology at the University of Washington in Seattle, by surprise. "I hadn't anticipated that the older people would improve more than the group in their 20s and 30s," he says.

The explanation, Levy believes, may involve improvement in the function of the mitochondria—spherical or rod-shaped structures in our cells that take glucose, protein, and fat from the food we eat and turn them into energy. In fact, scientists believe that most of the dramatic benefits we get from exercise can be traced to this improvement in the mitochondria. "Mitochondrial function naturally declines with age," explains Kevin Short, Ph.D., who studies mitochondria and exercise at the Mayo Clinic in Rochester, Minnesota. But exercise, he found, can reverse that decline.

When Short and his colleagues put 65 healthy nonexercisers ranging in age from 21 to 87 on a bicycle training program

11

three days a week, they found that everyone's maximum aerobic capacity had increased by about 10 percent after four months. When they studied thigh-muscle samples, they found out why: the mitochondria were pumping out more adenosine triphosphate (ATP), the fuel muscles use to move.

Now, if mightier mitochondria aren't enough to get you on your exercise bike each morning, this might be: it appears physical activity may also combat oxidative damage (see "Browning apples: oxidation at work". "During exercise there's a tremendous burst of oxidative agents that are injurious to tissue," says Abraham Aviv, M.D., director of the Center of Human Development and Aging at the University of Medicine and Dentistry of New Jersey.

The theory is that although you take in more oxygen while exercising, regular exercise slows your resting heart rate, thereby decreasing the amount of oxygen you need overall and reducing the rate at which you create harmful free radicals.

Finally, to all these substantial benefits of exercise add one more: Professor Tim Spector, director of the Twins UK registry at St. Thomas' Hospital in London, is conducting experiments to determine whether exercise slows down the rate at which our telomeres shrink. (Telomeres are DNA sequences, located on the ends of chromosomes, that shorten as we age—see "Telomeres: your body's biological clock". Although the results have not yet been published, preliminary findings suggest that in exercising and sedentary twin pairs, the twin who exercises has much longer telomeres "even when you adjust for differences in weight and smoking," says Spector.

In short, the evidence is clear: daily physical activity can transform your life. And it's never too late to start. "I started strength-training my father when he was 82," recalls Westcott. "He's six feet tall, but he was emaciated by the stress of my mother's death and weighed only 124 pounds. In a year and a half, he added 24 pounds of muscle. At 97, he's stronger than people half his age."

SUSAN CRANDELL is the author of *Thinking About Tomorrow: Reinventing Yourself at Midlife.*

Secrets to Longevity

In the four "blue zones" people live well for a very long time.

CATHY GULLI

On the island of Sardinia, less than 200 km west of mainland Italy, very old people are like celebrities. This is despite the fact that their days are mostly spent in bed or in their favourite chair. Otherwise, they eat, or on particularly active days, promenade through the village. A stop in any local *taverna* reveals just how much glory these seniors get. "Usually we see swimsuit calendars" inside North American sports bars, says Dan Buettner, but when he was in Sardinia, "it was Centenarian of the Month calendars."

As unsettling as a great-great-grandfather in a Speedo may sound, his fame—let alone his triple-digit age—provides one example of the differences between where most of us live and the world's "blue zones." These are places where people have the lengthiest lifespans. In a new book published by National Geographic, *The Blue Zone: Lessons for Living Longer from the People Who've Lived the Longest,* explorer Dan Buettner identifies four areas around the globe where this is happening: Sardinia; Okinawa, Japan; the Nicoya Peninsula in Costa Rica; and Seventh Day Adventists in Linda Loma, Calif. (He says two more may be announced later this year.) While "we don't live in the South Pacific or on a mountain" like the blue zone populations, says Buettner, "how we emulate what they do in our houses and communities can [stretch] our lifespan by 10 years."

Each blue zone offers distinct keys to prospering. In Sardinia, besides revering their elders, people drink daily two glasses of red wine rich in antioxidants. In Okinawa, family and friends form a *moai,* a network to care for one another. Along the Nicoya Peninsula, people eat a diet similar to what their ancestors ate for the last 3,500 years, comprised mainly of black beans, fruit, and a type of corn soaked in lime that infuses it with amino acids. "It's almost a perfect longevity diet," says Buettner. And in Linda Loma, the Adventists observe a weekly Sabbath "no matter how busy or stressed out they are, no matter what's happened in this 'CrackBerry' world," he enthuses. The result: women live nine years longer than other Californian females; Adventist men get 11 more years of life than their state counterparts.

Of course, if you asked any of the blue zone inhabitants their secrets to a long lifespan, they wouldn't have an answer.

"A 100-year-old no more knows how he got to be 100 than a tall man knows how he got to be tall," philosophizes Buettner. So, over a few years, he and his team of researchers identified blue zones using demographic data such as "life expectancy to centenary rate" (the proportion of a population that lives to be 100) or middle-aged mortality. Then they went to those places and observed the lifestyles of centenarians. Finally Buettner aggregated the information and distilled it into nine common denominators that he says make up the formula for longevity.

"The Power 9," as they're called, are assembled in a pyramid shape evocative of Abraham Maslow's Hierarchy of Needs. At the top is the "Move naturally" category, which says low-intensity physical activity should be part of a person's daily routine. Buettner suggests "de-conveniencing your house or office" to get more exercise in. Twenty minutes of gentle aerobic, balancing and muscle-strengthening movements four or five times a week should reduce mortality by 26 percent, and add three or four years to your life.

Below it, the "Belong to the right tribe" group focuses on the importance of healthy, supportive relationships between friends and family. Buettner says that if you're estranged from relatives then you should make amends, and if you don't have an encouraging friend then you'd better "go searching for one." There's also emphasis on joining a spiritual community. One meta-analysis of 42 studies examining the link between religion and longevity found that people who regularly participated in faith groups had a lower mortality by 29 percent. If you do all this, says Buettner, you could tack on four years of living.

To get eight more years of extra life, the next category is "Eat wisely." It is based in the credo of Okinawa elders to stop eating when you are 80 percent full—or feeling almost satisfied. The Sardinia standard of two glasses of red wine a day is also endorsed, as well as a diet light on meat and heavy on plants. Lastly, the base of the Power 9 pyramid is the "Right outlook" group, which can add four years to a person's lifespan if he can articulate his purpose in life, or as the Nicoyans say, "Why I wake up in the morning." Buettner points out that all these changes don't have a cumulative effect in adding years to lifespan, but rather work together to provide roughly a decade more longevity.

This is, obviously, hard stuff to do. On www.bluezones.com you can take the "Vitality Compass" test to determine your life expectancy and where you need to take particular care. Buettner, who's 47 and is predicted to live until he's 95 after adopting many of the Power 9, suggests beginning with the three changes that seem easiest to pull off. People should also attempt them with a partner who can offer motivation, and with whom they can hold one another accountable. And, Buettner writes in *Blue Zones,* reward yourself when you achieve any modifications.

One study indicated longevity is only 20 percent genetic—the rest is lifestyle

Slight improvements to the way you live should produce some results because, Buettner notes, a Danish study has indicated that longevity is only 20 percent genetic—the rest comes down to lifestyle. It's a controversial statement because daily discoveries reveal how DNA impacts our likelihood of developing various diseases. But Buettner says that blue zone populations don't have to endure the long, debilitated path to death so common in North America. "The average Canadian is going to have 2½ to three years of morbidity," he explains, compared to the blue zones where people suffer for six months. By living better, Buettner believes, "you're chopping off the worst of the worst years of your life."

"The goal," says Buettner, "is to live 90 or 95 really great years and die in our sleep"

How to Live Longer

Consider these recommendations, adapted from Dan Buettner's Power 9 Pyramid in *The Blue Zone.*

1. Add simple activities throughout your day like walking farther than you need to, doing gardening or home repairs yourself, or running around with your children or pets.
2. Try eating off of smaller plates to decrease your portion sizes and reduce calories.
3. Limit the number of servings of meat you eat in a week.
4. Drink a glass or two of red wine most evenings.
5. Know your passions in life and take time to enjoy them most days.
6. Take quiet time to relieve stress.
7. Belong to a spiritual community and gather with them regularly.
8. Make your family and loved ones a priority. Express that through your actions.
9. Surround yourself with friends who have healthy habits and support you in your goals.

If you are doing many of these things, you could add up to 10 good years to your life.

"The goal," he continues, "is to live 90 or 95 really great years and die in our sleep." And then Buettner adds, "Preferably after really great sex."

To calculate your life expectancy visit www.macleans.ca/howhealthy.

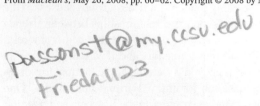

Will You Live to Be 100?

THOMAS PERLS, MD AND MARGERY HUTTER SILVER, EdD

After completing a study of 150 centenarians, Harvard Medical School researchers Thomas Perls, M.D., and Margery Hutter Silver, Ed.D., developed a quiz to help you calculate your estimated life expectancy.

Longevity Quiz

Score

1. Do you smoke or chew tobacco, or are you around a lot of secondhand smoke? Yes (−20) No (0)

2. Do you cook your fish, poultry, or meat until it is charred? Yes (−2) No (0)

3. Do you avoid butter, cream, pastries, and other saturated fats as well as fried foods (eg., French Fries)? Yes (+3) No (−7)

4. Do you minimize meat in your diet, preferably making a point to eat plenty of fruits, vegetables, and bran instead? Yes (+5) No (−4)

5. Do you consume more than two drinks of beer, wine, and/or liquor a day? (A standard drink is one 12-ounce bottle of beer, one wine cooler, one five-ounce glass of wine, or one and a half ounces of 80-proof distilled spirits.) Yes (−10) No (0)

6. Do you drink beer, wine, and/or liquor in moderate amounts (one or two drinks/day)? Yes (+3) No (0)

7. Do air pollution warnings occur where you live? Yes (−4) No (+1)

8. **a.** Do you drink more than 16 ounces of coffee a day? Yes (−3) No (0) **b.** Do you drink tea daily? Yes (+3) No (0)

9. Do you take an aspirin a day? Yes (+4) No (0)

10. Do you floss your teeth every day? Yes (+2) No (−4)

11. Do you have a bowel movement less than once every two days? Yes (−4) No (0)

12. Have you had a stroke or heart attack? Yes (−10) No (0)

13. Do you try to get a sun tan? Yes (−4) No (+3)

14. Are you more than 20 pounds overweight? Yes (−10) No (0)

15. Do you live near enough to other family members (other than your spouse and dependent children) that you can and want to drop by spontaneously? Yes (+5) No (−4)

16. Which statement is applicable to you? **a.** "Stress eats away at me. I can't seem to shake it off." Yes (−7) **b.** "I can shed stress." This might be by praying, exercising, meditating, finding humor in everyday life, or other means. Yes (+7)

17. Did both of your parents either die before age 75 of nonaccidental causes or require daily assistance by the time they reached age 75? Yes (−10) No (0) Don't know (0)

18. Did more than one of the following relatives live to at least age 90 in excellent health: parents, aunts/uncles, grandparents? Yes (+24) No (0) Don't know (0)

19. **a.** Are you a couch potato (do no regular aerobic or resistance exercise)? Yes (−7) **b.** Do you exercise at least three times a week? Yes (+7)

20. Do you take vitamin E (400–800 IU) and selenium (100–200 mcg) every day? Yes (+5) No (−3)

Score

STEP 1: Add the negative and positive scores together. Example: −45 *plus* +30 = −15. Divide the preceding score by 5 (−15 divided by 5 = −3).

STEP 2: Add the negative or positive number to age 84 if you are a man or age 88 if you are a woman (example: −3 + 88 = 85) to get your estimated life span.

The Science behind the Quiz

Question 1 Cigarette smoke contains toxins that directly damage DNA, causing cancer and other diseases and accelerating aging.

Question 2 Charring food changes its proteins and amino acids into heterocyclic amines, which are potent mutagens that can alter your DNA.

Questions 3, 4 A high-fat diet, and especially a high-fat, high-protein diet, may increase your risk of cancer of the breast, uterus, prostate, colon, pancreas, and kidney. A diet rich in fruits and vegetables may lower the risk of heart disease and cancer.

Questions 5, 6 Excessive alcohol consumption can damage the liver and other organs, leading to accelerated aging and increased susceptibility to disease. Moderate consumption may lower the risk of heart disease.

Question 7 Certain air pollutants may cause cancer; many also contain oxidants that accelerate aging.

Question 8 Too much coffee predisposes the stomach to ulcers and chronic inflammation, which in turn raise the risk of heart disease. High coffee consumption may also indicate and exacerbate stress. Tea, on the other hand, is noted for its significant antioxidant content.

Question 9 Taking 81 milligrams of aspirin a day (the amount in one baby aspirin) has been shown to decrease the risk of heart disease, possibly because of its anticlotting effects.

Question 10 Research now shows that chronic gum disease can lead to the release of bacteria into the bloodstream, contributing to heart disease.

Question 11 Scientists believe that having at least one bowel movement every 20 hours decreases the incidence of colon cancer.

Question 12 A previous history of stroke and heart attack makes you more susceptible to future attacks.

Question 13 The ultraviolet rays in sunlight directly damage DNA, causing wrinkles and increasing the risk of skin cancer.

Question 14 Being obese increases the risk of various cancers, heart disease, and diabetes. The more overweight you are, the higher your risk of disease and death.

Questions 15, 16 People who do not belong to cohesive families have fewer coping resources and therefore have increased levels of social and psychological stress. Stress is associated with heart disease and some cancers.

Questions 17, 18 Studies show that genetics plays a significant role in the ability to reach extreme old age.

Question 19 Exercise leads to more efficient energy production in the cells and overall, less oxygen radical formation. Oxygen (or free) radicals are highly reactive molecules or atoms that damage cells and DNA, ultimately leading to aging.

Question 20 Vitamin E is a powerful antioxidant and has been shown to retard the progression of Alzheimer's, heart disease, and stroke. Selenium may prevent some types of cancer.

Adapted from *Living to 100: Lessons in Living to Your Maximum Potential at Any Age* (Basic Books, 1999) by **THOMAS PERLS,** MD, and **MARGERY HUTTER SILVER,** EdD, with John F. Lauerman.

Faulty Fountains of Youth

Adult stem cells may contribute to aging.

PATRICK BARRY

Skin sags. Hair grays. Organs don't work quite like they used to. A gradual wearing out and running down of the body's tissues seems an inherent part of growing older. Rejuvenation of skin, muscles, and other body parts naturally declines with the passing years.

Scientifically speaking, however, this observation is much less self-evident. Some cells in a person's body can resist the tide of aging. Consider the reproductive cells a person carries that will become the cells of newborn children who have 80-plus years of life to look forward to. Generation after generation, these reproductive cells form an unbroken line stretching for millennia.

The reason that an otherwise healthy person grows old and dies remains a mystery. Scientists have suggested several suspects for why people's bodies wear out with age, including accumulated damage to DNA, free radicals, and the shortening of telomeres—the caps on the ends of chromosomes. While each of these factors may play a part, biologists acknowledge that their understanding of aging is incomplete.

Enter stem cells. Scientists have long known that people have small reservoirs of stem cells in some of their tissues, such as bone marrow. These stem cells are distinct from those found in newly fertilized embryos—the more controversial embryonic stem cells. The embryonic type can become any type of cell in the body.

Adult stem cells, in contrast, can normally generate new cells only for the tissue in which they're found: blood cells for blood, intestinal cells for the intestines. As old cells in these tissues are damaged or wear out, nearby stem cells can manufacture new ones to take their place. At the same time, the stem cells produce more copies of themselves, maintaining a seemingly indefinite pool of cells capable of churning out a stream of replacement cells.

Until recently, most scientists thought that adult stem cells existed only in tissues that need to constantly replace their cells, such as skin, blood, and the lining of the intestine. But over the past few years, researchers have found stem cells in many, perhaps most, of the body's organs and tissues. Even the brain, which scientists once thought never replaced its nerve cells during adulthood, is now known to have stem cells that make new nerve cells throughout life (*SN: 6/16/07, p. 376*).

With the realization that so much of the body contains self-renewing stem cells, scientists began wondering whether changes in these stem cells over time might contribute to aging.

Imagine that, as a person ages, these fountains of cellular youth might start to run dry. As the supply of fresh cells dwindles, tissues would gradually decline and show signs of age. "That was the initial model" of how stem cells could be involved in aging, says Norman E. Sharpless, a stem cell expert at the University of North Carolina in Chapel Hill. And some data support this idea.

Graying of hair, for example, could be caused by a decline in melanocyte stem cells that accompanies aging, as observed by Emi K. Nishimura and her colleagues at Dana-Farber Cancer Institute in Boston. Melanocytes make the hair pigment melanin, so depleting these stem cells eventually causes loss of hair color, the team reported in *Science* in 2005.

Elderly people also have diminished resistance to disease because their immune systems make fewer of the disease-fighting white blood cells known as lymphocytes. In mice, bone marrow stem cells produce fewer lymphocytes as the mice get older, Derrick J. Rossi, now at Harvard Stem Cell Institute in Cambridge, reported in 2005 in the *Proceedings of the National Academy of Sciences*.

Yet evidence is mounting that the connection between adult stem cells and aging is more complex. Some kinds of stem cell actually grow *more* abundant with age. And just as stem cells affect aging, the aging body affects stem cells.

Tinkering with Time

To untangle these effects, scientists led by Thomas A. Rando of Stanford University surgically joined pairs of mice like reconnected Siamese twins. The team linked the animals' circulatory systems so that blood from each member of a pair flowed through both mice. One mouse in each pair was old; the other was young.

Scientists knew that the ability of muscle stem cells (also called satellite cells) to repair damaged muscles declines substantially with age. Rando's team wanted to find out whether such declines should be attributed to changes in the satellite cells themselves or to changes in the cells' environment as the animals aged.

"There clearly is an effect of aging on stem cells," Rando says. "But I think the other question is . . . are those changes reversible or irreversible?"

Amazingly, the blood of the young mice completely restored the tissue-healing powers of the satellite cells in the older mice, Rando's team reported in 2005 in *Nature*. Exposure to the young blood reactivated a system of proteins inside the cells called the Notch signaling pathway, which is crucial for triggering the cells' muscle-repair functions. Notch signaling in satellite cells normally declines in old age, but Rando's experiment showed that this decline is a response to changes in the blood, not the result of an inherent wearing out of the satellite cells themselves.

This influence of the cells' environment is possible because all cells receive signals—including hormones and other messenger proteins—from their surroundings, and these signals allow the cells to behave appropriately for their context. So a change in these external messengers in aging mice could diminish the satellite cells' muscle-repair activity.

Stem cells' surroundings also wield an influence in fruit fly testes. Changes in the stem cell-harboring niche inside the testes contribute to a decline in the number of sperm-making stem cells with age, according to research by D. Leanne Jones of the Salk Institute for Biological Studies in La Jolla, Calif., and her colleagues. As the flies grew old, the niche produced less of a protein that activates a gene in the stem cells called *unpaired,* which triggers self-renewal of the cells, the team reported in the Oct. 11, 2007 *Cell Stem Cell.*

"We definitely see changes in the environment long before we start to see" signs of intrinsic aging, Jones says. In mice testes as well, "there seems to be evidence for the environment aging instead of the stem cells themselves."

In other cases, though, stem cell aging seems independent of context. Blood-forming stem cells from bone marrow age in an unusual way. When scientists transplant blood stem cells from an old mouse into a young mouse, allow the young mouse to grow old, and then repeat the process for several generations, the stem cells lose none of their ability to make copies of themselves. In fact, in some mouse strains, blood stem cells become even more numerous with age.

But that's not necessarily a good thing. While old age doesn't appear to affect blood stem cells' power of self-renewal, it does gum up their ability to make specialized offspring cells. Ideally, each time a stem cell divides, one of the daughter cells would remain a stem cell, and the other would continue dividing to produce a fresh crop of specialized cells to replenish the tissue. That way, the stem cell's lineage always contains only one stem cell at a time to replace the original, keeping the total number of stem cells constant.

For that number to increase, daughter cells must sometimes both become stem cells, decreasing production of tissue-replenishing cells.

Even when these elderly stem cells do spawn new lines of specialized cells, the process goes awry. Blood stem cells must give rise to a whole family of specialized cells: red blood cells, lymphocytes, monocytes, macrophages, and others. As the stem cells age, something goes wrong in this specialization process,

skewing it away from making lymphocytes. So the old-age slump in germ-fighting lymphocytes happens not because the stem cells peter out but because they charge ahead with their specialization machinery slightly broken. In mice, this misbehaving of blood stem cells occurs even when scientists repeatedly transplant the cells into young animals, leading them to conclude that the stem cells themselves become damaged with time.

Fighting Death with Aging

In trying to understand how stem cells in various organs deteriorate with age, scientists have run up against the perennial nemesis of cell biology: cancer.

"Having all these cells around that can divide all the time is quite dangerous for an organism," Sharpless says. Cells continually accumulate DNA damage, but copying and segregating the DNA during cell division is particularly hazardous. Every time a cell divides, there's some error of replication.

Most of these mistakes get fixed by repair enzymes, but certain lingering errors in DNA can cause a cell to begin growing and dividing out of control, which is how cancer arises. Cells have elaborate tools for detecting DNA damage early and either fixing it or shutting down the affected cell. Recent data suggest that these mechanisms for thwarting cancer could cause the body to cull some of its own stem cell supplies.

For example, researchers led by Sean J. Morrison of the University of Michigan in Ann Arbor found a link between the decline in nerve stem cells in mouse brains and the potent anticancer gene *p16*. This gene causes cells to enter a dormant state called senescence. Mice bred without *p16* retained significantly more of their nerve stem cells into old age than did mice that had the gene, Morrison's team reported in *Nature* in 2006.

The famous tumor-fighting gene *p53* also reins in damaged stem cells in old age. Blocking the activity of *p53* in stem cells restored populations of intestinal stem cells in elderly mice, K. Lenhard Rudolph of Hannover Medical School in Germany and his colleagues reported in the January 2007 *Nature Genetics.*

Whether the bodily declines that come with aging are due to the depletion of stem cells depends on which organ is in question—and on which scientist you ask. Most scientists agree that adult stem cells play an important role in aging; the other thing that they seem to agree about is that this role is complicated. "There's still a tremendous amount of debate about even the [blood stem cell] system, which is one of the best-studied systems," Jones says.

In blood and other tissues with high cell turnover, decline of stem cells may make a greater contribution to the signs of aging than it does in tissues with slower cell turnover.

In skin, which constantly produces new cells, a decline in stem cell vigor is expected by some scientists to play a big part in the sagging and poor elasticity of skin that comes with old age. For organs such as the brain and heart, which retain most of their cells throughout adulthood, signs of old age more likely come from traditional mechanisms of aging acting on the organs' mature, specialized cells.

But even this guideline may be too simple. Alzheimer's disease, a form of dementia that commonly occurs in the elderly, is characterized by plaques accumulating in the brain. Young people's brains make the plaque proteins as well, but some data suggest that immune cells called macrophages patrol the brain and clear out budding plaques. Macrophages are continuously being made by—you guessed it—blood stem cells. So even for organs in which cell renewal by stem cells proceeds very slowly, the declines of old age might be caused by the decline of adult stem cells elsewhere in the body.

Some aspects of aging will likely prove unrelated to stem cells, Sharpless says, but these cells now appear far more important for aging than scientists once thought. "I've stopped trying to predict which symptoms of aging are related to [stem cell] proliferation and which are not," Sharpless says. Scientists "used to be so confident about this 10 years ago. Now I'm prepared to be wrong."

From *Science News,* Vol. 173, February 9, 2008, pp. 88–89. Copyright © 2008 by Science Service Inc. Reprinted by permission.

UNIT 2

The Quality of Later Life

Unit Selections

Key Points to Consider

- How do the lifestyle choices that people make throughout their lives affect the quality of their later lives?

- What are the critical factors that Lou Ann Walker identifies as contributing to a long, healthy life?

- What can be done to combat the conditions that are associated with "failure to thrive" symptoms in older adults?

- What have past studies indicated about the dangers on a person's health of being overweight?

Student Website
www.mhhe.com/cls

Internet References

Aging with Dignity
   http://www.agingwithdignity.org
The Gerontological Society of America
   http://www.geron.org
The National Council on the Aging
   http://www.ncoa.org

Although it is true that one ages from the moment of conception to the moment of death, children are usually considered to be "growing and developing" while adults are often thought of as "aging." Having accepted this assumption, most biologists concerned with the problems of aging focus their attention on what happens to individuals after they reach maturity. Moreover, most of the biological and medical research dealing with the aging process focuses on the later part of the mature adult's life cycle. A commonly used definition of *senescence* is "the changes that occur generally in the postreproductive period and that result in decreased survival capacity on the part of the individual organism" (B. L. Shrehler, *Time, Cells and Aging,* New York: Academic Press, 1977).

As a person ages, physiological changes take place. The skin loses its elasticity, becomes more pigmented, and bruises more easily. Joints stiffen, and the bone structure becomes less firm. Muscles lose their strength. The respiratory system becomes less efficient. The individual's metabolism changes, resulting in different dietary demands. Bowel and bladder movements are more difficult to regulate. Visual acuity diminishes, hearing declines, and the entire system is less able to resist environmental stresses and strains.

Increases in life expectancy have resulted largely from decreased mortality rates among younger people, rather than from increased longevity after age 65. In 1900, the average life expectancy at birth was 47.3 years; in 2000, it was 76.9 years. Thus, in the last century, the average life expectancy rose by 29.6 years. However, those who now live to the age of 65 do not have an appreciably different life expectancy than did their 1900 cohorts. In 1900, 65-year-olds could expect to live approximately 11.9 years longer, while in 2000 they could expect to live approximately 17.9 years longer, an increase of six years. Although more people survive to age 65 today, the chances of being afflicted by one of the major killers of older persons is still about as great for this generation as it was for its grandparents'.

While medical science has had considerable success in controlling the acute diseases of the young—such as measles, chicken pox, and scarlet fever—it has not been as successful in controlling the chronic conditions of old age, such as heart disease, cancer, and emphysema. Organ transplants, greater knowledge of the immune system, and undiscovered medical technologies will probably increase the life expectancy for the 65-and-over population, resulting in longer life for the next generation.

Although people 65 years of age today are living only slightly longer than 65-year-olds did in 1900, the quality of their later

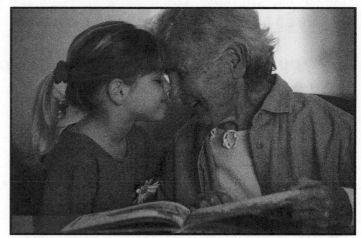

© Creatas/PictureQuest

years has greatly improved. Economically, Social Security and a multitude of private retirement programs have given most older persons a more secure retirement. Physically, many people remain active, mobile, and independent throughout their retirement years. Socially, most older persons are married, involved in community activities, and leading productive lives. While they may experience some chronic ailments, most people 65 or older are able to live in their own homes, direct their own lives, and involve themselves in activities they enjoy.

The articles in this section examine health, psychological, social, and spiritual factors that affect the quality of aging. All of us are faced with the process of aging, and by putting a strong emphasis on health—both mental and physical—a long, satisfying life is much more attainable. In "Failure to Thrive: Interventions to Improve Quality of Life in the Older Adult," the author points out how being lonely, bored, and depressed leads to health problems and a failure to thrive for older persons. In "Overweight and Mortality among Baby Boomers—Now We're Getting Personal," Tim Byers points out the dangers of being overweight on the lives and health of older persons. "Lifetime Achievements" explains that Americans are healthier and live longer than ever before. A short quiz developed by Harvard Medical School shows the correlation between health risks and life expectancy. Finally, Lou Ann Walker gives specific recommendations for what the individual can do to improve his or her chances of aging well in "We Can Control How We Age."

Failure to Thrive

Interventions to Improve Quality of Life in the Older Adult

BECKY DORNER, RD, LD

The term *failure to thrive* (FTT) is used to describe infants and young children with failure to grow or gain weight at the expected rate. Possible causes include physical and emotional deprivation, poor appetite and diet, and medical problems.[1] It is this type of syndrome of physical and emotional deprivation that so often applies to the older person who was once active and is now lonely, bored, and possibly depressed. This deprivation and depression can easily lead to social withdrawal and poor food intake, which can result in malnutrition and unintentional weight loss, followed by weakness, functional decline, and other complicating factors.

Geriatric FTT is a common enough term to have its own ICD code (783.4), yet it is a controversial term in practice. In 1991, the Institute of Medicine described FTT late in life as "a syndrome manifested by weight loss greater than 5% of baseline, decreased appetite, poor nutrition, and inactivity, often accompanied by dehydration, depressive symptoms, impaired immune function, and low cholesterol levels."[2]

FTT in the older adult may be the result of multiple issues, including chronic disease and functional decline. As clinicians, we first notice the symptoms of poor food and fluid intake, unintentional weight loss, malnutrition, and inactivity. The adverse outcomes of this syndrome follow and include malnutrition, depression, cognitive impairment, and impaired physical function.

Robertson notes, "Failure to thrive should not be considered a normal consequence of aging, a synonym for dementia, the inevitable result of a chronic disease, or a descriptor of the later stages of a terminal disease."[1]

Woolley notes that physicians should take caution when applying the geriatric FTT label. FTT should not be treated as a diagnosis or disease or equated with frailty, and it should not signal the withdrawal of efforts to find and treat underlying causes. Instead, it should be viewed as unexpected and significant change in normal health status and a decline in vigor, weight, and function that can affect even the healthiest of older people. For older individuals who exhibit unintentional reduction of food intake and weight loss, decline in ability to provide self care, decline in cognitive function, and a general decline in interest in daily life, the term *failure to thrive* should trigger a thorough evaluation to determine possible reversible underlying causes.[3]

Identification and Assessment

FTT affects anywhere from 5% to 35% of community-dwelling elders and 25% to 40% of nursing home residents.[1] Prevalence of the syndrome appears to increase with age. Studies indicate that it is associated with decreased immunity and increased rates of infection, incidence of hip fractures, pressure ulcers, surgical mortality, mortality rates, and medical costs.[1]

Because the decline is so gradual, loved ones often do not notice the subtle changes in condition. If they do observe changes, the older adult often denies there is anything wrong and treatment may be delayed until there is an acute illness or event (eg, fall, fracture, pneumonia). At the time of the assessment for the acute event, healthcare professionals and caregivers realize there has been a decline in condition, which usually includes unintentional weight loss.

Initial assessment should include a total review of mental and physical health, functional ability, and social/environmental factors. This total assessment should include a review of chronic diseases, possible medication interactions, a nutritional assessment, and appropriate laboratory and radiological evaluations individualized to the patient's specific needs. An alcohol and substance abuse screening is also recommended.[1]

Common medical conditions associated with FTT include cancer, congestive heart failure (CHF), chronic lung disease, chronic renal insufficiency, chronic steroid use, cirrhosis, cerebrovascular accident, depression or other mental disorders, diabetes, hepatitis, hip or large bone fracture, inflammatory bowel disease, history of gastrointestinal surgery, M. incognitus, recurrent urinary tract infections, recurrent pneumonia, rheumatologic disease (eg, rheumatoid arthritis, lupus), systemic infection, and tuberculosis.[1]

Common medications associated with FTT include anticholinergic drugs, antiepileptic drugs, benzodiazepines, beta blockers, central alpha antagonists, diuretics in high-potency combinations, glucocorticoids, neuroleptics, opioids, selective serotonin reuptake inhibitors, tricyclic antidepressants, and more than four prescription medications.[1]

Four main areas of assessment and treatment for FTT syndrome have been identified:

- impaired physical function or status;
- undernutrition or malnutrition (including unintentional or significant weight loss);
- depression or depressive symptoms; and
- cognitive impairment or decline.[1,4]

Impaired Physical Function or Status

It is important to assess the individual's ability to perform activities of daily living. This can be achieved using the Katz ADL scale to assess ability in six areas: eating, dressing, toileting, transferring, continence, and bathing. A physician can administer a simple test called the "Up and Go." The physician asks the patient to rise from a chair, walk 10 feet, turn, and return to the chair to sit down. If the patient can easily achieve this task in less than 20 seconds, he or she is generally competent to perform basic transfers. Those who take more than 30 seconds to complete the test generally need more assistance and have a higher risk for falls.[1]

Undernutrition or Malnutrition

One of the most common symptoms of FTT is unintentional weight loss. Malnutrition may result if the patient is not treated. In the nursing home setting, residents are assessed by the dietetics professional and appropriate interventions are determined and implemented. In the outpatient setting, The Mini Nutritional Assessment (MNA) is a validated nutrition assessment tool that may be used to identify malnutrition.[5] However, a more commonly used tool in the outpatient and home care setting is the DETERMINE Your Health Checklist.[6]

Depression or Depressive Symptoms

Depression is common with FTT and may be either a cause or a result of the syndrome. Depression can be a major cause of unintentional weight loss, and if left untreated, it is associated with increased morbidity and mortality in FTT patients. It is imperative to screen for depression. The Geriatric Depression Scale is a commonly used tool for assessment of depression.[7]

Cognitive Impairment or Decline

The Mini-Mental State Examination is the most common and valid screening tool to assess cognitive disorders.[8] Cognitive impairment may be the result of factors such as abuse or neglect, lack of support, recent personal loss, medications, chronic disease, malnutrition, electrolyte imbalances, and dehydration. Cognitive status should be evaluated frequently due to potential ongoing changes in overall health status and condition in an older adult with FTT.[1]

In addition to an in-depth evaluation of the above four factors, a thorough medical evaluation should determine any underlying medical problems. Undiagnosed health problems such as diabetes, hypertension, or acute issues such as urinary tract or upper respiratory infections can result in rapid declines in older adults. A review of medications is also pertinent. Drug nutrient interactions, drug-drug interactions, polypharmacy, and adverse reactions can all have devastating effects on an older person. Dentition, vision, hearing, continence, and gastrointestinal issues must also be addressed. Each patient should also be assessed for psychosocial, economic, spiritual, and emotional needs. Living situation, caregiver ability, potential abuse or neglect situations, isolation, and financial ability to purchase food and prescriptions can all have a dramatic effect on an older adult's ability to thrive.[4]

Treatment

The goal of medical interventions is to improve overall quality of life and functional abilities. Interventions for easily treatable causes of FTT (eg, poor nutritional intake) should be implemented immediately. Treatment is best achieved through a team approach: physician, nurse, dietitian, physical therapist, social worker, mental health professional, and/or speech pathologist, as dictated by individual need.[1]

Malnutrition

Nutritional status has a significant impact on a person's ability to resist infection; recover from illness, injury, or surgery; and have the strength and energy to rehabilitate. Malnourished older adults have diminished muscle strength, which can lead to weakness, decreased independence, and falls. They may also have slower recovery from illness or acute episodes, a tendency toward poor healing, increased risk of pressure ulcers, weight loss, infection, immune dysfunction, anemia, weakness, fatigue, and morbidity and mortality.

Low albumin and anemia are associated with lower survival rates, decreased ability for self care, depression, and cognitive impairment. Low albumin in FTT may be related to effects of chronic disease and inflammation or to "interactions between nutrition and illness."[9]

Sarcopenia

In addition to malnutrition, sarcopenia may exacerbate the difficulties challenging the health of an older adult. Sarcopenia is the excessive loss of muscle associated with aging. Generally, people start losing muscle at roughly 45 years of age and tend to continue losing muscle at a rate of approximately 1% per year. This muscle loss leads to reduced strength and ability to perform everyday tasks. In addition, unsteadiness may result in falls.

There are several key factors that accelerate loss of muscle mass, including decreased physical activity, testosterone and growth hormone deficiency, decreased neuronal endplate input into muscles, and possibly mild cytokine excess (severe cytokine excess leads to cachexia).[10] The stress response can create additional loss of lean body mass (LBM). The stress response can occur due to catabolic illness such as wounds, trauma, surgery, and infection. It is essentially a hormonal response to stress (a heightened "fight or flight" response) that increases energy needs, causes the body to break down proteins and LBM, and can lead to protein calorie malnutrition.

LBM makes up 75% of body weight, mostly in the form of muscle, bone, and tendon. This LBM provides the majority of the body's protein. Unfortunately, the rate of recovery of LBM is much slower during the recovery stage than the rate of loss during the inflammatory stage. Loss of just 10% of LBM decreases immune response and increases the risk of infection. A loss of 15% or more reduces the rate of wound healing and increases weakness. At 30% loss of LBM, pressure ulcers may develop and healing response is nonexistent. A 40% LBM loss usually results in death (often due to pneumonia).[11]

Medical Nutrition Therapy (MNT)

It is important to quickly and accurately identify older adults at risk of malnutrition. There are various tools available, including the DETERMINE Your Health Checklist, the Subjective Global Assessment, the MNA (www.mna-elderly.com), and the Malnutrition Universal Screening Tool.[12,13]

In addition to these standardized tools, some simple screening questions may also be practical in certain settings:

- Have you lost weight recently? If so, how much and in what period of time?
- Do you eat three meals per day?
- What do you typically eat for breakfast, lunch, dinner, and snacks (24-hour recall)?
- Do you consume at least three servings of dairy products and 5 ounces of meat per day?
- Are you taking any vitamin/mineral supplements? If so, what are you taking?
- Are you having any difficulty chewing or swallowing?

The goal of MNT should be to improve quality of life, stabilize or reverse weight loss and malnutrition, and treat any identified problems. Even if an older person is overweight, he or she may have a low LBM. Common nutritional problems of older adults include an inability to consume adequate calories and protein to meet needs, overly restrictive diets (liberalized diets can help to improve food intake), dysphagia, and depression.[14]

One of the most important interventions is to ensure adequate calorie and protein intake. This can be achieved using enhanced foods and oral nutritional supplements, ensuring adequate access to foods and a pleasant dining experience, offering favorite foods, providing adequate assistance, and starting enteral feeding, if necessary. Every bite counts for these frail individuals, so it is important to liberalize diets as much as possible.[14]

Nutrient Needs

General recommendations for calorie needs of older adults are as follows:

- 25 calories per kilogram for normal weight/nonstressed patients;
- 30 to 35 calories per kilogram for underweight or for pressure ulcers or stressed patients; and

- 40 calories per kilogram for more severe cases (stage 3/4, multiple pressure ulcers, or severe unintentional weight loss).[14–19]

It is important to ensure adequate protein intake to slow sarcopenia, decrease the loss of LBM, and avoid protein-energy malnutrition by following these recommendations:

- 1 to 1.2 grams per kilogram of body weight for nonstressed patients;
- 1.2 to 1.5 grams per kilogram of body weight for patients at high risk of pressure ulcers, with pressure ulcers, or those who are stressed; and
- 0.8 grams per kilogram of body weight for chronic renal failure (predialysis).[14,18,19]

Fluid needs for older adults may be met by following these general guidelines:

- 30 milliliters per kilogram of body weight;
- 35 milliliters per kilogram of body weight for dehydration;
- 25 milliliters per kilogram of body weight for CHF and renal failure; and
- 1 milliliter per calorie for enteral feeding.[14,18]

Some older adults need vitamin and mineral supplementation with calcium, folate, vitamin B_{12}, and vitamin B_6. Most will need vitamins D and E. Magnesium and zinc intake are sometimes inadequate. In general, a daily multivitamin and mineral supplement is suggested for most older adults.[10,19]

Individuals who experience anorexia, food aversions, or loss of appetite may benefit from alternative interventions such as appetite stimulants and/or anabolic steroids.[20]

Physical Activity

Falls are the leading cause of injuries, hospital admissions for trauma, and deaths due to injury. Estimates indicate that there are 360,000 to 480,000 fall-related fractures per year.[21] By age 65, 48% of all people in the United States do not participate in leisure time physical activity, and at 75-plus years of age, more than 61% do not participate. Inactivity contributes to an increase in body fat and a decrease in muscle mass, which in turn leads to reduced functional ability.

Nearly all older adults can benefit from resistive and strength training to increase muscle strength, improve functional ability, and prevent further decline.[4]

Four components of physical activity are important for a well-balanced exercise plan:

- endurance to improve cardiovascular and circulatory systems (low-impact exercises)
- strength to reduce sarcopenia, build muscles, and possibly prevent osteoporosis. (Strength training can include resistance training three times per week. Tylenol or a nonsteroidal anti-inflammatory agent may be needed prior to exercise to reduce postworkout pain from inflammation.[10] Alone and in combination with

nutritional supplementation, strength training increases strength and functional capacity.)[19]

- balance to prevent falls (Balance exercises may include Tai Chi, which improves balance, or something as simple as standing on one leg with eyes closed. Older adults may need to hold on to something.) and
- flexibility to recover from or prevent injuries. (Flexibility exercises such as yoga or stretching may help prevent falls.)[21]

A Winning Combination

Nutrition and exercise together have a synergistic effect that helps combat malnutrition, increase strength, and promote well-being. Patients need adequate energy and protein to meet needs and support muscle synthesis and repair.[19] Encourage physical activity to promote anabolism and suggest appropriate exercises (including strength training). Address protein losses if present and encourage adequate protein and caloric intake.[10] Refer to a physical therapist to assess range of motion, strength, and endurance and determine need for assistive devices (eg, canes, walkers, grab bars, shower chairs). Offer early physical therapy, strength training, and occupational therapy, if necessary. Encourage walking, and refer to social services for home environment assessment if necessary.[19]

By being aware of each individual's conditions, problems, and concerns in relation to nutrition and physical activity, you can provide the most appropriate interventions for each individual.

BECKY DORNER, RD, LD, is a speaker and on author who provides publications, presentations, and consulting services to enhance the quality of care for the nation's older adults. Visit www.beckydorner.com for free articles, newsletters, and information.

Overweight and Mortality among Baby Boomers—Now We're Getting Personal

TIM BYERS, MD, MPH

I am a baby boomer, and my body-mass index (BMI) is 27.3. I am also an epidemiologist, so for both personal and professional reasons, I have closely followed the sometimes divergent conclusions about the health risks associated with growing older and being a little overweight. As reported in this issue of the *Journal,* trials involving more than half a million Americans (Adams et al., pages 763–778) and more than a million Koreans (Jee et al., pages 779–787) are the latest in a series of cohort studies published in recent years on the risks associated with excess adiposity. Now that studies are beginning to describe the risk of death associated with even modest levels of adiposity among baby boomers, this issue is getting more personal for me.

At first glance, the new study involving members of the AARP (formerly the American Association of Retired Persons) looks reassuring for those of us who are not obese, but only overweight. Among the entire cohort of AARP members, the risk of death seems to be substantially increased only for those whose BMI is over 30, the cutoff defining obesity. However, we have learned in recent years that only studies of the relationship between adiposity and the risk of death that properly account for tobacco use and chronic medical conditions can be truly informative about the risk caused by lesser degrees of adiposity. The AARP study clearly shows that if the effects of smoking are set aside, at age 50, when the prevalence of chronic disease is low, there is also an elevated risk of death for persons whose BMIs are well below 30.

The study of adiposity and mortality among Korean adults also shows a graded relationship between BMI and death from atherosclerotic cardiovascular disease across a very wide range of BMI levels, including what would be regarded as only modest levels of adiposity in the United States. This finding is a sobering reminder that because obesity is now a worldwide problem, the phenomenon of "global fattening" will contribute to a pandemic of chronic diseases for many years to come.

What are we to do about the epidemic of adiposity, both collectively and personally? As health care providers, we are all touched by the personal dimensions of the problem, sometimes because we are ourselves overweight and sometimes because of the many personal issues that arise as we try to help our patients. The medical management of hypertension,

hyperlipidemia, and insulin resistance certainly helps, but the treatment of these mediating factors does not completely eliminate the excess risk associated with adiposity. Adverse consequences of adiposity are seen in even quite health-conscious cohorts, such as AARP members, insured Korean patients, American Cancer Society volunteers, and registered nurses.[1,2] Our inability to negate these health risks may be due to the irreversibility of some of the biologic harm, our inability to achieve perfect control over the known mediating factors, or the effects of other as-yet-uncontrollable factors, such as the chronic inflammatory state of adiposity, as is signaled by the association between white-cell counts and BMI in the Korean cohort study.

We baby boomers are now into the second half of our lives. How will our current excess weight, much of it gained after age 50 during the ongoing obesity epidemic, affect our health risks as we age? A 1999 study conducted in an American Cancer Society cohort of more than a million Americans[1] provides a clear answer: among nonsmokers without chronic medical conditions, the risk of death is elevated even among the modestly overweight, and this elevated risk persists as age advances (see graph). Observations that the risk of death expressed as a ratio (including the relative risk in the AARP cohort and the hazard ratio in the Korean cohort) diminishes with advancing age cannot be taken as evidence that the effects of adiposity diminish. In fact, the absolute degree of additional risk associated with excess adiposity (the difference in risk between overweight persons and those of normal weight) substantially increases with advancing age, according to the analysis of the American Cancer Society cohort. Risk ratios diminish with advancing age simply because the ratios are diluted by the many other causes of death associated with aging, which figure into both the numerator and the denominator of the ratio.

As we baby boomers move past 50, we will have to address the reality that excess adiposity substantially increases with advancing age. Fortunately, evidence points to a substantial health benefit from even small changes in weight trajectory, so the achievement of an ideal body weight need not be the primary goal. There are many ways that physicians can help patients to make the critical first step of stopping weight gain.[3] Small steps toward weight control, such as short bursts of activity and

A

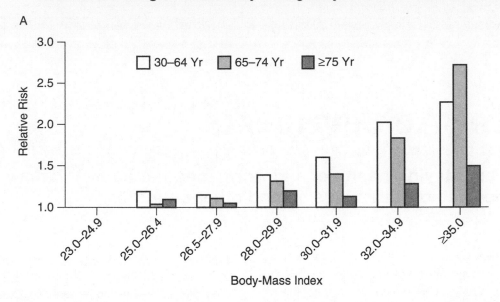

B

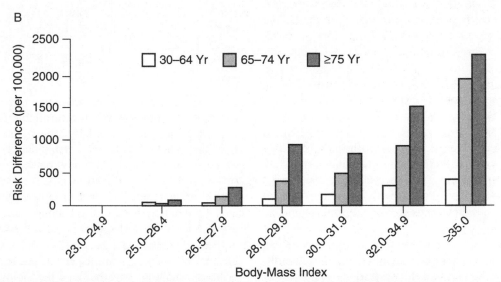

Risk of Death Associated with BMI among Male Nonsmokers without Chronic Health Conditions, According to Age. The annual risk of death is expressed as both the relative risk (Panel A) and the absolute amount of additional risk (risk difference) (Panel B) per 100,000 population, as reported in the American Cancer Society Cancer Prevention Study 2.[1] Even though the excess risk of death due to adiposity increased with age, the relative risk decreased with age because of dilution by the many other causes of death associated with increasing age.

discrete changes in eating habits, need not require major lifestyle modification.

In my own personal adiposity epidemic, small steps seem to help. When I turned 50, I began to gain weight, even though it seemed that my eating and activity habits had not changed. When I turned 55, I cut out powdered doughnuts and began to walk more. Now, at age 57, I am 10 pounds lighter, my wife is happier that there is less powdered sugar on the seat of the car, and I have a little more energy. As I reflect on my BMI of 27.3, however, I am now looking for more small steps. My office is located on the fourth floor of a building with both stairs and an elevator. Hmmm.

Notes

1. Calle EE, Thun MJ, Petrelli JM, Rodriguez C, Heath CW Jr. Body-mass index and mortality in a prospective cohort of U.S. adults. N Engl J Med 1999;341:1097–105.
2. Manson JE, Willett WC, Stampfer MJ, et al. Body weight and mortality among women. N Engl J Med 1995;333:677–85.
3. Manson JE, Skerrett PJ, Greenland P, VanItallie TB. The escalating pandemics of obesity and sedentary lifestyle: a call to action for clinicians. Arch Intern Med 2004; 164:249–58.

Dr. Byers, MD, MPH, is a professor of preventive medicine at the University of Colorado School of Medicine, Denver.

Lifetime Achievements

Americans are staying healthier and living longer than ever before, although the United States lags behind other countries.

Life-expectancy figures are statistical crystal balls that predict the average number of years a person of a given age, sex, and race can be expected to live. Expected age at death is the pessimistic way to express the same idea. According to the latest figures, life expectancy in the United States is 77.6 years, up considerably from 75.4 in 1990, although still quite a way behind the Japanese, who (on average) reach their 80s.

These figures represent life expectancy at birth—that is, how long today's newborns are expected to live. We adults are not going to make it to 2083 like today's babies. But the good news is that as you get older, your statistical chances of beating the current life expectancy at birth improve. Why? Because you've managed to dodge the mortal dangers that stalk younger lives: infant mortality, violence, car wrecks. There's also a healthy survivor effect: People with advantages derived from heredity or life circumstances are over-represented in any older population.

An American man celebrating his 65th birthday today can expect to live long enough to blow out candles on his 81st birthday cake. If he's 75, he can look forward to an 85th birthday bash, and at that party, his 90th (see Table 1).

In the United States and throughout the world, women outlive men, although the gap is closing. On average, a 65-year-old American woman can expect to live another 19½ years, surpassing her male contemporaries by three years and beating the current life expectancy at birth by almost five years (84.5 versus 80.1). And 75-year-old American women will, on average, live long enough to celebrate their 87th birthdays, and the 85-year-olds will live to almost 92.

We worry about tempting fate with glowing predictions, but there's good reason to believe that life expectancies for the old are going to get even longer. Mortality rates for the conditions that disproportionately affect older people—heart disease, cancer, stroke—are falling.

Moreover, we seem to be staying healthy much longer. Research shows that rates of disability and years of so-called functional decline among the American elderly are dropping. Experts have different theories about the "compression of morbidity." Vincent Mor, chair of the Department of Community Health at Brown University Medical School, has identified three factors that are squeezing illness and loss of independence into

Table 1   Age Has Its Benefits

The older you are, the longer your life expectancy

	Men	Women
At birth*	74.8	80.1
At 65	81.6	84.5
At 75	85.3	87.4
At 85	90.7	91.9

*At birth figures are for 2003; others are for 2002.
Source: National Center for Health Statistics.

fewer years at the end of life. First, older people have access to cars and are more likely to live in homes conducive to old age (fewer or no stairs, for example). As a result, older Americans can get around and fend for themselves. Second, as clouded as their futures may be with the coming wave of baby boomers, Social Security and Medicare have been a strong safety net for millions of older Americans. Last but not least, medical advances like cataract surgery, hip replacement, and medical management of heart conditions have buffered the biological impact of old age. All in all, it's a pretty good time to be growing older.

Yet relative to people in other countries, Americans aren't doing so well. American males and females rank 12th and 15th, respectively, in life expectancy at age 65. The World Health Organization publishes country-by-country statistics for healthy life expectancy, or HALE, to assess not just the years that people live, but the years they spend in good health. At age 60, American men have 15.3 years of healthy life expectancy, and women, 17.9. HALE rankings aren't readily available, but as with life expectancy, United States is out of the top 10 and behind Japan (17.5 for men and 21.7 for women) and several European countries.

In May, a study comparing the health of older middle-aged people (ages 55–64) in the United States and England received a great deal of attention. British researchers found that Americans were less healthy than their English counterparts, with higher rates of cancer, diabetes, heart disease, high blood pressure, lung disease, and stroke. Some of the gap might be explained by differences in screening and testing practices and how diseases are defined and diagnosed. But the Americans also came out worse on objective lab test results, such as C-reactive protein, "good" HDL cholesterol, and fibrinogen, a clotting factor.

The researchers say that's evidence that the health differences between the two countries are real, not just a question of better detection or broader definitions of disease in the United States.

Designing a Better Crystal Ball

But life-expectancy statistics are broad generalizations. Even when they're broken down by race, sex, and other categories, they are just overall averages that aren't intended to be applied to an individual. Researchers at the San Francisco Veterans Affairs Medical Center have come up with a quiz that gives a clearer picture of individual destiny—or, as they are calling it, a "prognostic index."

They used data collected in the Health and Retirement Survey (HRS), a large, federally funded study of the health and economic circumstances of Americans over age 50. In 1998, the HRS had about 20,000 people enrolled; by 2002, almost 12% of them had died. By combing through the large amount of data from this study and plugging some of it into statistical equations, the San Francisco researchers came up with 12 factors that correlated with death in that four-year interval. Then they tested their index against data from another cohort of the HRS to see whether it would accurately identify the people who died. It did. The results and the index, or quiz, were published in the Feb. 15, 2006, issue of the *Journal of the American Medical Association*.

Taking the Quiz

The quiz features 12 questions that address some of the usual suspects, including cancer, diabetes, and smoking.

Age, of course, is a big factor. An 85-year-old (7 points) non-smoking (0 points) woman (0 points) without diabetes (0 points) who has no difficulty walking several blocks (0 points) earns the same number of risk points (7) as a 60-year-old (1 point) woman (0 points) with congestive heart failure (2 points) who smokes (2 points) and can't walk several blocks without difficulty (2 points).

You may notice the last four questions on the quiz aren't strictly medical but involve coping with day-to-day life: bathing, managing money, and overall strength and mobility. With age, these functional indicators are as important as any lab test in assessing health.

The researchers said they wanted to keep their index as simple as possible so that it could be used inexpensively in a wide variety of circumstances. That's one reason why the questions have yes/no answers. And for most people, the questions can be answered from memory ("Has a doctor told you that you have congestive heart failure?") without knowledge of medical details or test results (blood pressure levels, cholesterol counts, and so on). The researchers wanted to avoid the high cost of reviewing medical charts or ordering new lab tests.

Curiously, a body mass index (BMI) that's less than 25 is a health debit in this quiz. Usually, a "normal" BMI (between 18.5 and 25) is considered a nice feather in the health cap. But assessing the health consequences of weight in old age gets

Mortality Quiz

Factor	Points		Your Score
Age	Under 60: **0**	75–79: **4**	
	60–64: **1**	80–84: **5**	
	65–69: **2**	85 and	
	70–74: **3**	over: **7**	
Sex	Female: **0**	Male: **2**	
Body mass index	25 and over: **0**	Under 25: **1**	
Has a doctor ever told you that you have diabetes or high blood sugar?	No: **0**	Yes: **1**	
Has a doctor told you that you have cancer or a malignant tumor, excluding minor skin cancers?	No: **0**	Yes: **2**	
Do you have a chronic lung disease that limits your usual activities or makes you need oxygen at home?	No: **0**	Yes: **2**	
Has a doctor told you that you have congestive heart failure?	No: **0**	Yes: **2**	
Have you smoked cigarettes in the past week?	No: **0**	Yes: **2**	
Because of a health or memory problem, do you have any difficulty with bathing?	No: **0**	Yes: **2**	
Because of a health or memory problem, do you have any difficulty with managing your money—such as paying your bills and keeping track of expenses?	No: **0**	Yes: **2**	
Because of a health problem, do you have any difficulty with walking several blocks?	No: **0**	Yes: **2**	
Because of a health problem, do you have any difficulty with pulling or pushing large objects like a living room chair?	No: **0**	Yes: **1**	

Mortality risk in the next 4 years
Point total

Your Total

0–5 ▬ 4%
6–9 ▬▬ 15%
10–13 ▬▬▬▬▬ 42%
14 and over ▬▬▬▬▬▬▬ 64%

Source: *Journal of the American Medical Association*, Feb. 15, 2006, pp. 801–8.

tricky because losing weight is often a sign of an underlying illness. On the other hand, being heavy if you're older may have some limited benefits that offset, if only partially, the increased risk for cardiovascular disease and cancer. Probably the clearest example is osteoporosis and hip fracture: Extra weight seems to protect women from these problems.

So What's the Use?

With the baby-boom bulge now edging into older age, experts are anticipating a surge in demand for late-life medical care. Prognostic indices like this one may help doctors and patients decide whether an operation, drug treatment, or test is worth it—injecting some objectivity into decisions that must be made in any case.

The researchers also envision health officials and fellow researchers using the index—or one like it—to "risk-adjust" outcome data for operations, hospital care, and so on. More of that kind of information is available these days, but there's worry that it can be misinterpreted if a doctor or hospital takes on harder cases involving sicker people. Reliable risk adjustment helps to level the playing field so outcome comparisons are fairer.

Some Limitations

No prognostic index is ever going to be perfect. This one is thought to be about 80% accurate, and its accuracy varies with the population. The San Francisco researchers deliberately left out people in nursing homes or other institutions because they envision the index being used for relatively healthy people living in the community. Whites are overrepresented in the data on which it's based, so the index may not be as accurate for African Americans or other groups. The yes/no questions don't take into account the severity of the various conditions and some other potentially significant information. Another question is how you set the clock: Factors that predict mortality in, say, the next 10 years aren't necessarily the same ones that are predictive over the four-year span used to formulate this quiz.

For the individual doctor and patient, this sort of assessment should feature a prominent "handle with care" warning. A short quiz can't take into account all a person's health issues and the relevant circumstances. So go ahead, take the quiz, but take the results with a grain of salt.

Excerpted from *Harvard Health Letter*, Vol. 31, no. 9, July 2006, pp. 1–3. Copyright © 2006 by the President and Fellow of Harvard College. Reprinted with permission. www.health.harvard.edu/health

A Practical Guide to Better Health

We Can Control How We Age

What does it take to age successfully—to maintain both a sound body and mind? A landmark Harvard study has followed individuals from their teens into their 80s.

Lou Ann Walker

How do some people age so successfully? Many of us assume it takes genes or dumb luck. So here's the surprise. Arguably the longest and most comprehensive study of human development ever undertaken is just revealing its final results: *We are very much in control of our own aging.* The secret to a long and happy life, it seems, does not lie as much in our stars as in ourselves.

The Study of Adult Development at Harvard Medical School comprises three projects begun in the 1920s, '30s, and '40s. These careful scientific studies analyze three very different demographic groups: one of Harvard men (the Grant Study), another of inner-city Boston men and the third of gifted California women. In all, 824 men and women have been followed from their teens into their 80s. Over the decades, these people were given psychological tests and asked to evaluate their lives and feelings. They responded to numerous questionnaires, interviews by psychiatrists and physical examinations by doctors.

The study is a medical rarity because it examines the lives of the well, not the sick. "Old age is like a minefield," the study's director, Dr. George E. Vaillant, told PARADE. "If you see footprints leading to the other side, step in them." These results show a clear path that Baby Boomers and Gen X-ers can follow to lead a long, happy life.

The study divides individuals between 60 and 80 years old into two main groups: (1) the "Happy-Well," those who are physically healthy and find life satisfying; and (2) the "Sad-Sick," those with various ailments who do not seem to enjoy life. And it analyzes those who died during the course of the study (the "Prematurely Dead").

Living with a Full Heart

The Harvard study found these four attributes vital to successful aging:

- Orientation toward the Future. The ability to anticipate, to plan and to hope.
- Gratitude, Forgiveness and Optimism. We need to see the glass as half-full, not half-empty.
- Empathy. The ability to imagine the world as it seems to the other person.
- The Ability to Reach Out. "We should want to do things *with* people, not do things *to* people or ruminate that they do things to us," says Dr. George E. Vaillant. In other words, we need to "leave the screen door unlatched."

It's *Not* in Our Genes . . .

A major finding was that good genes did not account for better aging. Nor did income. Good care obviously is important, said Dr. Vaillant, "but the trick is not going to the hospital in the first place."

The study disputes the assumption that with aging comes decay. When 30- and 55-year-old brains are compared, the older one is better developed. Advancing age impairs some motor skills, but maturation can make people sharper at emotional tasks.

Seven Keys to Aging Well
What Are the Secrets to a Long, Happy Life?

Dr. George E. Vaillant points out seven major factors that, at 50, predict what life's outcome will be at 80:

1 Not smoking or quitting early: Those who quit the habit before 50 were, at 70, as healthy as those who had never smoked. And heavy smoking was 10 times more prevalent among the Prematurely Dead than among the Happy-Well. "Smoking," said Vaillant, "is probably the most significant factor in terms of health."

Coping with Life's Stresses
Those who learn early how to roll with the punches are much happier in their later years, despite real problems.

2 The ability to take life's ups and downs in stride: If you can make lemonade out of lemons, then you have an adaptive coping style, also known as "mature defenses." Mature defenses don't actually ensure good health at an older age. But a person will suffer less from life's real problems if he or she has the ability to roll with the punches. "Life ain't easy," Vaillant said. "Terrible things happen to everyone. You have to keep your sense of humor, give something of yourself to others, make friends who are younger than you, learn new things and have fun."

An Active Lifestyle
The long-term results of regular exercise are both physical and psychological well-being.

3 Absence of alcohol abuse: "Abusing alcohol destroys both your physical and mental health," Vaillant noted. (He added that a partner's alcoholism can destroy a marriage, which also may have an impact on how one ages.)

4 Healthy weight: Obesity is a risk factor for poor health in later life.

A Strong Marriage
A good marriage contributes to a long and happy life. The study also found that, overall, marriages improved with time—if people were willing to work out the bumps.

5 A solid marriage: This is important for both physical and psychological health. Happy-Well people were six times more likely to be in good marriages than were the Sad-Sick.

6 Physical activity: The study specified that the Happy-Well usually did "some exercise." The benefits of fitness also extended to mental health.

Continuing Education
The more years of school people have, the more they tend to age successfully.

7 Years of education: Vaillant speculated that people to whom "self-care and perseverance" are important are also more likely to continue their educations. These individuals, he surmised, are able to take the long view. "People seek education because they believe it is possible to control the course of their lives," he said. In the study, people with less education also were more likely to be obese. Their physical health at age 65 was close to that of the more-educated group at 75.

People who had four or more of these seven factors at age 50 were one-third less likely to be dead by 80. People who had three or fewer of these factors at 50—even though they were in good physical shape—were three times as likely to die during the following 30 years.

. . . but in Ourselves

Many of the study's findings focus on psychological health. As we age, we should try to develop more mature coping styles, Vaillant concluded from the results. "Our defenses are always more mature when we are not hungry, angry, lonely, tired or drunk," he noted.

"Taking people inside oneself" emotionally is important, he said, adding, "Popular people can be extraordinarily lonely and depressed. The paradox is that they starve, yet there's plenty of food." He pointed to the example of Marilyn Monroe, who made Arthur Miller and others feel cared for yet was unable to feel that love within herself.

Although developmental psychologists often say that personality is formed by age 5, the study found otherwise. By 70, it's how we nurture ourselves throughout our lifetimes that takes precedence over nature. Interestingly, Vaillant discovered that many people who aged well unconsciously reinterpreted early events in their lives in a more positive light as they grew older. Those who clung to negative events were less happy adults. Forever blaming parents for a rotten childhood seems to impede maturity.

"What goes *right* in childhood predicts the future far better than what goes wrong," he noted. Especially important was a feeling of acceptance.

As one ages, remaining connected to life is crucial—as is learning the rules of a changing world. On the other hand, Vaillant said, "One task of living out the last half of life is excavating and recovering those whom we loved in the first half. The recovery of lost loves becomes an important way in which the past affects the present."

The study's results will be published by Little, Brown in January in a book titled *Aging Well: Surprising Guideposts to a Happier Life from the Landmark Harvard Study of Adult Development.* In addition to facts and figures, the book is filled with life stories of the men and women studied.

Vaillant, who has been called "a big, handsome, humorous psychiatrist," looks a decade younger than his 67 years. He and his wife of 30 years, Caroline, live in Vermont. In addition to his research, he maintains a small clinical practice at Boston's Brigham and Women's Hospital. He calls himself an "oppositional character" who loves "proving other people wrong."

I asked Vaillant what he hopes the results of this study will accomplish. "A heightened appreciation of the positive," he shot back. Then he added: "Worry less about cholesterol and more about gratitude and forgiveness."

UNIT 3

Societal Attitudes toward Old Age

Unit Selections

Key Points to Consider

- What are the prevalent images Americans have of older people?

- Why do most Americans fear getting old?

- What advantages go to the older person who does not hold any of the negative stereotypes of aging?

- Have current studies found older Americans to be lonely, isolated, and unhappy?

- As the workforce ages, what changes in employer attitudes toward older workers will have to take place in order to keep and maintain the critical skills of these workers?

Student Website

www.mhhe.com/cls

Internet References

Adult Development and Aging: Division 20 of the American Psychological Association
   http://www.iog.wayne.edu/APADIV20/APADIV20.HTM
American Society on Aging
   http://www.asaging.org/index.cfm
Canadian Psychological Association
   http://www.cpa.ca

There are a wide range of beliefs regarding the social position and status of the aged in American society today. Some people believe that the best way to understand the problems of the elderly is to regard them as a minority group, faced with difficulties similar to those of other minority groups. Discrimination against older people, like racial discrimination, is believed to be based on a bias against visible physical traits. Since the aging process is viewed negatively, it is natural that the elderly try to appear and act younger. Some spend a tremendous amount of money trying to make themselves look and feel younger.

The theory that old people are a minority group is weak because too many circumstances prove otherwise. The U.S. Congress, for example, favors its senior members, and delegates power to them by bestowing considerable prestige. The leadership roles in most religious organizations are held by older persons. Many older Americans are in good health, have comfortable incomes, and are treated with respect by friends and associates.

Perhaps the most realistic way to view the aged is as a status group, like other status groups in society. Every society has some method of "age grading," by which it groups together individuals of roughly similar age. ("Preteens" and "senior citizens" are some of the age-grade labels in American society.)

Because it is a labeling process, age grading causes members of the age group, as well as others, to perceive them in terms of the connotations of the label. Unfortunately, the tag "old age" often has negative connotations in American society.

The readings included in this section illustrate the wide range of stereotypical attitudes toward older Americans. Many of society's typical assumptions about the limitations of old age have been refuted. A major force behind this reassessment of the elderly is that there are so many people living longer and healthier lives, and in consequence, playing more of a role in all aspects of our society. Older people can remain productive members of society for many more years than has been traditionally assumed.

Such standard stereotypes of the elderly as frail, senile, childish, and sexually inactive are topics discussed in this section. Mary Pipher, in "Society Fears the Aging Process," contends that young people often avoid interacting with older persons because it reminds them that someday they too will get old and die. She further argues that the media most often portray a negative and stereotypical view of the elderly.

Lea Winerman in "A Healthy Mind, a Longer Life" asserts that accepting the negative stereotypes of aging is not good for the older person's physical or mental health. She believes that

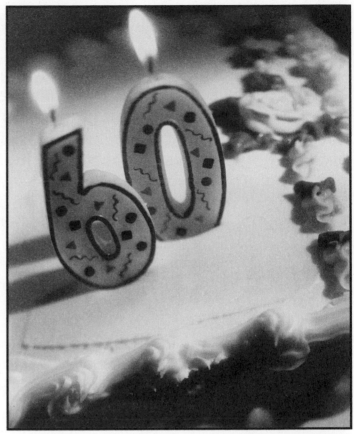

the ability to discard the negative stereotypes and adopt a more positive view of later life would appreciably improve the lives and health of older persons. In "Research: Oldest Americans Happiest," Lindsey Tanner points out that the stereotype view of the older Americans being lonely, isolated, and unhappy was not proven to be the reality that was found in a number of different studies on this subject. Robert J. Grossman, in "The Under-Reported Impact of Age Discrimination and Its Threat to Business Vitality," believes that the legal system is slanted toward the employers who perpetuate many of the negative stereotypes and views of the older workers. He sees age discrimination in the workplace as a more serious problem in the future, when labor shortages will make older workers and their skills more critical and in demand.

Society Fears the Aging Process

Americans fear the processes of aging and dying, Mary Pipher contends in the following viewpoint. She claims that younger and healthier adults often avoid spending time around the aging because they want to avoid the issues of mortality and loss of independence. In addition, she contends that negative views of the aging process are portrayed in the media and expressed through the use of pejorative words to describe the elderly. Pipher is a psychologist and author of several books, including *Another Country: Navigating the Emotional Terrain of Our Elders,* the book from which this viewpoint was excerpted.

MARY PIPHER

W e segregate the old for many reasons—prejudice, ignorance, a lack of good alternatives, and a youth-worshiping culture without guidelines on how to care for the old. The old are different from us, and that makes us nervous. Xenophobia means fear of people from another country. In America we are xenophobic toward our old people.

How Greeting Cards Reflect Culture

An anthropologist could learn about us by examining our greeting cards. As with all aspects of popular culture, greeting cards both mirror and shape our realities. Cards reflect what we feel about people in different roles, and they also teach us what to feel. I visited my favorite local drugstore and took a look.

There are really two sets of cards that relate to aging. One is the grandparent/grandchild set that is all about connection. Even a very dim-witted anthropologist would sense the love and respect that exist between these two generations in our culture. Young children's cards to their grandparents say, "I wish I could hop on your lap," or, "You're so much fun." Grandparents' cards to children are filled with pride and love.

There is another section of cards on birthdays. These compare human aging to wine aging, or point out compensations. "With age comes wisdom, of course that doesn't make up for what you lose." We joke the most about that which makes us anxious. "Have you picked out your bench at the mall yet?" There are jokes about hearing loss, incontinence, and losing sexual abilities and interest. There are cards on saggy behinds, gray hair, and wrinkles, and cards about preferring chocolate or

sleep to sex. "You know you're getting old when someone asks if you're getting enough and you think about sleep."

Fears of Aging and Dying

Poking fun at aging isn't all bad. It's better to laugh than to cry, especially at what cannot be prevented. However, these jokes reflect our fears about aging in a youth-oriented culture. We younger, healthier people sometimes avoid the old to avoid our own fears of aging. If we aren't around dying people, we don't have to think about dying.

We baby boomers have been a futureless generation, raised in the eternal present of TV and advertising. We have allowed ourselves to be persuaded by ads that teach that if we take good care of ourselves, we will stay healthy. Sick people, hospitals, and funerals destroy our illusions of invulnerability. They force us to think of the future.

Carolyn Heilbrun said, "It is only past the meridian of fifty that one can believe that the universal sentence of death applies to oneself." Before that time, if we are healthy, we are likely to be in deep denial about death, to feel as if we have plenty of time, that we have an endless vista ahead. But in hospitals and at funerals, we remember that we all will die in the last act. And we don't necessarily appreciate being reminded.

When I first visited rest homes, I had to force myself to stay. What made me most upset was the thought of myself in a place like that. I didn't want to go there, literally or figuratively. Recently I sat in an eye doctor's office surrounded by old people with white canes. Being in this room gave me intimations of mortality. I thought of Bob Dylan's line: "It's not dark yet, but it's getting there."

We know the old-old will die soon. The more we care and the more involved we are with the old, the more pain we feel at their suffering. Death is easier to bear in the abstract, far away and clinical. It's much harder to watch someone we love fade before our eyes. It's hard to visit an uncle in a rest home and realize he no longer knows who we are or even who he is. It's hard to see a grandmother in pain or drugged up on morphine. Sometimes it's so hard that we stay away from the people who need us the most.

Our culture reinforces our individual fears. To call something old is to insult, as in *old hat* or *old ideas*. To call something young is to compliment, as in *young thinking* or *young acting*. It's considered rude even to ask an old person's age. When we meet an adult we haven't seen in a long time, we compliment her by saying, "You haven't aged at all." The taboos against acknowledging age tell us that aging is shameful.

Many of the people I interviewed were uncomfortable talking about age and were unhappy to be labeled old. They said, "I don't feel old." What they meant was, "I don't act and feel like the person who the stereotypes suggest I am." Also, they were trying to avoid being put in a socially undesirable class. In this country, it is unpleasant to be called old, just as it is unpleasant to be called fat or poor. The old naturally try to avoid being identified with an unappreciated group. . . .

The Elderly Are Treated Poorly

Nothing in our culture guides us in a positive way toward the old. Our media, music, and advertising industries all glorify the young. Stereotypes suggest that older people keep younger people from fun, work, and excitement. They take time (valuable time) and patience (in very short supply in the 1990s). We are very body-oriented, and old bodies fail. We are appearance-oriented, and youthful attractiveness fades. We are not taught that old spirits often shimmer with beauty.

Language is a problem. Old people are referred to in pejorative terms, such as *biddy, codger,* or *geezer,* or with cutesy words, such as *oldster, chronologically challenged,* or *senior citizen.* People describe themselves as "eighty years young." Even *retirement* is an ugly word that implies passivity, uselessness, and withdrawal from the social and working world. Many of the old are offended by ageist stereotypes and jokes. Some internalize these beliefs and feel badly about themselves. They stay with their own kind in order to avoid the harsh appraisals of the young.

Some people do not have good manners with the old. I've seen the elderly bossed around, treated like children or simpletons, and simply ignored. Once in a cafe, I heard a woman order her mother to take a pill and saw the mother wince in embarrassment. My mother-in-law says she sees young people but they don't see her. Her age makes her invisible.

In our culture the old are held to an odd standard. They are admired for not being a bother, for being chronically cheerful. They are expected to be interested in others, bland in their opinions, optimistic, and emotionally generous. But the young certainly don't hold themselves to these standards.

Accidents that old drivers have are blamed on age. After a ninety-year-old friend had his first car accident, he was terrified that he would lose his license. "If I were young, this accident would be perceived as just one of those things," he pointed out. "But because I am old, it will be attributed to my age." Now, of course, some old people are bad drivers. But so are some young people. To say "He did that because he's old" is often as narrow as to say, "He did that because he's black" or "Japanese." Young people burn countertops with hot pans, forget appointments, and write overdrafts on their checking accounts. But when the old do these same things, they experience double jeopardy. Their mistakes are not viewed as accidents but rather as loss of functioning. Such mistakes have implications for their freedom.

Media Stereotypes

As in so many other areas, the media hurts rather than helps with our social misunderstandings. George Gerbner reported on the curious absence of media images of people older than sixty-five. Every once in a while a romantic movie plot might involve an older man, but almost never an older woman. In general, the old have been cast as silly, stubborn, and eccentric. He also found that on children's programs, older women bear a disproportionate burden of negative characteristics. In our culture, the old get lumped together into a few stereotyped images: the sweet old lady, the lecherous old man, or the irascible but softhearted grandfather. Almost no ads and billboards feature the old. Every now and then an ad will show a grandparent figure, but then the grandparent is invariably youthful and healthy.

In *Fountain of Age,* Betty Friedan noted that the old are portrayed as sexless, demented, incontinent, toothless, and childish. Old women are portrayed as sentimental, naive, and silly gossips, and as troublemakers. A common movie plot is the portrayal of the old trying to be young—showing them on motorbikes, talking hip or dirty, or liking rock and roll. Of course there are exceptions, such as *Nobody's Fool, On Golden Pond, Mr. and Mrs. Bridge, Driving Miss Daisy, Mrs. Brown,* and *Twilight.* But we need more movies in which old people are portrayed in all their diversity and complexity.

The media is only part of much larger cultural problems. We aren't organized to accommodate this developmental stage. For example, being old-old costs a lot of money. Assisted-living housing, medical care, and all the other services the old need are expensive. And yet, most old people can't earn money. It's true that some of our elders are wealthy, but many live on small incomes. Visiting the old, I heard tragic stories involving money. I met Arlene, who, while dying of cancer, had to fear losing her house because of high property taxes. I met Shirley, who lived on noodles and white rice so that she could buy food for her cat and small gifts for her grandchildren. I met people who had to choose between pills and food or heat.

The American Obsession with Independence

Another thing that makes old age a difficult stage to navigate is our American belief that adults need no one. We think of independence as the ideal state for adults. We associate independence with heroes and cultural icons such as the Marlboro man and the Virginia Slims woman, and we associate dependence with toxic families, enmeshment, and weakness. To our post-modern, educated ears, a psychologically healthy but dependent adult sounds oxymoronic.

We all learn when we are very young to make our own personal declarations of independence. In our culture, *adult* means "self-sufficient." Autonomy is our highest virtue. We want relationships that have no strings attached instead of understanding, as one lady told me, "Honey, life ain't nothing but strings."

These American ideas about independence hurt families with teens. Just when children most need guidance from parents, they turn away from them and toward peers and media. They are socialized to believe that to be an adult, they must break away from parents. Our ideas about independence also hurt families with aging relatives. As people move from the young-old stage into the old-old stage, they need more help. Yet in our culture we provide almost no graceful ways for adults to ask for help. We make it almost impossible to be dependent yet dignified, respected, and in control.

As people age, they may need help with everything from their finances to their driving. They may need help getting out of bed, feeding themselves, and bathing. Many would rather pay strangers, do without help, or even die than be dependent on those they love. They don't want to be a burden, the greatest of American crimes. The old-old often feel ashamed of what is a natural stage of the life cycle. In fact, the greatest challenge for many elders is learning to accept vulnerability and to ask for help.

If we view life as a time line, we realize that all of us are sometimes more and sometimes less dependent on others. At certain stages we are caretakers, and at other stages we are cared for. Neither stage is superior to the other. Neither implies pathology or weakness. Both are just the results of life having seasons and circumstances. In fact, good mental health is not a matter of being dependent or independent, but of being able to accept the stage one is in with grace and dignity. It's an awareness of being, over the course of one's lifetime, continually interdependent.

Rethinking Dependency

In our culture the old fear their deaths will go badly, slowly, and painfully, and will cost lots of money. Nobody wants to die alone, yet nobody wants to put their families through too much stress. Families are uneasy as they negotiate this rocky terrain. The trick for the younger members is to help without feeling trapped and overwhelmed. The trick for older members is to accept help while preserving dignity and control. Caregivers can say, "You have nurtured us, why wouldn't we want to nurture you?" The old must learn to say, "I am grateful for your help and I am still a person worthy of respect."

As our times and circumstances change, we need new language. We need the elderly to become elders. We need a word for the neediness of the old-old, a word with less negative connotations than *dependency*, a word that connotes wisdom, connection, and dignity. *Dependency* could become mutuality or

interdependency. We can say to the old: "You need us now, but we needed you and we will need our children. We need each other."

However, the issues are much larger than simply which words to use or social skills to employ. We need to completely rethink our ideas about caring for the elderly. Like the Lakota, we need to see it as an honor and an opportunity to learn. It is our chance to repay our parents for the love they gave us, and it is our last chance to become grown-ups. We help them to help ourselves.

We need to make the old understand that they can be helped without being infantilized, that the help comes from respect and gratitude rather than from pity or a sense of obligation. In our society of disposables and planned obsolescence, the old are phased out. Usually they fade away graciously. They want to be kind and strong, and, in America, they learn that to do so means they should ask little of others and not bother young people.

Perhaps we need to help them redefine kindness and courage. For the old, to be kind ought to mean welcoming younger relatives' help, and to be brave ought to mean accepting the dependency that old-old age will bring. We can reassure the old that by showing their children how to cope, they will teach them and their children how well this last stage can be managed. This information is not peripheral but rather something everyone will need to know.

Further Readings

Henry J. Aaron and Robert D. Reischauer. *Countdown to Reform: The Great Social Security Debate.* New York: Century Foundation Press, 2001.

Claude Amarnick. *Don't Put Me in a Nursing Home.* Deerfield Beach, FL: Garrett, 1996.

Dean Baker and Mark Weisbrot. *Social Security: The Phony Crisis.* Chicago: University of Chicago Press, 1999.

Margret M. Baltes. *The Many Faces of Dependency in Old Age.* Cambridge, England: Cambridge University Press, 1996.

Sam Beard. *Restoring Hope in America: The Social Security Solution.* San Francisco: Institute for Contemporary Studies, 1996.

Robert H. Binstock, Leighton E. Cluff, and Otto von Mering, eds. *The Future of Long-Term Care: Social and Policy Issues.* Baltimore: Johns Hopkins University Press, 1996.

Robert H. Binstock and Linda K. George, eds. *Handbook of Aging and the Social Sciences.* San Diego: Academic Press, 1996.

Jimmy Carter. *The Virtues of Aging.* New York: Ballantine, 1998.

Marshall N. Carter and William G. Shipman. *Promises to Keep: Saving Social Security's Dream.* Washington, DC: Regnery, 1996.

Martin Cetron and Owen Davies. *Cheating Death: The Promise and the Future Impact of Trying to Live Forever.* New York: St. Martin's Press, 1998.

William C. Cockerham. *This Aging Society.* Upper Saddle River, NJ: Prentice-Hall, 1997.

Peter A. Diamond, David C. Lindeman, and Howard Young, eds. *Social Security: What Role for the Future?* Washington, DC: National Academy of Social Insurance, 1996.

Ursula Adler Falk and Gerhard Falk. *Ageism, the Aged and Aging in America: On Being Old in an Alienated Society.* Springfield, IL: Charles C. Thomas, 1997.

Peter J. Ferrara and Michael Tanner. *A New Deal for Social Security.* Washington, DC: Cato Institute, 1998.

Arthur D. Fisk and Wendy A. Rogers, eds. *Handbook of Human Factors and the Older Adult.* San Diego: Academic Press, 1997.

Muriel R. Gillick. *Lifelines: Living Longer: Growing Frail, Taking Heart.* New York: W. W. Norton, 2000.

Margaret Morganroth Gullette. *Declining to Decline: Cultural Combat and the Politics of the Midlife.* Charlottesville: University Press of Virginia, 1997.

Charles B. Inlander and Michael A. Donio. *Medicare Made Easy.* Allentown, PA: People's Medical Society, 1999.

Donald H. Kausler and Barry C. Kausler. *The Graying of America: An Encyclopedia of Aging, Health, Mind, and Behavior.* Urbana: University of Illinois Press, 2001.

Eric R. Kingson and James H. Schulz, eds. *Social Security in the Twenty-First Century.* New York: Oxford University Press, 1997.

Thelma J. Lofquist. *Frail Elders and the Wounded Caregiver.* Portland, OR: Binford and Mort, 2001.

Joseph L. Matthews. *Social Security, Medicare, and Pensions.* Berkeley, CA: Nolo, 1999.

E. J. Myers. *Let's Get Rid of Social Security: How Americans Can Take Charge of Their Own Future.* Amherst, NY: Prometheus Books, 1996.

Evelyn M. O'Reilly. *Decoding the Cultural Stereotypes About Aging: New Perspectives on Aging Talk and Aging Issues.* New York: Garland, 1997.

S. Jay Olshansky and Bruce A. Carnes. *The Quest for Immortality: Science at the Frontiers of Aging.* New York: W. W. Norton, 2001.

Fred C. Pampel. *Aging, Social Inequality, and Public Policy.* Thousand Oaks, CA: Pine Forge Press, 1998.

Peter G. Peterson. *Gray Dawn: How the Coming Age Wave Will Transform America—And the World.* New York: Times Books, 1999.

Peter G. Peterson. *Will America Grow Up Before It Grows Old?: How the Coming Social Security Crisis Threatens You, Your Family, and Your Country.* New York: Random House, 1996.

John W. Rowe and Robert L. Kahn. *Successful Aging.* New York: Pantheon Books, 1998.

Sylvester J. Schieber and John B. Shoven. *The Real Deal: The History and Future of Social Security.* New Haven, CT: Yale University Press, 1999.

Ken Skala. *American Guidance for Seniors—And Their Caregivers.* Falls Church, VA: K. Skala, 1996.

Max J. Skidmore. *Social Security and Its Enemies: The Case for America's Most Efficient Insurance Program.* Boulder, CO: Westview Press, 1999.

Richard D. Thau and Jay S. Heflin, eds. *Generations Apart: Xers vs. Boomers vs. the Elderly.* Amherst, NY: Prometheus Books, 1997.

Dale Van Atta. *Trust Betrayed: Inside the AARP.* Washington, DC: Regnery, 1998.

James W. Walters, ed. *Choosing Who's to Live: Ethics and Aging.* Urbana: University of Illinois Press, 1996.

David A. Wise, ed. *Facing the Age Wave.* Stanford, CA: Hoover Institutional Press, Stanford University, 1997.

Periodicals

W. Andrew Achenbaum. "Perceptions of Aging in America," *National Forum,* Spring 1998. Available from the Honor Society of Phi Kappa Phi, Box 16000, Louisiana State University, Baton Rouge, LA 70893.

America. "Keep an Eye on the Third Age," May 16, 1998.

Robert Butler. "The Longevity Revolution," *UNESCO Courier,* January 1999.

Issues and Controversies on File. "Age Discrimination," May 21, 1999. Available from Facts on File News Services, 11 Penn Plaza, New York, NY 10001-2006.

Margot Jefferys. "A New Way of Seeing Old Age Is Needed," *World Health,* September/October 1996.

Ann Monroe. "Getting Rid of the Gray: Will Age Discrimination Be the Downfall of Downsizing?" *Mother Jones,* July/August 1996.

Bernadette Puijalon and Jacqueline Trincaz. "Sage or Spoilsport?" *UNESCO Courier,* January 1999.

Jody Robinson. "The Baby Boomers' Final Revolt," *Wall Street Journal,* July 31, 1998.

Dan Seligman. "The Case for Age Discrimination," *Forbes,* December 13, 1999.

Ruth Simon. "Too Damn Old," *Money,* July 1996.

John C. Weicher. "Life in a Gray America," *American Outlook,* Fall 1998. Available from 5395 Emerson Way, Indianapolis, IN 46226.

Ron Winslow. "The Age of Man," *Wall Street Journal,* October 18, 1999.

A Healthy Mind, a Longer Life

Can the right attitude and personality help you live longer? Psychologists are trying to find out.

LEA WINERMAN

Thirty years ago, gerontologist Robert Atchley, PhD, contacted every resident over the age of 50 in the town of Oxford, Ohio. About two-thirds of them—more than 1,100 people—agreed to participate in Atchley's Ohio Longitudinal Study of Aging and Retirement.

The participants answered multitudes of survey questions about their physical and mental health, socioeconomic status, work life, family and other topics. Included in the questions were a few that measured the people's attitudes toward their own aging—they were asked to agree or disagree with statements such as "I am as happy now as I was when I was younger," and "As you get older, you get less useful."

Over the years, the participants returned several times to answer more questions, giving the researchers a detailed snapshot of the course of aging in late 20th-century America.

In the late 1990s, Yale University psychologist Becca Levy, PhD, realized that the aging-attitudes questions from the Ohio study could help her answer a research question she'd begun to consider: Could people's attitudes toward aging influence how long they lived?

Levy collected death records to find out whether each participant was still alive or the age at which they had died. When she matched up the records with the people's survey answers, she found that people with more positive views of their own aging lived, on average, 7.6 years longer than people with more negative views. This significant survival advantage remained after controlling for other relevant factors.

Levy's study, published in 2002 in the *Journal of Personality and Social Psychology* (Vol. 83, No. 2, pages 261–270), is one of many over the past several years that have begun to suggest that your personality, attitude toward aging and other psychosocial variables might help either grant you extra years or shorten your life. Personality and attitude may also influence your physical and mental abilities as you age.

If that's true, Levy says, the negative stereotypes of aging and the elderly that permeate our culture could have serious consequences that go beyond just making people feel bad. "Negative images of aging could be a public health issue," she says.

The Stereotype Threat

Levy, a social psychologist, first became interested in aging because she studied stereotypes, and she was curious about how negative stereotypes of aging influenced the elderly's physical and mental health. She explains that members of racial or ethnic minorities encounter stereotypes while their identities are still forming, and they develop defenses early on. In contrast, people encounter aging stereotypes while they are still young, so because the stereotypes don't apply to them yet, they don't challenge them. As a result, once people are older, they may be more inclined to accept negative views of their age group unquestioningly.

"By the time they become old, they've already internalized [the stereotypes]," Levy says.

In her earliest study on the topic, published in 1994 in the *Journal of Personality and Social Psychology* (Vol. 66, No. 6, pages 989–997), Levy found that elderly Chinese performed better on memory tasks than did elderly Americans—possibly, she hypothesized, because the Chinese tend to have more positive views of aging than Americans. Supporting this, she also found that older Americans who were deaf—another group that, she says, tends to hold the elderly in higher esteem than mainstream American culture—also performed better than hearing Americans on memory tests.

The Ohio longevity study followed up on this earlier work, and suggested that attitudes toward aging could affect not just discrete abilities like memory, but overall physical health.

In her most recent study, published in March in the *Journal of Gerontology: Psychological Sciences* (Vol. 61, No. 2, pages 82–87), Levy looked at another hallmark of old age—hearing loss. She found that seniors who held negative self-stereotypes about aging tended to lose more of their hearing over the course of three years than seniors with more positive views of aging.

Levy says that she and her colleagues still don't know the exact mechanism by which positive attitudes translate into better memory, sharper hearing and a longer life. But, she says, it may have something to do with the will to live—people's belief that the positive aspects of life outweigh the hardships. In the longevity study, for example, she found that the participants' will to live—as measured by descriptions of their lives as either hopeful or hopeless, worthless or worthy and empty or full—correlated with both their perceptions of aging and their lifespan.

Results like these show the power of negative aging stereotypes, according to University of Massachusetts Amherst psychologist Susan Krauss Whitbourne, PhD, who also studies aging and ageism.

"There are a lot of variations in how people look at their own aging process," she says. And in her research, she says, she's found that people who don't dwell on the negative changes that come with age generally seem to do best.

But, she adds, it's hard to avoid dwelling on those changes in a culture as saturated with ageism as ours.

"I hate the term 'senior moment'—I just hate it," she says. "Because if you start to use terms like that about yourself, even if you're kidding, it's going to have a negative impact on your self-esteem."

A Worrier's Advantage?

Of course, taking a positive and optimistic attitude toward aging does not mean being unrealistic or ignoring serious age-related problems. Howard Friedman, PhD, a psychology professor at the University of California, Riverside, studies personality characteristics associated with longevity and health. He's found that, contrary to popular belief, people who are extremely cheerful as children may actually die slightly younger than their less happy-go-lucky peers.

In a series of studies begun in 1993, he retrieved the mortality data for a group of children first studied by psychologist Lewis Terman in 1922. He found that on average the most cheerful children died earlier, and that their earlier deaths may have been

---

Plan Ahead for Retirement

APA's Committee on Aging has developed a pamphlet to help young, middle-aged and older psychologists plan for the challenges that can arise as they age. "Life Plan for the Life Span" offers guidance, advice and links to resources on financial, health, psychological, social and work/life issues. View the brochure and other aging resources at www.apa.org/pi/aging.

---

at least partially caused by a more careless attitude toward their health—they were somewhat more likely to drink, smoke and take other risks.

What's more, particularly conscientious children lived longer, healthier lives on average. This makes sense, Friedman says: A conscientious person will probably head to the doctor at the first sign of trouble, avoiding later, more serious problems.

Still, he adds, the associations between personality and longevity are complicated—even all of the mediating variables such as drinking, smoking and obesity didn't entirely explain the cheerfulness/early mortality link. And animal research has shown that individuals who are easily stressed may die earlier, due to the wear of frequently going through the startle response.

"People try to generalize and say a trait like cheerfulness or neuroticism is good or bad," he says. "But sometimes it's good to worry, and sometimes it's not—it depends on the situation."

Whitbourne agrees that when a positive attitude toward aging shades into a laissez-faire attitude toward health, it can go too far. "You don't want to overdo it; if you go into denial that's bad," she says. "It's good to have some anxiety about aging if it gets you moving and taking care of yourself, but it's bad if you become incapacitated by it."

From *Monitor on Psychology,* November 2006, pp. 42–44. Copyright © 2006 by American Psychological Association. Reprinted by permission. No Further distribution without permission from the American Psychological Association.

Research: Oldest Americans Happiest

LINDSEY TANNER

I t turns out the golden years really are golden.

Eye-opening new research finds the happiest Americans are the oldest, and older adults are more socially active than the stereotype of the lonely senior suggests. The two go hand-in-hand: Being social can help keep away the blues.

"The good news is that with age comes happiness," said study author Yang Yang, a University of Chicago sociologist. "Life gets better in one's perception as one ages."

A certain amount of distress in old age is inevitable, including aches and pains and the deaths of loved ones and friends. But older people generally have learned to be more content with what they have than younger adults, Yang said.

This is partly because older people have learned to lower their expectations and accept their achievements, said Duke University aging expert Linda George. An older person may realize "it's fine that I was a school-teacher and not a Nobel prize winner."

George, who was not involved in the new study, believes the research is important because people tend to think that "late life is far from the best stage of life, and they don't look forward to it."

Yang's findings are based on periodic face-to-face interviews with a nationally representative sample of Americans from 1972 to 2004. About 28,000 people ages 18 to 88 took part.

There were ups and downs in overall happiness levels during the study, generally corresponding with good and bad economic times. But at every stage, older Americans were the happiest.

While younger blacks and poor people tended to be less happy than whites and wealthier people, those differences faded as people aged.

In general, the odds of being happy increased 5 percent with every 10 years of age.

Overall, about 33 percent of Americans reported being very happy at age 88, versus about 24 percent of those age 18 to their early 20s. And throughout the study years, most Americans reported being very happy or pretty happy. Less than 20 percent said they were not too happy.

A separate University of Chicago study found that about 75 percent of people aged 57 to 85 engage in one or more social activities at least every week. Those include socializing with neighbors, attending religious services, volunteering or going to group meetings.

Those in their 80s were twice as likely as those in their 50s to do at least one of these activities.

Both studies appear in April's *American Sociological Review.*

"People's social circles do tend to shrink a little as they age—that is mainly where that stereotype comes from, but that image of the isolated elderly really falls apart when we broaden our definition of what social connection is," said study co-author Benjamin Cornwell, also a University of Chicago researcher.

The Under-Reported Impact of Age Discrimination and Its Threat to Business Vitality

The Age Discrimination in Employment Act (ADEA, 29 USCA, 621) is credited with helping eliminate many blatant forms of age discrimination in employment. For example, before the ADEA was enacted 37 years ago, it was common for employment ads to list age limitations, indicating people over 40 need not apply. Across the board, mandatory retirement policies went unchallenged. Despite advancements in these areas since the founding of the Age Discrimination in Employment Act, it remains to be seen whether the ADEA has completed the job it set out to do. Has it proven to be an effective tool for eliminating the unreasonable prejudices that make it difficult for older workers to achieve their full potential? Has it provided adequate compensation for victims of discrimination? The following article takes a snapshot of the current work environment to gain a perspective. Based on extensive interviews with academics, employment lawyers, advocates for older workers, and older workers themselves, it reveals the need for reforms. It finds that, in a legal environment slanted toward employers, older workers continue to face bias and stereotyping, that most victims of discrimination are not made whole, and that society's lack of concern for this type of discrimination may prove more costly in the future as employers look more to older workers to fill projected workforce gaps.

ROBERT J. GROSSMAN

1. The ADEA: An Introduction

Thirty-seven years ago, Congress passed the Age Discrimination in Employment Act (ADEA) which makes it illegal for an employer or union to discharge, refuse to hire, or otherwise discriminate on the basis of age. Looking back, it is easy to forget the overt discrimination faced by older workers at the time. It was common for employment ads prior to 1967 to list age limitations, indicating people over 40 need not apply. Mandatory retirement policies, applicable to almost everyone but Supreme Court Justices, went unchallenged. Although some states had antidiscrimination laws on the books, they were not enforced, giving employers a free hand to discriminate. But now, almost four decades later, it bears asking whether the ADEA has done more than address age discrimination in its most blatant manifestations. Is it really effective in preventing age bias? Has it been successful in "alleviating serious economic and psychological suffering of persons between the ages of 40 and 65 caused by unreasonable prejudice?" (Polstorff v. Fletcher [1978, ND Ala] 452 F Supp 17). What role has it played in transforming the U.S. culture to be more accepting and appreciative of older workers?

2. Stereotypes Survive

Despite protestations to the contrary, there seems to be little indication that attitudes have changed significantly since the enactment of the ADEA. The notion that older people have had their day and should make room for the next generation continues to be deeply ingrained. "We think maybe it's okay because it's an economic issue, not a civil rights issue," says Laurie McCann, Senior Attorney for AARP in Washington, D.C. "Until we view it as just as wrong and serious, we may not be making the inroads we need to address the intractable, subtle discrimination that is so pervasive. I don't think employers want to discriminate; they don't hate older workers. It's the stereotypes. They may not even know they harbor these biases, but they do" (McCann, 2003).

Such attitudes are evident in the case of Ann Klingert, a 64-year-old resident of the Bronx, who recalled with astonishment the public response to an article in a local New York City newspaper regarding an EEOC lawsuit she had filed. Klingert filed with the EEOC after she was fired by Woolworths and then prohibited from applying for newly created part-time jobs which were filled mostly by student applicants. "When the lawsuit was reported in a local New York City newspaper, *Our Town,* people were outraged," she said. "They wrote letters to the editor saying things like 'why don't you just retire and just take your social security and go away'" (Klingert, 2003).

Although most employers are sensitive to the issues of sexism and racism, "the idea that you cannot teach an old dog new tricks does not seem to carry the same taboo status in society and the workplace," says Todd Maurer, Associate Professor of Industrial-Organization Psychology at the Georgia Institute of Technology. Maurer says that generalizing is dangerous in the range of older workers; perhaps even more so than in other categories. "One size does not fit all," he says. "There can be older individuals who are both interested and able when it comes to learning. Research has found large differences within older groups in things like training performance and in abilities like memory and reaction time" (Maurer, 2003). However, too often, as in the case of Maryland resident Mort Beres, employers are influenced more by stereotypes than skills or experience. When Beres, then in his late 50s, lost his job, the prior owner of small businesses and successful salesman in the auto parts manufacturing industry knew he had skills that should have been in demand, yet he was turned away repeatedly. Any offers he did receive were salaried at much less than he had earned previously, and the positions were often demeaning in nature. Beres held on as long as he could, but admitted that, out of desperation, he took some sketchy jobs. "You take every jerky job you can get just to have some income; some of them make you nauseous" (Beres, 2003).

Eventually, Beres found his niche, working as a trainer and sales rep for Irvine, California-based BDS Marketing. Assigned to the Canon account at a Best Buy in Maryland, his job was to help store personnel sell Canon printers, for which he was paid a salary plus commission. After 5 years on the job, working with a series of regional supervisors, at age 67, Beres achieved a noteworthy record by helping his store become one of the top five in the territory. However, when a new supervisor took over, Beres's star began to fall. "He'd call me and make stupid comments about my age, like 'you're too old, I think it's time for a change.'" Finally, Beres got the axe. When he asked why he had been fired, the manager told him, "I'm not telling you and I don't have to." Beres recalls hanging up and thinking about what had happened. "I got angry; really angry. It was a little, unimportant job, but they had no right to treat me that way." *(BDS Marketing's Vice President for Human Resources, Jeffrey Sopko, refused to comment specifically but denied Beres's version of what happened and claimed that there were other reasons for Beres's dismissal.)*

Beres's plight is not uncommon, yet society appears to be less outraged at age bias than other types of discrimination. "It seems more politically correct to discriminate

Table 1 Workers Over Age 45 Reporting Presence of Age Discrimination ($n = 1500$)

Do not know	2%
No	31%
Yes	67%

Source: AARP Work and Careers Study Summary (2002).

against older people," says Mindy Farber, Managing Partner at Farber Taylor, LLC in Rockville, Maryland. Farber recalls hiring a new associate for the firm who was in her mid-fifties. "It was shocking. I was surprised how open people were about talking about the wisdom of my decision in light of her age. If I had hired an African American, they would have been silent. Here they told me straight out that I had made a mistake" (Farber, 2003).

3. Perspective: How Older Workers See It

From their perspectives, older workers see little evidence that they are competing on a level playing field. Sixty-seven percent of employed workers aged 45 to 74 surveyed by AARP in 2003's *Staying Ahead of the Curve* said that age discrimination is a fact of life in the workplace (AARP, 2003) (Table 1). This percentage is even higher among African Americans and Hispanics, both at 72%. Age is viewed as so critical to employees that respondents listed it, along with education, as more important in how workers are treated than are gender, race, sexual orientation or religion. Sixty percent said they believe that older workers are the first to go when employers make cuts.

A 2002 Conference Board survey of 1,600 workers aged 50 and older found that 31 percent of workers intending to retire within five years said they would stay on if given more responsibilities. Twenty-five percent said they were leaving because they were being held back or marginalized because of their age (The Conference Board, 2002). Linda Barrington, Labor Economist at The Conference Board, says the high percentage of dissatisfied workers is cause for concern. "It's twice as big as I might have expected," she says. Perceptions, of course, are not necessarily reality, but Barrington says that does not matter. "Perceptions affect the way you work; if you're feeling undervalued, that discouragement will affect your work. Is it perception or reality? Either way, it has to be dealt with" (Barrington, 2003).

It also bears noting that far fewer of the respondents said they have suffered personally from ageism. About 9% say they believe they have been passed up for a promotion because of their age, 6% said they were fired or laid off because of age, 5% said they were passed up for a raise because of age, and 15% attributed their not being hired for a job to their age. However, the survey only queried current workers and did not include individuals in the same age category who were no longer in the workforce.

4. Advantage: Employers

Compared to its sister statutes aimed at race, religion, gender, and disability, the ADEA offers less protection. Court interpretations have proven to be less rigorous and more employer-friendly, ceding to employers the right to make bonafide business decisions even when age is linked. In practice, instead of preventing discrimination, the law serves as a roadmap for employers, enabling all but the obtuse to avoid liability and shield all but the most egregious ageist actions from public scrutiny.

Under the ADEA, if there is a valid reason for an action, it is considered acceptable if age happens to be an accompanying factor. "If you can show you would have done it anyway, you're off the hook," says Harlan Miller, an employment attorney with Miller, Billips, and Ates (Miller et al., 2003) in Atlanta, Georgia. As a result, it is almost impossible to catch a crafty employer discriminating. "I can always get around it if I'm smart. Only idiots get nailed," agrees David Neumark, a nationally recognized expert on the ADEA and Senior Fellow at the Public Policy Institute of California in San Francisco (Neumark, 2003).

Employers are not infallible, however, and they still mess up on occasion. Often when they do, it is because of retaliation: reacting badly to an employee whose initial complaint does not rise above the threshold set by the ADEA. "We tell them to go back and complain about their treatment," says James Rubin, an employment attorney with Farber Taylor. "Then the employer does something really bad. It's not the original claim; it's the reprisal. You can bring an action based on the reprisal even if the original claim is weak" (Rubin, 2003).

Employers also get caught when the rationale for their business decision falls apart. "Typically, the employer comes in with some kind of bogus selection process that says they're trying to keep the most competent," Miller says. "Gulfstream Aerospace's decision to cut from 200 to 230 of its nearly 2000 management-level employees during the period from August through December, 2000, is a case in point. Gulfstream had a rating device based on flexibility and adaptability; code words for old or young . . . and not subject to any kind of objective analysis. Our analysis showed a complete correlation between age and those factors" (Miller et al., 2003).

On the other hand, if it is legitimate, an employer's business argument can carry the day. "Is it discrimination to fire someone if it is based on economic foundations?" asks Bob Smith, Professor of Labor Economics, ILR at Cornell University in Ithaca, New York. "It's not a slam dunk that

they've been mistreated just because they say they are. There may be good reasons why they're singled out. They often are paid too much and have shorter time to work, making them a poorer investment. Why should I expect my employer to invest more in me than someone who will be there longer? Just because they complain, doesn't mean there's discrimination" (Smith, 2003).

5. Avoiding Scrutiny

Employers' incentives to avoid litigation are compelling from financial and public relations perspectives. Generally, when employers get wind that employees are disgruntled and plan to complain or sue, they move to settle by enticing them into retirement with incentives and buyouts, awarded contingent upon their agreeing to confidentiality clauses that prevent discussion of the situation.

The Older Worker Protection Act clarified for employers what they need to say and do when they reach termination agreements with workers. The act requires an employer to give workers 21 days to consider a buyout proposal, to advise them of their right to seek legal counsel, and even to rescind the agreement 10 days after the fact if they have a change of heart. Until recently, a properly negotiated settlement would foreclose a former employee from further litigation. Now, there has been at least one case where the EEOC has been able to sue on behalf of workers who previously signed releases.

In a typical settlement, the employer denies discrimination, attributing the settlement to "business decisions." In a recent survey by Jury Verdict Research, plaintiffs' lawyers estimated that 84% of their clients' claims were settled, while defense lawyers reported 79% (Jury Verdict Research, 2002).

Often, employees are relieved to accept the face-saving exit. In reality, their options are meager. They are scared if they are still working or owed pensions, and lack money if they have been terminated. According to Howard Eglit, Professor of Law at Chicago-Kent College, it costs, on average, about $50,000 for a lawyer if cases go beyond early negotiations with an employer. Most attorneys will not handle such cases on a contingent basis because they know the chances of winning are slim. Employers, on average, can count on spending $100,000 in legal fees from the time a complaint is filed with the EEOC until trial (Eglit, 2003).

Although the amounts paid to ease workers into retirement or silence complaints are private, high-profile EEOC settlements reveal just how well workers actually do when they press the ADEA to the limit. In March, 2003, the EEOC announced a class action settlement with Gulfstream Aerospace, owned by General Dynamics, on behalf of 66 workers for $2.1 million dollars, an average of approximately $33,000 for each manager the EEOC claimed had been wrongfully terminated. Ninety-three percent, many of whom may never work again full-time, accepted the deal and faded away, careers in shambles.

As meager as the settlement proved to be, there would not have been a case without former Gulfstream Aerospace manager Eddie Cosper of Rincon, Georgia. His role suggests that, behind every major class action, there is an activist who serves as a catalyst in pushing for remediation.

When Gulfstream Aerospace cut more than 200 of its nearly 2000 management employees, most of whom worked in Savannah, it had not bargained on Cosper's pride and persistence. Aged 54 and with the company for 28 years, Eddie Cosper was proud, professional, and still moving up. "I was still ambitious. Every time I put out a fire, I kept getting a promotion," he recalls. However, Cosper reached a dead-end when General Dynamics took over the company in 1999. His seasoning suddenly turned sour. "The VP would tell me, 'You're like father time; you've been here forever. Wouldn't you like to retire and do something different?'" Soon Cosper found himself reassigned to nights, with responsibility for 40 people instead of the 300 he usually had. Then, 30 days later, he was terminated. "My performance reviews were all above average," he says. "I had the highest ranking of all the four managers in my category." How did he feel when his career went up in smoke? "It's like a burning sensation in your gut. You say, why me? I put my whole life into something and it's been taken away for no reason. In the beginning, I felt sorry for myself, then I got angry. I did the numbers and realized I wasn't the only older person being targeted. So I started talking to others and built a network and database." Communication was key. "People who don't have that network have no clue," he says. "Every Joe Blow could get hit cold and not know what's happening. Probably half the people in our suit were along for the ride. If I hadn't reached them, they wouldn't have realized they were discriminated against and would have gotten nothing."

The EEOC's settlement with Footlocker is another example of a remedy that fell short of the mark. When the company settled with 764 former Woolworth employees, the complainants, mostly low-paid hourly workers, walked off with an average of $4,000 per person. Overall, the $3.4 million was a small price to pay for a 40,000-worker retailing giant like Footlocker (EEOC, 2002). A tougher question is why they let the matter fester as long as they did. Many companies buy themselves out of trouble, right or wrong (Eglit, 2003). According to Jury Verdict Research, the median settlement for age cases from 1994 to 2000 was $65,000, $5,000 higher than the median reported for all types of discrimination, age included (Jury Verdict Research, 2002).

6. Complaints Grow

If age discrimination had been decreasing throughout the years, even allowing for more people being aware of their right to complain and more older workers proving their mettle to those who question their ability, it would be reasonable to expect the number of complaints to be trending down. Instead, there are more cases. The EEOC logged 19,921 age discrimination complaints in 2002, an increase of 14.5% from the previous year and accounting for 23.6% of all discrimination claims filed with the agency (U.S. Equal Employment Opportunity Commission, ADEA Charges, 2003).

Some EEOC complainants, either uncertain as to the true basis of the discrimination against them or believing there is more than one basis, file multiple charges. EEOC data reveals that instances of ADEA claimants who alleged an additional type of discrimination are declining. The data suggests there is no move on the part of complainants making their case on some other basis of discrimination (gender, race, religion, or national origin) to add age simply in order to bolster the case, even though it was not thought to be the primary or even substantial basis of the discrimination. For the 3-year period of 1997 to 1999, an average of 17.9% of ADEA claimants made an additional charge. From 2000 to 2003, the average percentage dropped to 15.8%. In addition, states Farber, private lawyers are seeing similar increases in age complaints in proportion to race, gender, and disability (Farber, 2003).

7. Profile

Overall, the majority of claimants tend to be white males, 55 and older at the middle management level. However, the number of women filing claims has doubled in the last few years, a trend that Eglit estimates will continue as women earn more, hold more desirable jobs, and can afford to hire counsel. "The ADEA offers two essential remedies: reinstatement and back pay. If you weren't getting much and your job wasn't worth much, why sue? Now, even with the glass ceiling, women have good jobs and can afford to hire an attorney and sue" (Eglit, 2003) (Table 2).

In 2002, 53% of the cases related to job loss; wrongful discharge, 8,741 and involuntary layoff, 1,463. "They're easier to prove," Eglit says. "If you've been working at a place for 20 years, look around and see five other people fired, you have a case" (Eglit, 2003). It happened in the Woolworth's/Footlocker case, says Michelle LeMoal-Grey, EEOC attorney. "When they were fired, workers spoke by phone and began to see a pattern forming in their store and beyond" (LeMoal-Grey, 2003).

Of the EEOC claimants between ages 40 and 69, 46% were in their fifties, 31% in their 60s and 23% in their 40s. About 25% of claims were based on failure to hire,

Table 2 Age Bias Charge Filings with EEOC Nationwide by Age Group of Charging Parties Fiscal Years 1999–2002[a]

Fiscal year/age	Age 40–49	Age 50–59	Age 60–69
1999	3367	5949	3526
2000	3941	6620	4609
2001	3779	7584	4603
2002	4219	8455	5686

Source: EEOC, Office of Communications and Legislative Affairs (2003).

[a]Note. The three age ranges combined do not comprise the total ADEA charge filings with the EEOC per year, as a small number of charges which are not listed are filed by individuals 70 and older.

an increase of 200% since 1999. As these cases are harder to prove and because damages are limited, it is difficult to find a private attorney for hire without having to pay up-front. "If you're not hired, how do you know what the reason was? It's not so easy to figure it out," Eglit observes (Eglit, 2003).

About 12% of the claimants cited harassment; antagonism, or intimidation, creating a hostile work environment; an increase of 31.5% since 1999. Constructive discharge would be an example, says Dorothy Stubblebine, an expert witness for both plaintiffs and defendants, and President of DJS Associates in Mantua, New Jersey. "Tyically, the older person is pushed out by giving him a really hard time. He's given the worst assignments 'til he can't take it any more" (Stubblebine, 2003) (Table 3).

8. Chances for Success

Whatever the claim and whomever the claimant, few gamblers would bet on the probability of prevailing in an ADEA suit. EEOC data reveals that for most claimants, the filing with the EEOC is a dead-end. Last year, of the cases before it, the agency found "reasonable cause" only 4.3% of the time, "no reasonable cause" 52% of the time, and closed cases for "administrative" reasons 33.5% of the time. Only 6.5% of cases were eventually settled. In contrast, for claimants charging all types of discrimination, age included, the EEOC found reasonable cause 7.2% of the time, found no reasonable cause 59.3% of the time, and closed cases for administrative reasons 26% of the time (U.S. Equal Employment Opportunity Commission, 2003) (Table 4 and Table 5).

For plaintiffs who win at trial, damages are legally limited to reinstatement, loss of pay, or, where there is a finding of willful discrimination, double the lost salary. In contrast, race and gender plaintiffs have the opportunity to be awarded more lucrative punitive damages. "Why shouldn't someone who's old be compensated for pain and suffering just like someone who's fired for their religion, race, or gender?"

Miller asks. "There's nothing worse than, after 30 years' service, to be fired at 58" (Miller et al., 2003).

The solution for many attorneys is to bypass the ADEA and, where possible, sue under local or state statutes. "Everybody tries to stay out of Federal Court," Farber says. "Plaintiffs get their audience but they lose before they can get to a jury. It's so bad that a fellow attorney once told me that if I went to Federal Court when there were other options available, I would be guilty of malpractice." Farber says a plaintiff's chances to reach a jury brighten considerably in state or local courts. Virtually everyone on a jury can identify with the plight of an older worker. "Everybody on the jury is getting older and has a mother and father" (Farber, 2003).

If they get to a state or federal jury, Jury Verdict Research in its study, *Employment Practice Liability: Jury Award Trends and Statistics,* reports a 78% success rate overall for age cases in 2000. In Federal District Courts, from 1994 to 2000, the median verdict was $269,350, tops for all types of discrimination. However, the chances of plaintiffs getting there with the EEOC in their corner are limited. The Office of General counsel states that during the 5-year period from 1997 to 2001, the EEOC filed 205 lawsuits based on the ADEA, leaving plaintiffs who push ahead with claims the EEOC determines are without merit with the risk and expense of proceeding toward litigation on their own (Office of General Counsel, 2002). Jury Verdict Research indicates that the median verdict for more numerous privately initiated state cases was about the same (Jury Verdict Research, 2002).

9. Justification

Critics point out that there may be valid reasons for determining that older workers are less desirable employees. There is no question that technological changes have significantly altered the way we work, especially in white-collar jobs, explains Camille Olson, Chair of the Labor and Employment Practice Group, Seyfeith Shaw, in Chicago, Illinois. "Persons in their 20s and 30s who are comfortable with technology are more responsive and more adaptable to change. Can people in their 40s and 50s without this background feel that they belong in the workplace? You feel that time has passed you by. Does that affect your motivation, your ability to do things? It does" (Olson, 2003).

"A lot of people who think they've been screwed over have it wrong," agrees AARP's McCann. "Though I'm an advocate, I'd be the first to admit that when someone gets fired or doesn't get promoted, they yell foul. An age discrimination claim is the last resort for older white males. "If you're a 55 year old male who's lost your $70,000 job, what do you do? The odds of finding any job, let alone a comparable job, are slim, so you fight" (McCann, 2003).

Table 3 Age Discrimination Charge Filings with EEOC Nationwide Fiscal Years 1998–2002

Year[a]	FY 1998	FY 1999	FY 2000	FY 2001	FY 2002
Discharge	7054	6733	6851	7376	8741
Harassment	1871	1758	1966	2146	2311
Hiring	1953	1647	1990	3116	4889
Layoff	1036	1149	1128	1107	1810
Promotion	1547	1590	1666	1623	1463
Terms of Employment	2510	2357	2610	3440	3181
TOTAL	15,191	14,141	16,008	17,405	19,921

Source: EEOC, Office of Communications and Legislative Affairs (2003).

[a] Fiscal years run from October 1 through September 30.

Table 4 EEOC Resolution of ADEA Claims Fiscal Years 1998–2002

	FY 1998	FY 1999	FY 2000	FY 2001	FY 2002
Total ADEA Claims	15,191	14,141	16,008	17,405	19,921
Settlements (%)	4.7	5.3	7.9	6.6	6.5
Withdrawals with benefits (%)	3.6	3.7	3.8	3.6	3.6
Administrative closures (%)	26.1	23.3	22.0	26.1	33.5
No reasonable cause (%)	61.7	59.4	58.0	55.3	52.1
Reasonable cause (%)	3.9	8.3	8.2	8.2	4.3

Source: EEOC, Office of Research, Information, and Planning (2003).

Table 5 EEOC Resolution of all Discrimination Claims Fiscal Years 1998–2002

	FY 1998	FY 1999	FY 2000	FY 2001	FY 2002
Total Claims	79,591	77,444	79,896	80,840	84,442
Settlements (%)	4.6	6.2	8.5	8.1	8.8
Withdrawals with benefits (%)	3.2	3.7	4.0	4.1	4.0
Administrative closures (%)	26.7	24.1	20.5	20.7	20.6
No reasonable cause (%)	60.9	59.5	58.3	57.2	59.3
Reasonable cause (%)	4.6	6.6	8.8	9.9	7.2

Source: EEOC, Office of Research, Information, and Planning (2003).

"If a person has lost a step or two and doesn't project or have the kind of energy to move forward, the fact that he isn't promoted may show that's where he belongs," explains Ed King, Executive Director of the National Senior Citizen Law Center, a former EEOC mediator in Hawaii. "The question is whether the employer is stereotyping or it is legitimate" (King, 2003).

It is undeniable that age has its advantages; plusses that advocates for older workers tend to downplay. "They do better; get paid more. Their employment rates are high and they get cared for in retirement," Neumark observes. However, he says, it is not all roses and caviar for workers in their 50s or 60s. Once they are unemployed, it is hard for them to find work. They are out of work longer, have difficulty finding jobs with comparable responsibilities and wages, and tend to become disheartened and "retire" (Neumark, 2003).

Adding to the debate is the difference of opinion as to whether age 40, which seemed appropriate in the 1960s, should still be the turning point for providing a person with ADEA coverage. Some experts ask, Why not? There needs to be some beginning point, and 40 is reasonable. Others disagree, arguing that 45 or 50 are more realistic ages when discriminatory treatment is most likely to occur. Whatever the threshold, it has been clear until recently that all people from 40 on up had to be treated similarly, but no longer.

In an opinion issued February 24, 2004, on General Dynamics Land Systems versus Cline, the U.S. Supreme Court held that the ADEA does not prevent an employer from favoring older employees over younger employees. The court upheld an agreement between General Dynamics and the United Auto Workers union that provided for continued retirement health benefits for employees then over 50 years of age but eliminated that benefit for all other employees. The plaintiffs were between the ages of 40 and 50, and were denied the benefits available only to workers over the age of 50.

10. No Special Treatment

Should an employer invest extra to help support an older worker? Offer more and different training? Provide less stressful assignments? The issue, Olson says, is whether under the ADEA an employer needs to take affirmative efforts to assist individuals who do not naturally have the same skills, while at the same time paying them more. Clearly, Olson says, the law never contemplated affirmative action. The law is there only to make sure older people are not treated differently (Olson, 2003).

"The ADEA is about equal treatment, not about preferential treatment," agrees Lynn Clemens, Attorney, Office of Legal Counsel at EEOC. "There are no affirmative obligations on the employer's part. That notion goes against the act." Regardless, advocates are making the case that there are other benefits to be gained by retaining older workers anyway, although they are paid more and have fewer skills. Olson says she does not buy it unless there is a compelling business case. "The issue is whether you need to invest in targeted training, making older workers more productive because you need them to stick around" (Olson, 2003).

11. Call for Action

Meanwhile, William Rothwell, Professor of Workforce Education and Development at Penn State University observes that Bureau of Labor Statistics projections show that while 13 percent of American workers today are 55 and older, that figure will increase to 20% by the year 2015. At the same time, the nation is expected to experience a drop in the percentage of younger workers aged 25 to 44.

With this information in mind, Rothwell says the current economic slump is the calm before the storm. When the economy turns around and there is more demand for products and services, the worker shortage will be the number

one issue. "Employers in the U.S. will be forced to go back to their retiree base and deploy it more effectively than ever before. If we can't get labor from anywhere else, we'll look to the most obvious population who knows everything about our business" (Rothwell, 2003).

Unless we get serious about addressing the stereotypes and focus on reducing the alienation that older workers feel, these workers, as well as retirees, may be unreceptive and unprepared to step up when the market finally swings in their favor. Reforming the ADEA is the first step. To better combat age discrimination, we must move quickly to put more teeth into the law. If we do not, when we go to the well, it may just be dry.

References

AARP. (2003). *Staying ahead of the curve.*

Barrington, L. (2003 April 10). Telephone interview. New York, NY.

Beres M. (2003 April 22). Telephone interview. Rockville, MD.

EEOC Press Release. (2002, November 15). *EEOC settles major age bias suit; Foot Locker to pay $3.5 million to former Woolworth employees.*

Eglit, H. (2003 April 10). Telephone interview. Chicago, IL.

Farber, M. (2003 April 21). Telephone interview. Rockville, MD.

Jury Verdict Research. (2002). *Employment practice liability verdicts and settlements: Jury award trends and statistics.*

King, E. (2003 April 15). Telephone interview. Washington, D.C.

Klingert, A. (2003 May 1). Telephone interview. Bronx, NY.

LeMoal-Grey, M. (2003 April 28). Telephone interview. New York, NY.

Maurer, T. (2003 April 17). Telephone interview. Atlanta, GA.

McCann, L. (2003 April 17). Telephone interview. Washington, D.C.

Miller, Harlan, Principal, Miller, Billips & Ates. (2003). Atlanta, GA. (18 April).

Neumark, D. (2003 April 8). Telephone interview. San Francisco, CA.

Office of General Counsel. (2002, August 13). The U.S. Equal Employment Opportunity Commission. *Study of the litigation program fiscal years 1997–2001,* Table 2.

Olson, C. (2003 April 10). Telephone interview. Chicago, IL.

Rothwell, W. (2003 April 17). Telephone interview. University Park, PA.

Rubin, J. (2003 April 21). Telephone interview. Rockville, MD.

Smith, B. (2003 April 17). Telephone interview. Ithaca, NY.

Stubblebine, D. (2003 April 4). Telephone interview. Mantua, NJ.

The Age Discrimination in Employment Act of 1967. (1967). Pub. L. 90–202, as amended. Volume 29 of the United States Code beginning at section 621.

The Conference Board. (2002). *Voices of experience: Mature workers in the future workplace.*

United States Supreme Court. (2004, February 24). *General Dynamics Land Systems v. Cline,* No. 02–1080.

U.S. Equal Employment Opportunity Commission. (2003). *Age discrimination in employment act charges,* FY 1992-FY 2002.

From *Business Horizons*, vol. 48, issue 1, January/February 2005, pp. 71–78. Copyright © 2005 by Foundation for the Kelley School of Business at Indiana University. Reprinted by permission of Elsevier Science Ltd via Rightslink. www.elsevier.com

UNIT 4

Problems and Potentials of Aging

Unit Selections

Key Points to Consider

- What are some of the things in the areas of diet, nutrition, and lifestyle that might be done to reduce the individual's risk of Alzheimer's disease?

- Does Barbara Basler believe that stem cells could be a possible cure for different kinds of cancers?

- Why might older persons be reluctant to turn over their finances and their property to their children?

- What is the relationship between frequent abuse and the health of older women?

Student Website

www.mhhe.com/cls

Internet References

Alzheimer's Association
http://www.alz.org
A.P.T.A. Section on Geriatrics
http://geriatricspt.org
Caregiver's Handbook
http://www.acsu.buffalo.edu/~drstall/hndbk0.html
Caregiver Survival Resources
http://www.caregiver.com
AARP Health Information
http://www.aarp.org/bulletin
International Food Information Council
http://www.ific.org
University of California at Irvine: Institute for Brain Aging and Dementia
http://www.alz.uci.edu

Viewed as part of the life cycle, aging might be considered a period of decline, poor health, increasing dependence, social isolation, and—ultimately—death. It often means retirement, decreased income, chronic health problems, and death of a spouse. In contrast, the first 50 years of life are seen as a period of growth and development.

For a young child, life centers around the home, and then the neighborhood. Later, the community and state become a part of the young person's environment. Finally, as an adult, the person is prepared to consider national and international issues—wars, alliances, changing economic cycles, and world problems.

During the later years, however, life space narrows. Retirement may distance the individual from national and international concerns, although he or she may remain actively involved in community affairs. Later, even community involvement may decrease, and the person may begin to stay close to home and the neighborhood. For some, the final years of life may once again focus on the confines of home, be it an apartment or a nursing home.

Many older Americans try to remain masters of their own destinies for as long as possible. They fear dependence and try to avoid it. Many are successful at maintaining independence and the right to make their own decisions. Others are less successful and must depend on their families for care and to make critical decisions. However, some older people are able to overcome the difficulties of aging and to lead comfortable and enjoyable lives.

In "Alzheimer's—The Case for Prevention," the author points out what could be done in the areas of diet, nutrition, and lifestyle to reduce the individual's risk of developing Alzheimer's disease. In "Brain Cancer: Could Adult Stem Cells Be the Cause—and the Cure?" the author points out the current research efforts in attempting to locate the stem cells that could be both the cause and the cure for a variety of different cancers.

In "Trust and Betrayal in the Golden Years," the author addresses the problems confronted by many older persons

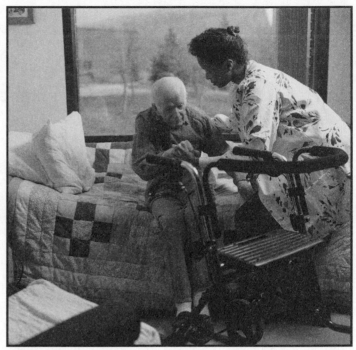

© Photodisc Collection/Getty Images

when they turn over control of their finances and property to their children. In addition, the almost insurmountable difficulties that older persons encounter when trying to resolve these problems are pointed out.

In "The Extent and Frequency of Abuse in the Lives of Older Women and Their Relationship with Health Outcomes," the authors review the extent of the abuse of older women and the negative impact of abuse on their health.

Article 15

Alzheimer's—The Case for Prevention

Are we losing our minds? And could something as simple and inexpensive as diet and lifestyle prevent it from happening?

OLIVER TICKELL

Alzheimer's and other dementias are dreadful diseases. They are also expensive. Just how expensive was revealed by the Alzheimer's Society in its *Dementia UK* report in February. The cost to the UK is £17 billion a year, or around £25,000 a year for each of the 700,000 sufferers of late-onset dementia. The number of sufferers is projected to rise: to 940,110 by 2021, and to 1,735,087 by 2051.

In response to the looming crisis, the Society makes seven sound recommendations. But something essential is missing: prevention. There are many cost-effective, scientifically robust steps that could dramatically reduce the incidence of dementia and enable elderly people to retain their cognitive faculties, especially in the areas of diet, nutrition and lifestyle. Applied systematically, these measures have the potential to transform the entire Alzheimer's risk landscape.

The brain is a fatty organ, and works best when fed the right kinds of oil and fat. It responds especially badly to the industrial trans fats found principally in hydrogenated oil. A 2003 study in the *Archives of Neurology,* which surveyed 815 people over 65, found that the 20 percent with the highest trans fat consumption were four times more likely to develop Alzheimer's than the 20 percent with the lowest trans fat consumption.

The same study found that the 20 percent with the lowest consumption of polyunsaturated vegetable oils were five times likelier to develop Alzheimer's than the 20 percent with the highest consumption. Combine these effects, and someone eating a diet high in trans fat and low in polyunsaturated fat is nine times more susceptible to Alzheimer's than someone eating a low trans fat, high polyunsaturated fat diet.

A 1999 study in the journal *Neurology* is one of many to show the benefit of mono-unsaturated oil, especially the oleic acid in olive oil. It suggests that, as people age, their brain chemistry may need more monounsaturated fat to prevent degeneration: 'High MUFA [monounsaturated fatty acid] intake *per se* could suggest preservation of cognitive functions in healthy elderly people. This effect could be related to the role of fatty acids in maintaining the structural integrity of neuronal membranes.'

Omega-3 oils, especially the long-chain EPA and DHA essential fatty acids, are a prerequisite of a healthy brain function and have successfully treated depression, attention deficit hyperactivity disorder (ADHD) and other mental conditions. Evidence published in the *Journal of Neuroscience* in 2005 shows that these oils reduce build-up of the amyloid plaque linked with Alzheimer's in mice, and may also help humans.

This supposition was supported in an October 2006 study in the *Archives of Neurology.* The one-year study of 204 Alzheimer's sufferers showed that the decline of very early-stage patients was significantly slowed by taking Omega-3 supplements. 'It seems that not only is DHA an important structural component of brain cells but DHA and its metabolites seem to exert a preventive effect against development of brain cell death,' commented the authors. 'These positive findings now indicate that early treatment with Omega 3 can help to reduce memory decline in patients experiencing the early symptoms of Alzheimer's.'

The risk of dementia is strongly correlated with higher levels of homocysteine—a rogue amino acid associated with low levels of folic acid and vitamin B12—as noted in the *American Journal of Clinical Nutrition,* February 2007. Treatment with B12 is protective: 'Higher plasma vitamin B12 may reduce the risk of homocysteine-associated dementia or CIND (cognitive impairment without dementia).'

Vitamin D also protects against dementia, as shown in a 2006 study of 80 participants, half with mild Alzheimer's and half without. It concluded: 'Vitamin D deficiency was associated with low mood and with impairment on two of four measures of cognitive performance.'

Protection is also conferred by the polyphenol antioxidants in fruit and vegetables, as shown in a 2006 paper in the *American Journal of Medicine,* based on a study of 1,836 Japanese Americans. Those who drank juice at least thrice weekly were a quarter as likely to contract Alzheimer's as those who drank juice less than once a week: 'Fruit and vegetable juices may play an important role in delaying the onset of Alzheimer's disease, particularly among those who are at high risk of the disease.'

Turmeric, the base spice of every curry, is strongly protective. It is rich in the oily chemical curcumin, which triggers our defence mechanisms against free radicals, a cause of cellular damage and a keypart of the ageing process. There's a host of evidence for curcumin's benefits, not just in Alzheimer's but in a broad range of pathologies from Crohn's disease to psoriasis. This is supported by the low incidence of Alzheimer's in India. One 2001 study in *Neurology* of a rural population at Ballabgarh, India, found a 0.3 percent incidence, 'among the lowest ever reported'—and roughly a quarter of that of a reference US population.

The same dietary changes that reduce the risk of Alzheimer's would also strongly benefit cardiovascular health, reducing heart disease and stroke. Mental and cardiovascular health are strongly correlated, as shown by a 21-year study of 1,500 Finns by Miia Kivipelto of the Karolinska Institute, Stockholm. 'Midlife obesity, high total cholesterol level, and high systolic blood pressure were all significant risk factors for dementia', each doubling the risk, 'and they increased the risk additively', so that people with all three risk factors were 6.2 times more likely to succumb to dementia.

Another vital dementia-prevention strategy is to stay lively and mentally active. In June 2003 the *New England Journal of Medicine* published a study of 269 healthy adults between 75 and 85 over a 21-year period, which found that 'reading, playing board games, playing musical instruments, and dancing were associated with a reduced risk of dementia'—a 75 percent reduced risk, for those who were most mentally active. 'It seems that remaining mentally agile makes the brain more healthy and more likely to resist illness, just as physical exercise can protect the body from disease,' said lead author Dr Joe Verghese. Numerous other studies have confirmed these findings.

Loneliness is another important factor, as a study by Professor Robert Wilson, professor of neuropsychology at Rush University Medical Centre, revealed in February 2007. His study of 823 older people in the Chicago area found that the risk of Alzheimer's 'was more than doubled in lonely persons' compared with those who were not lonely. 'Loneliness was associated with lower level of cognition at baseline and with more rapid cognitive decline during follow-up,' his team also found.

In recent months the Alzheimer's Society has accepted the need to assess the potential benefits of low-cost preventative measures. But the vast majority of its efforts are still aimed at securing drug therapies (many of dubious efficacy and with undesirable side effects) and adequate care for sufferers. Disproportionate medical research funding is also applied to patentable genetic technologies such as the role of inherited genetic predispositions, and the use of genetically modified cell transplants to produce Nerve Growth Factor.

The greatest disgrace is that the growing compendium of medical knowledge has had no policy response from the Government.

But the greatest disgrace is that the growing compendium of medical knowledge about diet, nutrition, lifestyle and dementia has produced no policy response from the Government. It is hard not to question whether it suits the Government to have the elderly population die relatively young. All the measures that would slow or prevent the onset of dementias would also extend life, especially through improved cardiovascular health, and thus increase pension, benefit, housing and other health costs.

But with the cost of Alzheimer's and other dementias projected to rise to alarming levels in the absence of preventative action, a rethink should (sooner or later) be on the way. Meanwhile, all of us can try, in our own lifestyles, to stay out of the dementia danger zone.

OLIVER TICKELL is a writer and campaigner on health and environmental issues. He is the founder of the tfX campaign against trans fats (www.tfx.org.uk) and architect of the Kyoto2 proposals for an effective climate protocol (www.kyoto2.org).

Brain Cancer
Could Adult Stem Cells Be the Cause—and the Cure?

BARBARA BASLER

It was national news when Sen. Edward Kennedy of Massachusetts was diagnosed with brain cancer last May. Then, just weeks later, veteran political columnist Robert Novak also was found to have a malignant brain tumor. Suddenly, the public was awash in a flood of stories about this deadly form of cancer. The fresh focus on this disease comes at a critical time, as scientists explore a new theory that could unlock the mystery of brain cancer—and other cancers as well.

Paradoxically, adult stem cells may be both the cause of cancer and a cure for it.

That theory, barely discussed even five years ago, has captivated the country's leading researchers, including Alfredo Quiñones-Hinojosa, M.D., a 40-year-old one-time farm worker from Mexico who now heads the Brain Tumor Center at the Johns Hopkins Bayview Medical Center in Baltimore.

Quiñones is a researcher with a difference. Dressed in his green scrubs and fresh from the second of what will be three brain surgeries that day, Quiñones puts in punishing 16-hour shifts, working not just in the operating room but in a brain cancer research lab as well. "The surgery can be perfect, a beautiful work of art," he says. "But I still know that no matter what I do, these patients will eventually succumb to this disease. So how can I not look for a cure when I see my patients and their families and the suffering this cancer causes?"

It's that work and passion that last year led *Popular Science* to name Quiñones to its annual Brilliant Ten list of "the most creative, the most groundbreaking, the most brilliant young scientists in the country."

Quiñones is convinced that adult stem cells act as triggers for brain cancer. (Unlike the use of embryonic stem cells, which requires the creation and destruction of an embryo, the use of adult stem cells found in children and adults is not politically controversial.)

Stem cells become new cells to maintain and repair tissue. Neural stem cells, for example, create new brain cells, while hematopoietic stem cells create new blood cells.

New studies suggest that cancer of the brain—along with cancer of the breast, prostate, colon, pancreas, lung and a host of other organs—grows from adult stem cells present in many tissues.

It's not clear how stem cells may cause cancer, but investigators theorize that rogue cancer stem cells have an uncanny ability to repair damage to their DNA and are therefore able to withstand standard radiation and chemotherapy treatments. Quiñones and his colleagues hope that by targeting these cells, they can destroy the cancer and prevent its return.

"We were once taught that brain cells die and can't be replaced," Quiñones says. "We now know that the mammalian brain has the ability to regenerate through adult neural stem cells. What we are exploring—and this is the great leap—is whether normal neural stem cells can lose their ability to self-regulate and become dangerous stem cells that create tumors.

"We are just beginning to understand this link between stem cells and cancer," he stresses. "We have to prove that brain cancer stem cells exist. But I think the potential here is real."

Close to 44,000 people will be diagnosed this year with tumors that originate in the brain; half of the tumors will be malignant. Another 170,000 patients will learn that cancers from other parts of their body have spread to their brain.

Brain cancer is one of the most intractable. In the last 30 years the median length of survival for patients with cancer that originates in the brain has increased by only four months—to 14.6 months.

"I think of this as the worst cancer, and if we can make progress with brain cancer I assure you that many other cancers will benefit, too," says Quiñones.

Along with his stem cell research, Quiñones runs a lab that is analyzing the medical records of thousands of brain cancer patients, looking for clues to more effective treatments. So far he's found that patients with high glucose levels and patients who are clinically depressed have much worse outcomes than other patients.

"Now, when I meet a patient, I want to know his glucose level and whether he is clinically depressed, because we can treat those conditions and improve his chances for survival," he says.

Quiñones' pursuit of a cure for brain cancer is marked by the same grit and determination that have shaped every facet of his life. This is a doctor, after all, whose life here began one cold, dark January night when, as a frightened 19-year-old, he climbed a chainlink fence along the border between Mexico and the United States. The first time he clambered over the fence he was caught and sent back across the border. Just hours later he was back. This time he made it over and escaped into the night.

An undocumented immigrant, Quiñones spoke no English and had no job skills. He labored as a farm worker in California. "One day a friend said to me, 'You will always be a migrant worker,' and something inside me just snapped. I just couldn't accept that," he says.

Quiñones, who lived in a dilapidated trailer, took English lessons and enrolled at a community college while juggling jobs as a painter and welder. He won a scholarship to the University of California, Berkeley. From there, he went on to medical school at Harvard University. He became a citizen.

Now, his office walls at Hopkins are covered in awards.

Quiñones "won't take no for an answer. He's an inspired scientist."

"This is a man who won't take no for an answer," says Henry Brem, MD, chair of neurosurgery at Hopkins. "He's an inspired scientist, and an extraordinarily hard-working one."

Today, standard procedures for brain tumors, like Kennedy's, call for removing as much of the tumor as possible, followed by radiation and chemo. But excising all the cancer lacing surrounding tissue is difficult, and 90 percent of the tumors grow back. It may be, Quiñones says, that just a few cancer stem cells left behind after surgery renew the tumor.

"We have isolated cells from human brain tumor samples that in a petri dish act like brain cancer stem cells," Quiñones says. "We're still not sure that they actually behave that way in the brain, but there is some very good data to suggest they do."

The first evidence for brain cancer stem cells was reported in a study published in 2004. Scientists in Canada isolated tumor cells with a genetic mutation they believed identified the cells as brain cancer stem cells. When they injected 100 of these cells into the brains of mice, the mice developed brain tumors. They also injected tens of thousands of other brain tumor cells without the mutation into mice—and all failed to produce tumors.

It appears that cancer stem cells may make up only a tiny portion of the brain tumor, which means that if they do trigger tumor growth, scientists may have been studying the wrong cells 95 percent of the time.

"Stem cells are a new paradigm," says Quiñones. "Imagine a world where we know which cells are responsible for the cancer and we understand how they work—and how to turn them off. That's the world I want. If it's there, we have to find it."

New Theories and Therapies

The theory that adult stem cells in the body may trigger brain cancer growth is revolutionary, exciting—and still very much unproven. In the meantime, scientists say that genetic discoveries and other cancer research are now yielding new information that may bring new therapies.

Just two months ago, scientists working on the Cancer Genome Atlas, a project funded by the National Institutes of Health, released a genetic map of 20,000 genes in glioblastoma, the most common form of brain tumor and the kind diagnosed in Sen. Edward Kennedy. Experts say the research uncovered a dozen genetic pathways, or networks, of genes, which control the spread and growth of the tumor.

"These pathways represent targets we can attack to damage the tumor," says Henry Friedman, MD, co-deputy director of the Brain Tumor Center at Duke University in Durham, N.C., where Kennedy was treated. "We already have some drugs to attack some of these pathways, so this really gives us something to work with."

One of the most exciting therapies in the pipeline involves using antibodies with isotopes that can be injected into the tumor to deliver high doses of radiation from within. The treatment is in Phase III clinical trials, Friedman says.

Joachim Baehring, MD, director of the Yale Brain Tumor Center in New Haven, Conn., says in the past 10 years he's seen an "explosion" in the number of experimental drugs for brain cancer, from vaccines to agents that target a tumor's ability to grow new blood vessels. He says while the stem cell theory is only a hypothesis, it's still useful. Although scientists haven't yet been able to identify the genetic changes in these tumors, he says, "studying cancer cells that behave like stem cells gives us a promising focus for our genetic studies."

Paul Watson of Baltimore, who lost his 19-year-old son, Aaron, to brain cancer last year, says this gifted surgeon with the warm, engaging manner "is a man of passion and great understanding. From the moment we met him, he was there for us, through three operations."

Despite the operations and the best treatment available, Aaron died 18 months later, and Quiñones went to his young patient's funeral.

"Dr. Quiñones held my hand and said that Aaron should not be dead," Watson says. "He said we have to find a cure for this disease."

Trust and Betrayal in the Golden Years

Just when they're needed most, a growing number of children are turning on aging parents—taking away their nest eggs and their independence.

KYLE G. BROWN

Concerned about her mother's mental health, Sarah took decisive action. She helped 82-year-old Celia move to a retirement community, she set up accounts for her at a local health-food store and an upscale clothing boutique. She also took over her financial affairs.

But at the mention of her daughter, Celia says: "I swear to God, she should be in jail."

Since 2004, when an Alberta court granted her daughter guardianship of her mother and control of her $400,000 in savings and stocks, Celia claims Sarah has taken almost all of her possessions—and left her without a bank account, or even identification. (Both of their names have been changed to protect their privacy.) While her daughter claims to be acting in her best interests, Celia feels betrayed and helpless.

And she is hardly alone. Toronto lawyer Jan Goddard, who has worked on elder-abuse issues for 17 years, says financial exploitation of seniors is now "endemic across the country." This can range from snatching a few dollars from grandma's purse to transferring property.

Brenda Hill, the director of the Kerby Rotary House Shelter in Calgary, agrees. "We've had people who have had their homes sold, who have been virtually on the street with no food and no money because their children have taken all their assets," she says. "It happens quite often."

And the problem is likely to get worse before it gets better. People 65-plus are the fastest-growing segment of the Canadian population—but cuts to health services in the 1990s have meant that fewer seniors are living in public institutions.

This, in turn, has placed increased pressure on family members, which a Statistics Canada report in 2002 suggested could lead to a rise in the abuse of older adults.

South of the border, taking money from mom and dad is also seen as a serious issue. So much so, that the Elder Financial Protection Network predicts that it will become the "crime of the century."

Ageism is partly to blame. As is a culture of entitlement—where the money parents spend can be seen as a "waste" of the child's future inheritance.

Charmaine Spencer, a gerontologist at B.C.'s Simon Fraser University, says both are particularly prevalent in North America. Although she adds, "I have not seen a single culture in which abuse of the elderly does not take place—it's financial and psychological abuse, and when that doesn't work, it's physical."

But addressing such exploitation is anything but straightforward. How do legal and medical professionals determine when adult children are taking advantage of aging parents—and when they are enforcing necessary restrictions on those no longer able to care for themselves? How do they intervene, either to stop abuse or to help elderly parents cope with newly dependent roles, when seniors are enmeshed in painful power struggles with grown sons and daughters?

Take one of Ms. Goddard's eightysomething clients. The increasingly frail woman complained that she needed more support than her son—who lives in her house—was providing. She decided to revoke his power of attorney.

But, according to Ms. Goddard, when the woman told her son about the meeting, he was furious. The next day, she called Ms. Goddard to cancel everything. As she spoke nervously on the phone, Ms. Goddard could hear the woman's son in the background, telling her what to say.

Though lawyers like Ms. Goddard can call in the police in such situations, getting seniors to make formal complaints against their children can be difficult. Ultimately, she says, clients have to face the repercussions of confronting their families and "keep wavering whenever they go back home."

Seniors' own shame can also keep them from reporting that their children are taking advantage of them. Although abuse seems to cut across socio-economic lines (even New York socialite Brooke Astor made headlines recently because of her son's alleged neglect), older adults often feel guilty talking publicly about private matters.

As for those who do brave action against their children, many do not make it very far. While money is in their children's hands, victims of financial abuse cannot afford the fees to take a case to court—which can run at a minimum of $10,000. And legal aid is rarely awarded to seniors involved in civil cases.

Ms. Hill tells the story of a Calgary widow who sold her house and moved into her daughter's home. Her children transferred money from her account to theirs, borrowed her bank card and charged her for "services" such as rides and errands.

A few months later, the woman fled to the Kerby Rotary House Shelter with a small fraction of her savings. But at the age of 87 she could not face the idea of spending what little time and money she had left in the courts. Now, she resides in a seniors' lodge with just enough cash to live out her days—though her daughter will never be brought to justice.

Dr. Elizabeth Podnieks, the founder of the Ontario Network for the Prevention of Elder Abuse, conducted the first national survey on elder abuse in 1990. She says that even when lawyers do take seniors' cases, complainants have difficulty convincing the court that they are the victims of theft and exploitation. For example, their memory is often called into question, as they struggle to recall "giving" money to defendants.

Family members who question their parents' ability to look after their finances may consult a capacity assessor—a health professional with special training in assessing mental capacity.

Tests vary from province to province, but Larry Leach, a psychologist at Toronto's Baycrest centre for geriatric care, says they generally set out to answer the tricky question of whether elderly adults "appreciate all the risks of making an investment and giving gifts to people."

If a parent is deemed incapable, the government may then become the guardian of property until a family member applies to the courts to gain guardianship.

This is what soured the relationship between Celia and her daughter. In 2004, Celia was diagnosed with dementia and deemed "unable to care for herself." Her daughter then won guardianship over Celia's affairs.

Celia hotly disputes the doctor's findings—but now the onus is on her to prove that she is mentally fit or to appoint a new guardian.

Meanwhile, she is no longer speaking to Sarah. Once in charge of her own health-food store, she feels humiliated taking "handouts" from her daughter. "I can't do anything. Where can I go with no money?" she says.

As for more cut and dried cases, where neither dementia nor family dynamics is in play, Dr. Podnieks says: "Older people don't understand why the police can't just 'go in and get my money back.' They know it's a crime, you know it's a crime, the abuser knows it's a crime—so where is the law, where is the protection?"

Detective Tony Simioni, who is part of the Edmonton Police Force's Elder Abuse Intervention Team, says senior abuse is about 20 years behind child abuse, both in terms of public awareness and government and police resources. "Financial-abuse cases rarely see the top of the agenda," he says. "It's low on the totem pole of crimes."

Still, Judith Wahl, who has been working at the Advocacy Centre for the Elderly in Toronto for more than 20 years, remains optimistic. She believes that public education campaigns on elder abuse are making an impact. The rising number of reported incidents, she says, is partly due to a growing willingness to talk openly about abuse.

A 75-year-old Winnipeg woman is a case in point. She was coerced for years into paying her daughter's bills, rent and grocery tabs.

"I would come home and cry and sort of tear my hair, and think, 'Where do I turn to for help? Who do I go to?'" she says.

But eventually her friends encouraged her to contact a seniors support centre. With their help, she gained the confidence to confront her daughter—and to grant her son power of attorney.

These days, she gives gifts to her granddaughter, but when her daughter asks her for more, she tells her to talk to her "attorney."

KYLE G. BROWN is a freelance writer based in Calgary.

The Extent and Frequency of Abuse in the Lives of Older Women and Their Relationship with Health Outcomes

Purpose: This study assessed the extent of different types of abuse, repeated and multiple abuse experiences among women aged 60 and older, and their effects on the women's self-reported health. **Design and Methods:** A cross-sectional study of a clinical sample of 842 community-dwelling women aged 60 and older completed a telephone survey about type and frequency of abuse, self-reported health status and health conditions, and demographic characteristics. Bivariate and multivariate analyses were performed using SPSS 11.5 and STATA 7.0. **Results:** Nearly half of the women had experienced at least one type of abuse—psychological/emotional, control, threat, physical, or sexual—since turning 55 years old. Sizable proportions were victims of repeat abuse. Many women experienced multiple types of abuse and experienced abuse often. Abused older women were significantly more likely to report more health conditions than those who were not abused. Women who experienced psychological/emotional abuse—alone, repeatedly, or with other types of abuse—had significantly increased odds of reporting bone or joint problems, digestive problems, depression or anxiety, chronic pain, and high blood pressure or heart problems. **Implications:** It is important that health care and service providers acknowledge psychological/emotional, control, threat, physical, and sexual abuse against older women and understand their health implications. In addition, it is important for providers to be trained in both aging and domestic violence services and resources.

BONNIE S. FISHER, PhD AND SAUNDRA L. REGAN, PhD

Researchers' understanding of psychological, physical, or sexual abuses against women and their relationship with physical and mental health conditions is derived almost exclusively from the experiences of teenage girls and pre-menopausal women. Generally, violence-against-women researchers and aging service providers have overlooked older women (Fisher et al., 2003). Even among the most steadfast advocates, only a handful of initiatives and collaborations promoting the intersection of abuse and aging exist (Brandl, 1997; Fisher, Zink, Pabst, Regan, & Rinto, 2004; Vinton, 2003; Wilke & Vinton, 2003).

Recently, however, there has been a renewed interest in examining the extent and nature of abuse against older women. Researchers and advocates from a variety of disciplines have reported that older women experience intimate-partner and domestic violence well into old age (Grossman & Lundy, 2003; Rennison & Rand, 2003; Teaster & Roberto, 2004). It should not be too surprising that, given the paucity of older women abuse studies, our understanding of the health consequences for abused older women is woefully limited. The issues of abuse and its health consequences will not retreat anytime soon. Older women are a fast-growing population as the baby boomers enter into old age and their life expectancy continues to lengthen.

Using data from a clinical sample of 842 community-dwelling women aged 60 and older, this study makes four contributions to researchers' understanding of the extent and nature of abuse against older women and the associated health conditions. First, we measured the extent of abuse experiences in late life—that is, since age 55—to capture the experiences of women who had reached a mature stage of their life cycle. Second, we expanded upon the types of abuse examined in previous studies to include control and threat abuses. Third, we examined not only the extent of abuse but also the extent of repeat abuse and multiple abuses and their respective frequencies. Last, we investigated the relationships between type of abuse (including repeat abuse) and older women's self-reported general health, number of health conditions, and specific psychological and physical health conditions.

The Extent of Abuse against Older Women

The estimation of the extent of abuse against older women is a young field of inquiry. Only two national-level studies have been conducted since Pillemer and Finkelhor's (1988) pioneering study revealed that older women had experienced physical violence and verbal aggression since turning 65 years old.

First, results from the National Elder Abuse Incidence Study (National Center on Elder Abuse, 1998) reported that 76.3% of surveyed women aged 60 and older had experienced emotional/psychological abuse and 71.4% were victims of physical abuse. Second, the National Crime Victimization Survey estimated that 118,000 intimate-partner victimizations were committed against women 55 years and older during a 9-year period (1993–2001; Rennison & Rand, 2003).

Only a handful of single-state studies have examined the extent of abuse suffered by older women (Grossman & Lundy, 2003; Teaster & Roberto, 2004). To illustrate, using data from the Women's Health Initiative in San Antonio, Texas, Mouton and colleagues (2004) reported that 11% of postmenopausal women had reported abuse within the past year. At the 3-year follow-up, 5% of the women had reported new experiences with abuse.

Collectively these studies reveal that older women are abuse victims into their old age, yet many questions about women's abuse later in life remain largely unanswered. These questions include: (a) What types of abuse do older women experience in their later years? (b) Are these women repeatedly abused, and, if so, which type of abuse do they repeatedly experience? (c) Do these women experience multiple types of abuse, and, if so, what are the patterns? and (d) How often does abuse occur? By better understanding the extent and frequency of abuse against older women, researchers can determine whether linkages exist between the abuse older women experience and their health-related outcomes.

The Associations between Abuse and Health-Related Outcomes

Researchers have documented that abused women are at risk for several negative health-related consequences.

Self-reported general health status. Three studies are illustrative of the association between abuse and general health status. First, Koss, Koss, and Woodruff (1991), using a 16-item measure of criminal victimization, reported that victimized women aged 19–69 years old perceived themselves as less healthy than nonvictimized women (i.e., as having more somatic complaints and less physical and mental well-being). Second, investigating a sample of women aged 21–55 years old, Campbell and colleagues (2002) reported that twice as many women who had experienced intimate-partner violence over a 9-year period rated their health as fair to poor compared with women who had never experienced such abuse. And third, Coker and colleagues (2002) reported that women aged 18–65 years old who had experienced lifetime intimate-partner physical, sexual, or psychological abuse were significantly more likely than nonabuse victims to self-report current poor health.

Number of self-reported health problems or conditions. Researchers have also shown that women who have experienced abuse are more likely to suffer more health problems compared with nonabused women. This includes suffering from more physical and mental health conditions and chronic health problems (see Sutherland, Bybee, & Sullivan,

2002). Campbell and colleagues (2002) reported that abused women had a higher rate of total physical health problems and central nervous system, gynecological, and chronic-stress symptoms compared with women who had never been abused.

Specific chronic health problems or conditions. There is mounting evidence that different types of abuse and their co-occurrence are related to specific short- and long-term mental and physical health problems and conditions (Sutherland et al., 2002). The list of negative health effects includes depression, fear, chronic pain, osteoarthritis, gastrointestinal disorders, chronic stress, gynecological symptoms, chest pains, and cardiac problems (Campbell et al., 2002; Coker et al., 2002).

Repeat and multiple abuse. For many women, abuse is not an isolated event; abuse happens repeatedly. Women who suffer repeated abuse experience two or more incidents of the same type of abuse within a specified time period—for some, this is daily (Tjaden & Thoennes, 1998). Women also experience different types of abuse (i.e., multiple forms of abuse). Campbell and colleagues (2002) reported that 33% of the abused women surveyed experienced both physical and sexual abuse.

Research suggests that repeat and multiple abuses take a negative toll on women's health, possibly even more negative than the abuse-nonabuse distinction that is commonly used in the abuse literature. First, there is evidence that women who experience multiple types of abuse report having poor health (Koss et al., 1991). Second, the frequency of different types of abuse may affect some health outcomes but not others. Coker and colleagues (2002) also found that increased psychological intimate-partner-violence scores were strongly associated with self-reported current poor health status. Physical or sexual intimate-partner violence, however, was not related to current poor health status. Further clarifying the relationship between repeat abuse and type of health condition, Coker and associates reported that the frequency of a certain type of abuse was related to specific health conditions. That is, higher psychological intimate-partner-violence scores were significantly related to both the development of a chronic disease and current depressive symptoms. Higher physical or sexual intimate-partner-violence scores were significantly related only to current depressive symptoms.

There is evidence to suggest that experiencing multiple abuses—a combination of two types of abuse—has negative health-related consequences. Hegarty, Gunn, Chondros, and Small (2004) reported that "probably" depressed women were more likely to have experienced physical abuse and emotional abuse or harassment than "not" depressed women.

Overall, the results from these studies suggest that abuse has negative effects on women's health. There is room for further research, including the examination of the abuse–health-consequences relationship for older women. To date, no published research has examined this relationship using a sample of women aged 60 years and older, and only a few published studies have examined abuse that happened after age 55 and its relationship to women's health (see Mouton, 2003; Zink, Fisher, Regan, & Pabst, 2005).

Methods

Sample

In March 2003, we obtained patient lists of women aged 55 and older from five adult primary care clinics affiliated with an academic institution in southwestern Ohio and serving Indiana, Ohio, and Kentucky. We arranged the patient lists into three groups of phone numbers stratified by age: 55–64 years, 65–74 years, and 75 years and older. Trained female interviewers called each woman on the list between March and June 2003. We had obtained a total of 4,261 phone numbers. Each woman, aged 55–90, was called at least three times at different times on different days before being taken out of the sample.

Women gave verbal consent by agreeing to participate in the Women's Health and Relationship Survey (WHRS). Of the 4,261 available numbers, 44% of the women ($n = 1,852$) were not available (answering machine or no answer). In addition, 7% ($n = 297$) of the numbers had been disconnected, and 6% ($n = 261$) were wrong numbers. Approximately 2% ($n = 67$) of the women were deceased, 1% ($n = 45$) were too sick to answer, and 0.4% ($n = 15$) of the women had family members who intercepted the call and would not allow them to participate. Of the 1,724 women reached by phone, 40% ($n = 695$) refused to participate, 1.5% ($n = 26$) were unable to answer the three mental competency questions correctly (their age, birth date, and the current year) to assess their mental status, and 0.5% ($n = 8$) refused to answer the abuse questions. This resulted in 995 usable surveys and an adjusted response rate of 58% (995 out of 1,698).

Only women aged 60 and older ($n = 842$) were included in the current study. All of the women in the sample were community dwelling. None lived in institutional settings, such as a nursing home.

Instrument

The WHRS was adapted from validated instruments and included questions about mental status (Lachs & Pillemer, 1995), health conditions (Tjaden & Thoennes, 1998), abuse (Shepherd & Campbell, 1992; Tjaden & Thoennes) and sociodemographics. The survey administration took 20–45 minutes, depending on whether the woman had experienced abuse.

Measures

Type of abuse. The WHRS measured five different types of abuse: (a) psychological/emotional, (b) control, (c) threat of physical abuse, (d) physical, and (e) sexual. The abuse measures combined the uniform definitions regarding intimate-partner violence recommended by the Centers for Disease Control and Prevention with definitions housed within the elder abuse framework recognized by the U.S. National Academy of Sciences (Bonnie & Wallace, 2002; Saltzman, Fanslow, McMahon, & Shelley, 1999/2002).

We measured each of these five types of abuse by using multiple items. A principal components factor analysis performed on the six psychological/emotional and control abuse items confirmed two distinct factors. Three items loaded on one factor, psychological/emotional abuse (.85, .82, and .52); and three other items loaded on a second factor, control abuse (.81, .70, and .66).

Psychological/emotional abuse was a 3-item measure (Cronbach's $\propto$ = .64). Control abuse was a 3-item measure (Cronbach's $\propto$ = .59). Threat abuse was a 2-item measure (Cronbach's $\propto$ = .52). Physical abuse was a 4-item measure (Cronbach's $\propto$ = .72). Sexual abuse was a 3-item measure (Cronbach's $\propto$ = .71). For each abuse item, women were asked if they had experienced the behavior "since you turned 55."

Extent of abuse. We created three variables to measure the extent to which women in the sample experienced the five types of abuse. First, we created a dichotomous variable, abuse victim, which measured whether a respondent had experienced any of the five types of abuse since she had turned 55 years old.

Second, we created a measure of repeated abuse. Repeated abuse was a count of the number of women who had experienced two or more abusive behaviors that comprised a specific type of abuse (i.e., the same type of abuse). To illustrate, three behaviors comprise psychological/emotional abuse. Women who reported having experienced two or more of these behaviors were coded as having been repeatedly psychologically/emotionally abused since age 55.

Third, multiple abuse was a measure of the number of women who had experienced any combination of at least two types of abuse. For example, a woman was coded as a victim of multiple abuse if she had experienced either both sexual and physical abuse, or both control and physical abuse.

Frequency of abuse. In order to measure the frequency with which abuse occurred, interviewers asked women how often different forms of abuse had happened to them since they had turned 55 years old. Responses were: never, rarely, occasionally, frequently, or very frequently. Of the respondents who had experienced at least one form of abuse within a specific type of abuse, those who reported "rarely" were coded as the Rarely group and those who reported "occasionally, frequently, or very frequently" were coded as the Often group. For example, a woman who had experienced any form of psychological/emotional abuse frequently was coded as often psychologically/emotionally abused. If, within the same type of abuse, she reported one form as having happened rarely and another form as having happened frequently, she was coded using the "highest" frequency category; in this case, coded as being in the Often group.

Health-related consequences. Because one of the primary aims of this study was to examine the relationship between abuse experience and health-related consequences, we used several measures of health outcome. First, we created a dichotomous measure of the status of a woman's health. Interviewers asked respondents to assess their health on a 5-point scale ranging from poor to excellent. For ease of analysis, we collapsed the "poor" and "fair" categories into one category and collapsed "good," "very good," and "excellent" categories into a second category to create the dichotomous measure of self-reported health status. We found that 55% ($n = 429$) of the women rated their health as good to excellent, and 45% ($n = 378$) rated their health as poor or fair.

The second dependent variable, number of self-reported health conditions, was a count of the number of health conditions that a doctor had told each woman that she currently had. The 10 items included: high blood pressure or heart problems; lung problems (e.g., asthma or chronic obstructive pulmonary disease); diabetes or thyroid problems; bone or joint problems (e.g., osteoporosis or arthritis); depression or anxiety; digestive problems (e.g., irritable bowel syndrome or heartburn); stroke or nerve problems (e.g., Multiple Sclerosis or Parkinson's disease); blood problems (e.g., anemia); chronic pain (e.g., migraines or back pain); and any type of cancer. Respondents averaged 3.3 ($SD = 1.8$) health conditions.

Third, we created a dichotomous measure of whether respondents currently had or did not have a specific health condition by asking questions that required respondents to identify which health conditions a doctor had told them they had. These were the 10 health conditions listed in the preceding paragraph. More than half of the respondents reported having high blood pressure or heart problems (75%) or bone or joint problems (65%). Less than half reported having diabetes or thyroid problems (37%), chronic pain (36%), digestive problems (31%), depression or anxiety (30%), lung problems (24%), cancer (13%), stroke or nerve problems (12%), or blood problems (12%).

Control variables. Similar to Coker and colleagues (2002) and Campbell and associates (2002), we employed several sociodemographic characteristics as control variables in the multivariate health-related consequences models. Using aged 75 and older (34%, $n = 285$) as the reference group, we created two age dummy variables for 60–64 years old (23%, $n = 191$), and 65–74 years old (44%, $n = 366$; percentages may equal greater than 100% due to rounding). Race/ethnicity was measured as a dichotomy: Black/African American or Other (45%, $n = 373$) and White (reference group, 55%, $n = 453$). Using less than high school education (36%, $n = 297$) as the reference group, we measured respondents' level of education with two dummy variables: high school diploma (31%, $n = 255$), and some college to college graduate (34%, $n = 281$). Using being married/common law (32%, $n = 336$) as the reference group, we measured current marital status with three dummy variables: divorced/separated (18%, $n = 152$), widowed (41%, $n = 342$), and single/never married (9%, $n = 72$). Using less than $20,000 (47%, $n = 389$) as the reference group, we measured annual household income with three dummy variables: $20,000–$40,000 (15%, $n = 128$), more than $40,000 (10%, $n = 84$), and refused to answer or did not know (28%, $n = 228$). Given the Appalachian heritage in southwest Ohio, we included a dichotomous measure of whether a woman was of Appalachian decent (9%, $n = 79$) or not (91%, $n = 717$).

Data Analysis

Descriptive statistics and bivariate and multivariate data analyses are reported here. Appropriate tests of significance are presented for the bivariate analyses. In order to examine the relationship between type of abuse and health-related consequences, we estimated several multivariate models. Depending on the distribution of the dependent variable, we estimated either a logit model or an analysis of covariance model. We estimated all of the multivariate logit models using STAT A, version 7.0 (Stata-Corp, 2001). We calculated the descriptive statistics and estimated the analysis of covariance models with SPSS 11.5 for Windows (SPSS Inc., 2002).

Results
The Extent and Frequency of Abuse and Repeat Abuse

Nearly half (47%, $n = 393$) of all women aged 60 and older had experienced at least one type of abuse since the age of 55. Table 1 presents the descriptive results for the extent and frequency of abuse among older women. As is shown in Table 1, a substantial percentage (45%) of older women had experienced psychological/emotional abuse since turning 55 years old. Nearly 12% of older women had been threatened. Less than 5% of women had been victims of control abuse (4%), physical abuse (4%), or sexual abuse (3%).

However, the results on type of abuse experienced mask a more telling result once we look at the extent of repeat abuse. Of women who had experienced a specific type of abuse, between 21% (sexual abuse) and 47% (psychological/emotional abuse) had been victims of repeat abuse. For example, 32% of the physical abuse victims had been victims of repeat physical abuse. This means that these women had experienced two or more forms of physical abuse since turning 55 years old (i.e., any combination of the four different forms of physical abuse, such as being pushed and slapped, being slapped and choked, or being pushed, slapped, or choked).

The frequency of the occurrence of abuse also reveals noteworthy patterns. Of the older women who had experienced a specific type of abuse, in the case of 4 of the 5 types of abuse, more than 45% of the women had experienced abuse often since age 55: control abuse (88%), psychological/emotional abuse (57%), threat abuse (48%), and sexual abuse (46%). Slightly less, but still a substantial proportion (41%), had experienced physical abuse often since age 55.

Asking who perpetrated the abuse also revealed interesting results (not presented here). Interviewers did not ask respondents about the identity of the perpetrator of psychological/emotional abuse due to their concern for the respondent's discomfort with answering the first set of experience questions about psychological/emotional abuse. Interviewers did ask respondents about different categories of perpetrators (i.e., spouse/boyfriend, relative, or non-relative) for the other types of abuse. Almost three-fourths of the women (73%, $n = 66$) reported that a relative—child, grandchild, or other relative—had threatened them, compared with 21% of women who had been threatened by a spouse/boyfriend and 14% by a non-relative. A majority of the women reported that their spouse/boyfriend had perpetrated control abuse (56%, $n = 19$) and sexual abuse (73%, $n = 19$). Physical abuse did not exhibit the same pattern as to who was the perpetrator. Of the physically abused women, 45% ($n = 14$) reported that a relative had been the perpetrator, compared

Table 1 Abuse Since 55 Years Old: Types of Abuse and Extent and Frequency of Abuse of Women 60 and Older

Type of Abuse Specific Behavior[a]	Extent of Abuse		
	Abuse Victim, % (n)[b]	Repeat Abuse Victim, % (n)	Abuse Occurring Often, % (n)[c]
Psychological/emotional	44.6 (372)	47.3 (176)	57.3 (212)
Called you a name or criticized you	30.2 (245)		
Shouted or swore at you	25.3 (209)		
Been possessive or jealous of someone close to you	17.6 (139)		
Control	4.1 (34)	29.4 (10)	88.2 (30)
Routinely checked up on you in a way that made you afraid	2.5 (21)		
Put you on an allowance	1.7 (14)		
Not letting you go to work or social activities or see or talk with your friends	1.3 (12)		
Threat	11.7 (98)	23.5 (23)	48.0 (47)
Said things to scare you	6.0 (50)		
Threw, hit, kicked, or smashed something	8.5 (71)		
Physical	3.8 (38)	31.6 (12)	40.6 (13)
Pushed, grabbed, or shoved you	2.6 (22)		
Slapped, hit, or punched you	1.7 (14)		
Hit you with an object	1.0 (8)		
Choked or attempted to drown you	0.7 (6)		
Sexual	3.4 (28)	21.4 (6)	46.4 (13)
Pressured you to have sex in a way you did not like or want	2.9 (24)		
Physically forced you to have sex	1.1 (9)		
Attacked the sexual parts of your body	0.5 (4)		

[a]The items listed under each type of abuse are the specific behaviors that comprise the respective type of abuse measure.

[b]Respondents who refused to answer or reported "don't know" to a form of abuse question were not included in the forms of abuse calculations. Only those who refused to answer or reported "don't know" to all the forms of abuse questions within a respective type of abuse were excluded from the type of abuse estimates.

[c]Percent represents those women who responded that at least one form of abuse within the specific type of abuse happened occasionally, frequently, or very frequently.

with 39% (n = 12) who reported that their spouse/boyfriend had. Almost 20% (n = 6) of these women reported that a non-relative had physically abused them.

The Extent and Frequency of Multiple Abuses

Table 2 presents additional insight into the multiple-abuse experiences of older women who had experienced two different types of abuse (i.e., had been victims of multiple abuse). The diagonal in bold shows the unconditional percentages, or the percentage of women who had been victims of the specific type of abuse listed in each column (same percentages as reported in Table 1). The conditional likelihood for women who had been abused in the specific manner as noted in the columns is presented in the off diagonal. For example, among the women who had been physically abused, 69% had been threatened, 44% reported having experienced control abuse, and 31% reported having been sexually abused. In more than half of the conditional likelihoods (13 out of the 20 pairs), 25% or more women had experienced

multiple types of abuse. It appears that multiple abuses were characteristic of the type of abuse from which these victimized women suffered.

Two additional noteworthy multiple-abuse patterns are evident in Table 2. First, psychological/emotional abuse co-occurred with other types of abuse for a large number of older women. Among those older women who had experienced a specific type of abuse, between 86% (threat) and 97% (physical abuse) had experienced psychological/emotional abuse. Second, the conditional likelihoods (in the off diagonal) exceed the unconditional likelihoods in their respective rows. This suggests that many older women were more likely to have experienced multiple types of abuse than one type of abuse. To illustrate, 12% of the women had been threatened, yet from twice (of those who had been psychological/emotionally abused, 23% had also been threatened) to more than five times (of those who had been physically abused, 69% had also been threatened) as many women had experienced multiple abuse in which they had also been threatened.

Table 2 The Extent of Multiple Abuse

	Conditional Type of Abuse				
Type of Abuse	Psychological/Emotional, % (n)	Control, % (n)	Threat, % (n)	Physical, % (n)	Sexual, % (n)
Psychological/emotional	**44.6 (372)**	91.2 (31)	85.7 (84)	96.9 (31)*	89.3 (25)
Control	8.4 (31)	**4.1 (34)**	18.4 (18)	43.8 (14)*	32.1 (9)*
Threat	22.6 (84)	52.9 (18)	**11.7 (98)**	68.8 (22)*	50.0 (14)
Physical	8.4 (31)	42.4 (14)*	22.7 (22)	**3.8 (38)**	35.7 (10)
Sexual	6.8 (25)	27.3 (9)	14.4 (14)	31.3 (10)*	**3.4 (28)**

Notes. Unconditional likelihoods are shown in the main diagonal in bold. The highest value in each row is indicated by an asterisk. The conditional type of crime is not necessarily temporally prior to the type of row abuse.

Extent and Frequency of Abuse Measures Refined

Two noteworthy results convinced us to refine our measures of extent and frequency of abuse. First, the extent of abuse results suggests that many older women had experienced repeat abuse and multiple types of abuse. The results in Table 2 suggest that psychological/emotional abuse occurred in conjunction with other types of abuse (control, threat, physical, or sexual). Nearly 30% (28.7%, n = 110) of abuse victims were multiple-abuse victims who had suffered from psychological/emotional abuse. The remaining abuse victims had experienced only one type of abuse. The majority of older abused women (67%, n = 262) had experienced *only* psychological/emotional abuse, and 5% (n = 21) had experienced *only* control, threat, physical, or sexual abuse since age 55. The analysis of those women who had *only* experienced control, threat, physical, or sexual abuse is not reported here due to the small number of cases.

In order to measure the possible effects that each of these three types of abuse experience may have had on health outcomes, we created two dummy variables that refined the extent-of-abuse measures in light of the multiple-abuse results. These new variables measured whether a woman had experienced (a) only psychological/emotional abuse, and no control, threat, physical, or sexual abuse, or (b) multiple abuses (psychological/emotional abuse plus any another type of abuse). Women who had not experienced any type of abuse since turning 55 years old were the reference group.

To measure repeat abuse, we created a nonrepeat-/repeat-abuse measure for those women who had experienced psychological/emotional abuse. As is shown in Table 1, 176 women (21% of the entire sample) had experienced repeated psychological/emotional abuse. Given the very small number of repeat victims within the other abuse categories, we did not create a nonrepeat-/repeat-abuse measure for these types of abuse.

Second, as the results on frequency of abuse presented in Table 1 suggest, a substantial proportion of older women had experienced abuse often. Taking into account the effects of the frequency with which these women had experienced psychological/emotional abuse or multiple types of abuse (psychological/emotional plus another type of abuse), we created four dummy variables. We further dichotomized each of the two dummy

variables for specific type of abuse into two frequency groups: Rarely or Often. We found that 51% of the psychologically/emotionally abused women and 81% of the multiple-abuse victims experienced abuse often.

Bivariate and Multivariate Results: Type and Frequency of Abuse and Health Outcomes

Demographic correlates of type of abuse. To examine the bivariate effects of the demographic characteristics used as control variables in the multivariate models, we examined their relationship with the type of abuse (psychological/emotional, repeated, and multiple abuse). The results of the chi-square test of independence showed that, of the demographic variables used as control variables in the multivariate analyses, only race was not significantly associated with any of the measures of abuse: abuse victimization ($\chi^2 = .434$, $df = 1$, $p = 0.51$), repeated psychological/emotional abuse ($\chi^2 = 0.272$, $df = 1$, $p = 0.60$), or multiple abuses ($\chi^2 = .346$, $df = 1$, $p = 0.56$). Level of education was not significantly related to experiencing multiple abuse ($\chi^2 = 0.367$, $df = 3$, $p = 0.94$). Being of Appalachian descent was not related to repeated abuse ($\chi^2 = 0.340$, $df = 1$, $p = 0.59$) or multiple abuse ($\chi^2 = 1.18$, $df = 1$, $p = 0.28$). Marital status was not related to multiple abuse ($\chi^2 = 4.89$, $df = 4$, $p = 0.30$). All of the relationships between the other control variables (e.g., age, income, and marital status) and the type of abuse were significant at $p < .05$ (the exception being the relationship between level of education and multiple abuse). A significantly larger percentage of younger older women (60–64 years old) had been abuse victims, victims of repeated abuse, and victims of multiple abuse compared with women older than age 65.

Type of abuse and health outcomes. Table 3 presents the effects of experiencing different types of abuse since age 55 on health outcomes. There are several noteworthy results. First, none of the abuse measures were significantly related to older women's self-reported poor health status. Second, older women who had experienced abuse were significantly more likely than nonvictims to self-report more health conditions, on average. Third, regardless of how psychological/emotional abuse

Table 3 Types of Abuse Since 55 Years Old and Health-Related Consequences

	Type of Abuse			
Variable	Abuse Victim, AOR[a] (95% CI)	Single Type of Abuse Victim: Psychological/ Emotional, AOR (95% CI)	Repeat Psychological/ Emotional Victim, AOR (95% CI)	Multiple Types of Abuse Victim: Psychological/ Emotional and Other Types,[b] AOR (95% CI)
Health-related consequence				
Self-reported poor health status	0.96 (0.73–1.25)	1.03 (0.73–1.45)	0.86 (0.58–1.29)	0.83 (0.51–1.32)
No. of self-reported health conditions	3.6***[c] (1.7)	3.7*** (1.6)	3.7*** (1.6)	3.6*** (1.9)
Current health conditions				
Depression or anxiety	2.24*** (1.70–2.96)	1.74*** (1.25–2.44)	1.93*** (1.32–2.82)	1.85** (1.17–2.92)
Digestive problems (e.g., irritable bowel, ulcer, heartburn)	1.60** (1.22–2.09)	1.70*** (1.23–2.37)	1.45* (1.10–2.10)	0.97 (0.61–1.56)
Chronic pain (e.g., back pain, migraines)	1.65*** (1.28–2.15)	1.60*** (1.16–2.22)	1.51* (1.04–2.18)	1.09 (0.69–1.72)
High blood pressure or heart problems	1.22 (0.91–1.64)	1.52* (1.04–2.23)	1.32 (0.85–2.06)	0.72 (0.43–1.20)

Notes. AOR = adjusted odds ratio. Significance of the Wald statistic: *$p < .05$; **$p < .01$; ***$p < .001$.
[a]Adjusted for age, race and ethnicity, education, marital status, income, and Appalachian descent.
[b]Other types include control, threat, physical, and sexual abuse.
[c]The mean has been adjusted for age, race and ethnicity, education, marital status, income, and Appalachian decent. The standard deviation is reported in parentheses. The mean for nonvictims is 3.1 ($SD = 1.8$).

was operationalized—as occurring alone, repeatedly, or with other types of abuse—this type of abuse took a negative toll on women's current health. Women who had been psychologically/ emotionally abused reported significantly more health conditions, on average, than did women who had not been abused in this manner.

Looking at the effects of abuse on current health conditions reveals that, overall, psychological/emotional abuse, again regardless of how it was operationalized, had negative effects on abused women. First, all types of abuse increased the odds of women reporting depression or anxiety by a factor of almost 2. Second, women who had experienced only psychological/ emotional abuse had increased odds of having digestive problems, high blood pressure or heart problems, or chronic pain. Third, repeated psychological/emotional abuse was associated with increased odds of digestive problems and chronic pain. Fourth, women who had experienced any abuse were not significantly more likely to have reported lung, diabetes or thyroid, stroke or nerve, or blood problems, or cancer ($p > .05$; results not shown here).

Frequency of abuse. Table 4 presents the effects of the frequency of different types of abuse since age 55 on health outcomes. These results show some noteworthy patterns supportive of those reported in Table 3.

First, in this study, frequency of abuse did not significantly predict women's self-reported poor health status. Second, abuse regardless of frequency or type was significantly associated

with a number of self-reported health conditions. Women who had experienced either psychological/emotional abuse or multiple abuse reported significantly more health conditions, on average, than nonvictims. Third, having experienced psychological/emotional abuse, regardless of how often, increased women's odds of having digestive problems or chronic pain. Fourth, women who experienced psychological/emotional abuse often had increased odds of having bone or joint problems, depression or anxiety, or high blood pressure or heart problems. Fifth, regardless of the frequency or type of abuse experienced, women's odds of reporting depression or anxiety significantly increased. Notably, for women who had often experienced multiple abuse, the odds of reporting depression or anxiety increased by a factor of 4. Last, the frequency of neither psychological/emotional nor multiple abuse was significantly related to having lung, diabetes or thyroid, stroke or nerve, or blood problems, or cancer ($p > .05$; results not shown here).

Discussion

These results shed insight on the extent and nature of different types and patterns of abuse against older women. The findings revealed that a substantial proportion, nearly half, of older women had experienced psychological/emotional, control, threat, physical, or sexual abuse since turning 55 years old. Second, the largest percentage of women had experienced psychological/emotional abuse. Third, a notable percentage of women had experienced multiple types of abuse. Fourth, many

Table 4 Frequency of Type of Abuse Since 55 Years Old
and Health-Related Consequences

Variable	Single Type of Abuse Victim: Psychological/Emotional, AOR[a] (95% CI)				Multiple Types of Abuse Victim: Psychological/Emotional and Other Types, AOR[b] (95% CI)			
	Rarely		Often		Rarely		Often	
Health-related consequence								
Self-reported poor health status	0.91	(0.57–1.47)	1.07	(0.69–1.67)	0.51	(0.17–1.52)	0.92	(0.53–1.58)
No. of self-reported health conditions	3.3[*c]	(1.6)	3.8***	(1.5)	3.6*	(2.0)	3.6***	(1.9)
Current health conditions								
Bone or joint problem (e.g., arthritis or osteoporosis)	1.08	(0.70–1.67)	1.58*	(1.01–2.47)	1.62	(0.56–4.70)	1.12	(0.66–1.88)
Depression or anxiety	1.76*	(1.10–2.82)	2.61***	(1.69–4.03)	2.34**	(1.37–3.98)	4.06**	(1.52–10.87)
Digestive problems (e.g., irritable bowel, ulcer, heartburn)	1.77**	(1.13–2.76)	1.62***	(1.19–2.79)	1.41	(0.51–3.92)	1.21	(0.70–2.07)
Chronic pain (e.g., back pain, migraines)	1.70*	(1.09–2.64)	1.81**	(1.19–2.75)	1.46	(0.54–3.97)	1.38	(0.82–2.34)
High blood pressure or heart problem	1.24	(0.76–2.03)	1.77*	(1.03–3.02)	0.59	(0.19–1.90)	0.87	(0.49–1.56)

Notes. AOR = adjusted odds ratio. Significance of the Wald statistic: $*p < .05; **p < .01; ***p < .001$.
[a]Adjusted for age, race and ethnicity, education, marital status, income, Appalachian descent, and single control, threat, physical or sexual abuse, and multiple abuses.
[b]Adjusted for age, race and ethnicity, education, marital status, income, Appalachian descent, and single psychological/emotional abuse and single control, threat, physical or sexual abuse.
[c]The mean has been adjusted for age, race and ethnicity, education, marital status, income, Appalachian descent, and as per the respective abuses noted in footnotes a and b. The standard deviation is reported in parentheses. The mean for nonvictims is 3.1 ($SD = 1.8$).

older women had experienced abuse repeatedly and often. Lastly, there does seem to be a relationship between abuse and health problems among older women.

As the literature review stated, the effect of abuse on younger women's health is becoming well documented. However, researchers have only begun to unravel the effects of abuse on the health of older women; more study is needed. Within the broader elder abuse literature, researchers have reported that older people who suffer abuse or mistreatment experience a much higher incidence of depression (Pillemer & Finkelhor, 1988; Pillemer & Prescott, 1989); and that experiencing elder abuse or mistreatment is a risk factor for nursing home placement in the older population (Lachs, Williams, O'Brien, & Pillemer, 2002) and higher mortality rates (Lachs, Williams, O'Brien, Pillemer, & Charlson, 1998). The present results are supportive of researchers' overall conclusion: Abuse takes a negative toll on the quality of life of older persons. The current results suggest that both the physical and mental health of older women are negatively affected by abuse.

This study has three main implications for people who serve the health care needs of older women. First, with regard to those practitioners in the health care arena who provide care to older women, it is important that providers acknowledge that abuse is happening and that it is affecting the health of these older women. The present results are a first step toward aiding in the understanding that women who are experiencing abuse may not report lower general health compared with women who are

not being abused, yet are more likely to experience detrimental effects to their health if one examines for specific health conditions. Second, because older women who are being abused are more likely than nonvictims to report a higher total number of health conditions and to experience certain health conditions such as depression, anxiety, digestive problems, and chronic pain, these conditions may serve as red flags to health providers to screen for possible abuse within intimate-partner and interpersonal relationships. Third, the type of abuse most frequently experienced by the older women in this study was psychological/emotional abuse. This confirms findings by Harris (1996) that physical and sexual abuse decreases with age, whereas psychological abuse remains. Although great progress has been made in the elder abuse and domestic violence arenas to come to a consensus on uniform definitions of abuse, it is important to continue to define different categories of abuse (e. g., psychological, emotional, and control) because older women may have a more difficult time identifying this behavior as abuse. Zink, Regan, Jacobson, and Pabst (2003), in a qualitative study of abused women, found that in many cases women did not even identify psychological/emotional abuse as abuse. Or women reported that things in their marriage were okay now that it was *only* psychological/emotional abuse and that the physical and sexual abuse had decreased or stopped. However, in the present study, we found that, for those women who were experiencing abuse, the likelihood that they were experiencing different kinds of abuse was high. Consequently, if an older woman does admit to one type of abuse, it is likely that she is experiencing or has experienced other types of abuse as well, and that she experiences abuse more than once and possibly often.

This study also has implications for individuals who provide social services for older women. First, it is important for providers to be trained to look for signs of psychological/emotional abuse in older women, as the present results suggest that (a) this is the type of abuse that is most likely to occur, and (b) this type of abuse is most likely to co-occur with other more severe forms of abuse. It is common for providers who suspect abuse to make referrals to agencies such as adult protective services. However, in the case of domestic abuse, this may be an inappropriate referral. In many states, adult protective services is only allowed to intervene if the victim is physically or mentally impaired, which may not be the case in every instance. Consequently, neither the cause nor the effects of the abuse will be addressed. Many people who provide services to the elderly are taught to think only about caregiver stress as a possible cause of abuse. In such cases, they may make referrals to get aging service providers into the home. In some situations this may exacerbate an already abusive situation. Advocates such as Brandl (1997) and researchers (Fisher et al., 2003; Vinton, 2003) have suggested that professionals in the aging field need to be more informed about the resources available for the victims of domestic violence. Similarly, professionals in the domestic violence field need to become more familiar with the resources available on aging (Fisher et al., 2004; Grossman & Lundy, 2003). As women who are being abused continue to age and live longer, it will become increasingly imperative that more and more crosstraining take place between these two fields. Lastly, this study found that control, threat, physical, and sexual abuse is perpetrated by many people who are routinely involved in their victim's lives. The perpetrator can be a spouse or boyfriend, other relative, or non-relative. Consequently, health care and social service providers need to insist, if possible, for a few minutes alone with the older woman to question her about possible abuse and even the identity of the abuser.

This study is not without limitations. First, this is a cross-sectional study, which limits our ability to make causal inferences about the effects of health and abuse. We are unable to ascertain if abuse is the cause of the increase in health conditions or if having more health conditions puts women at more risk for being abused. Second, many of the potential survey respondents were never reached, and, because of the Health Insurance Portability and Accountability Act regulations, we were unable to find out any information on non-responders. Third, the abuse and health information is uncorroborated self-report and could not be confirmed through medical record review. The abuse is also self-report; however, because women are unlikely to report abuse, the abuse reported for this study may actually be an underreporting of the abuse taking place. Fourth, interviewers asked women to recall events that may have happened several years ago. It must also be kept in mind that the marital status and abuse relationship is one that must be viewed with caution. Respondents were asked about their current marital status—not their marital status at the time of the abuse. A respondent may have been abused by her spouse a year ago, and the spouse has since died.

Despite its limitations, this study is an important first step in documenting the existence of the different types of abuse happening to older women, its repetitive nature and frequency, and its effect on health. It is imperative that health care and service providers be aware of the health implications of abuse and understand the need for identification and training in both aging and domestic violence. As the population continues to age, awareness of resources available through both aging and domestic violence networks will become necessary.

References

Bonnie, R., & Wallace, R. (Eds.). (2002). *Elder abuse: Abuse, neglect and exploitation in an aging America.* Washington, DC: The National Academies Press.

Brandl, B. (1997). *Developing services for older abused women.* Madison: Wisconsin Coalition Against Domestic Violence.

Campbell, J., Jones, A. S., Dienemann, J., Kub, J., Schollenberger, J., O'Campo, P., et al. (2002). Intimate partner violence and physical health consequences. *Archives of Internal Medicine, 162,* 1157–1163.

Coker, A. L., Davis, K. E., Arias, I., Desai, D., Sanderson, M., Brandt, H. M., et al. (2002). Physical and mental health effects on intimate partner violence for men and women. *American Journal of Preventive Medicine, 23,* 260–268.

Fisher, B. S., Zink, T., Pabst, S., Regan, S., & Rinto, B. (2004). Service and programming for older abused women: The Ohio experience. *Journal of Elder Abuse & Neglect, 15*(2), 67–83.

Fisher, B. S., Zink, T., Rinto, B., Regan, S., Pabst, S., & Gothelf, E. (2003). Overlooked during the golden years: Violence against older women. *Violence Against Women, 12,* 1409–1416.

Grossman, S., & Lundy, M. (2003). Use of domestic violence services across race and ethnicity by women 55 and older: The Illinois experience. *Violence Against Women, 12,* 1442–1452.

Harris, S. (1996). For better or for worse: Spouse abuse grown old. *Journal of Elder Abuse & Neglect, 8*(1), 1–33.

Hegarty, K., Gunn, J., Chondros, R., & Small, R. (2004). Association between depression and abuse by partners of women attending general practice: Descriptive, cross-sectional survey. *British Medical Journal, 328,* 621–624.

Koss, M. P., Koss, P. G., & Woodruff, W. J. (1991). The deleterious effects of criminal victimization on women's health and medical utilization. *Archives of Internal Medicine, 151,* 342–347.

Lachs, M., & Pillemer, K. (1995). Abuse and neglect of elderly persons. *New England Journal of Medicine, 332,* 437–443.

Lachs, M., Williams, C., O'Brien, S., & Pillemer, K. (2002). Adult protective service use and nursing home placement. *The Gerontologist, 42,* 734–739.

Lachs, M., Williams, C., O'Brien, S., Pillemer, K., & Charlson, M. (1998). The mortality of elder mistreatment. *Journal of the American Medical Association, 280,* 428–432.

Mouton, C. (2003). Intimate partner violence and health status among older women. *Violence Against Women, 12,* 1465–1477.

Mouton, C., Rodabrough, R., Rovim, S., Hunt, J., Talamantes, M., Brzyski, R., et al. (2004). Prevalence and 3-year incidence of abuse among postmenopausal women. *American Journal of Public Health, 94,* 605–612.

National Center on Elder Abuse. (1998). *The National Elder Abuse Incidence Study.* Washington, DC: The Administration for

Children and Families and the Administration on Aging, U.S. Department of Health and Human Services.

Pillemer, K., & Finkelhor, D. (1988). The prevalence of elder abuse: A random sample survey. *The Gerontologist, 28,* 51–57.

Pillemer, K., & Prescott, D. (1989). Psychological effects of elder abuse: A research note. *Journal of Elder Abuse & Neglect 1*(1), 65–74.

Rennison, C., & Rand, M. (2003). Non-lethal intimate partner violence: Women age 55 or older. *Violence Against Women, 12,* 1417–1428.

Saltzman, L., Fanslow, J., McMahon, P., & Shelley, G. (2002). *Intimate partner violence surveillance: Uniform definition and recommended data elements, version 1.0.* Atlanta, GA: National Center for Injury Prevention and Control, Centers for Disease Control and Prevention. (Original work published in 1999)

Shepard, M., & Campbell, J. (1992). The abusive behavior inventory: A measure of psychological and physical abuse. *Journal of Interpersonal Violence, 7,* 291–305.

SPSS, Incorporated. (2002). *SPSS 11.5 for Windows.* Chicago: Author.

StataCorp. (2001). *Stata Statistical Software: Release 7.0.* College Station, TX: Author.

Sutherland, C., Bybee, D., & Sullivan, C. (2002). Beyond bruises and broken bones: The joint effects of stress and injuries on battered women's health. *American Journal of Community Psychology, 30,* 609–636.

Teaster, P., & Roberto, K. (2004). Sexual abuse of older women living in nursing homes. *The Gerontologist, 44,* 788–796.

Tjaden, P., & Thoennes, N. (1998). *Prevalence, incidence and consequences of violence against women: Findings from the National Violence Against Women survey* (NCJ172837).

Washington, DC: U.S. Department of Justice, National Institute of Justice and Centers for Disease Control and Prevention.

Vinton, L. (2003). A model collaborative project toward making domestic violence centers elder ready. *Violence Against Women, 12,* 1504–1513.

Wilke, D., & Vinton, L. (2003). Domestic violence and aging: Teaching about their intersection. *Journal of Social Work Education, 39,* 225–235.

Zink, T., Fisher, B. S., Regan, S., & Pabst, S. (2005). The prevalence and incidence of intimate partner violence in older women in primary care practice. *Journal of General Internal Medicine, 20,* 884–888.

Zink, T., Regan, S., Jacobson, C. J., & Pabst, S. (2003). Cohort, period and aging effects: A qualitative study of older women's reasons for remaining in abusive relationships. *Violence Against Women, 9,* 1429–1441.

BONNIE S. FISHER, PhD: Division of Criminal Justice, University of Cincinnati, OH and **SAUNDRA L. REGAN,** PhD: Department of Family Medicine, University of Cincinnati, OH.

Address correspondence to Bonnie S. Fisher, PhD, Division of Criminal Justice, University of Cincinnati, P.O. Box 210389, Cincinnati, OH 45221-0389. E-mail: Bonnie.Fisher@uc.edu

This research was supported under award R605H23525 from the Attorney General of Ohio, Betty Montgomery. The points of view in this article are those of the authors and do not necessarily represent the official position of the office of Ohio Attorney General. Thanks to Dr. Therese Zink, Dr. Amy Cassedy, Stephanie Pabst, Barbara Rinto, and Elizabeth Gothelf for their enthusiasm and thoughtfulness as members of the research team. Thank you also to the anonymous reviewers who provided us with the opportunity to improve our research.

UNIT 5

Retirement: American Dream or Dilemma?

Unit Selections

Key Points to Consider

• What steps should be taken by a person throughout his or her adult life to ensure an adequate retirement income?

• Upon arriving at retirement age, why do some workers choose to continue to work either full-time or part-time?

• What are the advantages of employing older workers?

• What are the uncertainties about having an adequate retirement income for workers who have a 401(k) defined contribution plan as a means of saving for their retirement?

• Given different choices of lifestyles between work and retirement, which older Americans are most satisfied during their later years?

Student Website

www.mhhe.com/cls

Internet References

American Association of Retired People
   http://www.aarp.org
Health and Retirement Study (HRS)
   http://www.umich.edu/~hrswww

Since 1900, the number of people in America who are aged 65 years and over has been increasing steadily, but a decreasing proportion of that age group remains in the workforce. In 1900, nearly two-thirds of those over the age of 65 worked outside the home. By 1947, this figure had declined to about 48 percent (less than half), and in 1975, about 22 percent of men aged 65 and over were still in the workforce. The long-range trend indicates that fewer and fewer people are employed beyond the age of 65. Some people choose to retire at age 65 or earlier; for others, retirement is mandatory. A recent change in the law, however, allows individuals to work as long as they want with no mandatory retirement age.

Gordon Strieb and Clement Schneider (*Retirement in American Society,* 1971) observed that for retirement to become an institutionalized social pattern in any society, certain conditions must be present. A large group of people must live long enough to retire; the economy must be productive enough to support people who are not in the workforce; and there must be pensions or insurance programs to support retirees.

Retirement is a rite of passage. People can consider it either as the culmination of the American Dream or as a serious problem. Those who have ample incomes, interesting things to do, and friends to associate with often find the freedom of time and choice that retirement offers very rewarding. For others, however, retirement brings problems and personal losses. Often, these individuals find their incomes decreased; they miss the status, privilege, and power associated with holding a position in the occupational hierarchy. They may feel socially isolated if they do not find new activities to replace their previous work-related ones. Additionally, they might have to cope with the death of a spouse and/or their own failing health.

Older persons approach retirement with considerable concern about financial and personal problems. Will they have enough retirement income to maintain their current lifestyle? Will their income remain adequate as long as they live? Given the current state of health, how much longer can they continue to work?

The next articles deal with changing Social Security regulations and changing labor demands that are encouraging older

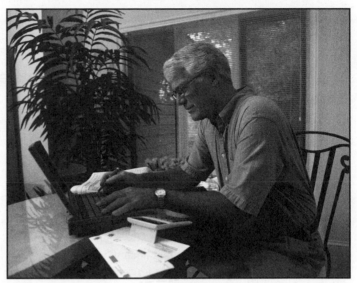

© Imagestate Media (John Foxx)/Imagestate

persons to work beyond the age of 65. *Consumer Reports* in "Retire Right" surveyed 6,700 retirees about their retirement decisions and what did or did not work well for them in their retirement years. Jane Bryant Quinn in "Money for Life" outlines and explains the five steps that a person should take throughout his or her adult life to ensure an adequate retirement income. In "Keep Pace with Older Workers," the author points out the advantage to the business community of employing older workers. In "Color Me Confident: Why Many Americans May Be Working When They Retire," the author discusses the problem of having an adequate retirement income with the new 401(k) defined contribution plans that most businesses have now implemented. And in "Work/Retirement Choices and Lifestyle Patterns of Older Americans," the authors examine six different work, retirement, and leisure patterns that older people may choose to determine which is most satisfying to the individual.

Retire Right

In a surprising new survey, 6,700 retired readers share their dos and don'ts.

What's the secret to a successful retirement? Our retired readers turned out to be a good group to ask. In a recent survey, a stunning 93 percent of them told us they were satisfied overall with their retirement, with 32 percent saying they were completely satisfied. Forty-one percent said retirement had actually been better than they expected. Only 5 percent said it had been worse.

If there was one widely shared regret, it was that they didn't have even more money to enjoy themselves. About 35 percent told us that, looking back, they wished they'd started saving earlier, and 30 percent said they would have put away more each year. Eight percent said they should have retired earlier, but the same percentage wished they had done it later. More than a third, when asked about their regrets and given a list to choose from, checked the box for "None of the above."

The Consumer Reports National Research Center surveyed 17,877 subscribers to ConsumerReports.org, ages 55 to 75. Some told us they were fully retired, some semi-retired, and others still working full-time in their main career.

Most of the retirees could probably have stayed in the workforce longer and piled up more savings had they chosen to do so. A third retired between the ages of 55 and 59, and another 38 percent between 60 and 64. Only 18 percent waited until 65 or later. The median age at which the group had retired was 60.

The group that was still working full-time expected to retire later. Forty-eight percent of that group told us they planned to retire between 65 and 69, with 14 percent saying they expected to wait until age 70 or later. That jibes with other research showing that today's workers expect to retire later, either because they enjoy what they do or simply because they can't afford to stop doing it.

For this report we focused our analysis on the 6,723 readers in the retired group. To be sure, our retired readers might not be representative of the U.S. population as a whole. For example, they are likely to be somewhat better educated and more affluent than the average American. However, they're apt to be a lot like other CONSUMER REPORTS readers. In other words, you.

Retirees Reveal Best & Worst Moves

Carol A. Quartana

Smartest move: Started buying employer's stock at age 25. Maxed out 401(k) plan.

Biggest mistake: Put too large a proportion of her retirement assets in that one stock.

Elvin Chong

Smartest move: Both he and his wife worked for an employer with a generous pension plan.

Biggest mistake: Invested in a real-estate limited partnership in the '70s.

Mary Kathryn Pickle

Smartest move: Invested in a 403(b) at work then rolled it into a balanced portfolio with the help of an adviser.

Biggest mistake: Invested in a mutual fund with low returns.

Savings Secrets

What exactly did the retirees do right? For one thing, they put money aside in a variety of vehicles toward the eventual day. When we asked them how they had gone about it, here's what they said:

- 67 percent had participated in a 401(k) or 403(b) plan at work.
- 60 percent had an IRA.
- 59 percent had built up equity in their homes.
- 43 percent owned stock outside of a retirement account.
- 38 percent owned mutual funds outside of a retirement account.
- 37 percent had a savings account or CD.

All of those are smart moves, in our view, with one possible caveat. Given the current state of the housing market, individuals planning for retirement today will probably not want to count on their homes being the cash machines they've *been for preceding generations.*

However, the broader lesson here, of saving through a variety of vehicles, is a solid one. In general, the more ways that our readers told us they saved, the more likely they were to be satisfied with their retirement.

Smaller percentages of readers told us they had saved for retirement via a whole-life insurance policy, an annuity, or gold or other precious metals. We agree with the majority there; none of those should represent a substantial part of a person's retirement savings in most cases.

As to when they started saving seriously for retirement, 32 percent told us they'd begun in their 30s, while 34 percent had waited until their 40s. A precocious few (15 percent) had started in their 20s. Only 11 percent had put it off until their 50s and 1 percent until their 60s. Seven percent told us they had never seriously saved. Perhaps not surprisingly, the sooner the person had started to save, the more satisfied he or she was with retirement.

One difference that's often cited between today's generation of retirees and tomorrow's is that the former group is more likely to have money coming in from a defined-benefit pension, the kind that is typically funded by an employer and pays a regular monthly benefit during retirement. Such pensions have been disappearing in recent years, as many employers abandoned them in favor of defined contribution plans, such as 401(k)s, which shift more of the burden of saving to the employee. Our survey found scant evidence of that so far. Among the retirees, 55 percent reported receiving money from a defined-benefit pension. Among the still-working full-timers, 53 percent said they had a defined-benefit plan with their current employer.

What You Can Do

Obviously none of us can start saving in our 30s if our 30s are behind us. But there are some changes many of us can still make, drawing on the lessons of this survey.

Don't invest too cautiously or wildly. A solid majority—57 percent—of the retired respondents characterized themselves as moderate risk-takers. That's also borne out in their choice of savings and investment vehicles, as previously listed. For most people that means not avoiding solid stocks and stock funds

How to Max out Your Retirement Plans

Here are the limits for some common plans, including extra catch-up contributions for anyone 50 and over. The first three are available from mutual fund companies and other institutions, the rest through employers. You still have until April 15, 2008, to fund an IRA for 2007.

Plan	Tax Year 2007 Maximum	Catch-Up for 50 and Over	Tax Year 2008 Maximum	Catch-Up for 50 and Over
Traditional IRA	$ 4,000	$1,000	$ 5,000	$1,000
Roth IRA	4,000	1,000	5,000	1,000
SEP-IRA	45,000*	NA	46,000*	NA
SIMPLE IRA	10,500	2,500	Same as '07	Same as '07
401(k) and Roth 401(k)		15,500	5,000	Same as '07	Same as '07
403(b) and Roth 403(b)	15,500	5,000	Same as '07	Same as '07
457	15,500	5,000	Same as '07	Same as '07

*Or 25 percent of compensation, whichever is less.

on the one hand or chasing after speculative, get-rich-quick schemes on the other.

Save even more if you can. The table at the top of this page shows the maximums for typical retirement plans.

Plan your transition. While 74 percent of the retirees immediately stopped working once they retired, about one in four told us they had continued to work reduced hours in their field, had worked part-time elsewhere, or had gone into business for themselves. There was no correlation between overall satisfaction and how people had made the transition, so whether you leap into retirement headfirst or ease into it one toe at a time is a matter of preference. That decision is likely to depend on your financial needs and what other dreams you have for your time.

The retirees we surveyed cited such motivations as hobbies, travel, and spending more time with their spouses or companions for bidding the workforce goodbye. Postponing retirement has a long list of financial advantages. But as our retired survey respondents told us, a well-planned retirement has a lot going for it, too.

Money for Life

JANE BRYANT QUINN

Retirement experts used to talk about finances as a three-legged stool: Social Security, pensions, and personal savings. That's not enough to stand on anymore. For one thing, the pension leg has collapsed entirely at many companies. As I think about my own retirement (someday!), I see a five-legged stool: Social Security (it will be there for our generation), personal savings, freedom from debt, health insurance (for retirees under 65), and realistic work goals. If you have a pension, congratulations—that's icing on the cake. But none of these legs can be taken for granted or strengthened without thought. Good retirements take good planning. Here are some tips for getting started:

1. Plan to Get out of Debt

When talking to people about their retirement experiences, I'm always struck by the amount of debt they're struggling to pay off. Often, it's medical debt, which can be hard to avoid. But other debts are preventable:

- Quit borrowing against your house. Bend all your efforts toward paying off your home equity lines and reducing your primary mortgage, too. If you find that you can't retire mortgage-free, think about selling your house and buying something smaller for cash.
- Get rid of consumer debt. It was never smart in the first place.
- Control your spending. You'll need to learn to live on a smaller amount of money once your paychecks stop. Start practicing well before retirement. Try putting half or more of your disposable income toward repaying debt and live on what's left. It's educational!
- Help your children only as a last resort. Too many parents are using needed retirement funds to bail their children out of various problems. Sometimes help is essential—say, for critical medical care. But preserving your retirement nest egg is more important than putting grandchildren through college. One way or another, the kids can work that out themselves.

2. Plan for Health Insurance

If at all possible, don't retire without health insurance before you have Medicare. It's tough to find an affordable policy in middle age—that is, if you're insurable at all. Take these steps:

- Evaluate your current coverage. Corporate early retirees often get health insurance until 65, when they qualify for Medicare. Your premium and copayment may increase over the years, but your coverage will almost certainly stick. If you don't get retiree health benefits, scout for an individual policy before you retire. If you're unsuccessful, COBRA coverage keeps you in the company plan for 18 months, at your expense.
- For individual policies, check eHealthInsurance.com and also work with an insurance agent. Your most affordable choice will carry a high deductible—say, $2,500 to $5,000 per year. If you remain healthy, you won't have to use that deductible before Medicare clicks in.
- Quit smoking, lose weight, and exercise. You must stay as healthy as you can, not only for the pleasure of it but to keep yourself out of medical debt. Even if you have insurance, it may not cover all your costs.

3. Plan Your Social Security

Deciding when to start taking benefits depends, of course, on your personal circumstances.

- If you have to retire early and are short of cash or are in poor health, you'll probably start at 62—the earliest age possible. But that cuts your personal benefit by at least 25 percent and your spousal benefit by at least 30 percent—for life. (The spousal benefit provides payments to a husband or wife who hasn't built a substantial account of his or her own.)
- If you can delay taking your benefit, you should. For each year you wait after your full retirement age, your starting check rises by 8 percent—a splendid, guaranteed "return." If you die, you'll also leave a larger benefit for your spouse. After age 70, the initial benefit stops going up.
- There's an exception for married people in good health when one of them has a small Social Security benefit. Typically, that's the wife. If she retires first, she should start her individual benefit at 62. When her husband retires, she'll switch to the spousal benefit. By using her own account first, she taps a benefit that otherwise would have gone to waste.

4. Plan for Retirement Savings

By the time you reach the end of your working life, you should be saving 15 percent or more of your gross income, in addition to anything your employer contributes to your 401(k) or similar plan. Here's what else to do:

- Those with an old-fashioned lifetime pension are lucky dogs. It's an income you'll never outlive. If you're offered a lump sum in lieu of a monthly income, consider the following: (1) Could you use the lump sum to buy yourself an immediate annuity that pays more per month? If not and you want a fixed income, the company pension is the better deal. (2) Are you worried that your company might fail, taking your pension with it? If so, take the lump sum and roll it into an immediate annuity (if you want fixed income) or an individual retirement account invested in stock and bond mutual funds. Company pensions are insured by the Pension Benefit Guaranty Corp., but perhaps for a lower amount than you'd otherwise get. (3) Don't roll the money into a tax-deferred variable annuity. The expenses are high (and often hidden), which means that long-term performance will generally be sub-par. If you need more than a modest amount of the money, you'll pay a penalty to take it out during the first seven to 10 years, and you'll owe ordinary income taxes on the gains.

- Those with 401(k)s and similar plans should be setting aside the maximum the law allows from their pay. Invest the money in well-diversified stock and bond funds—maybe 60 percent stocks, 40 percent bonds. (The bonds protect you in case of a catastrophe in stocks. If you also have a pension, however, you can put more into stocks.)

- When you retire, you can generally leave the money in the 401(k) or else roll it into an IRA. The 401(k) advantage: You're familiar with the funds in the plan and your money is usually managed at low cost. The IRA advantage: You have a broader investment choice. If you die, your spouse can roll the money from either plan into an IRA of his or her own and let it accumulate tax-deferred. It's a little trickier for other heirs. They have to open what's called an "inherited IRA" and are not allowed to let the money accumulate untouched. They can, however, stretch out withdrawals over their lifetime. This option is always available when they inherit an IRA. Starting this year, it's potentially available if they inherit a 401(k)—but only if the plan documents allow it. So you have to check. Inherited IRAs and 401(k)s are a highly technical area where a lot of heirs and their advisers are making mistakes. If heirs other than a spouse try to roll the money into an IRA of their own, rather than following the inherited-IRA rules, the money becomes taxable all at once.

- Those without company plans should be saving in pre-tax IRAs (if you work for an employer) and SEP-IRAs or individual 401(k)s (if you're self-employed). If you've maxed out on your contribution, save in regular, after-tax accounts. Make these savings automatic—with contributions taken from your bank account each month.

- Spend your savings frugally. You may have 30 or more years to live in retirement, and you don't want to outlive your money. Your spending target should be no more than 4 percent of your total financial assets (stocks, bonds, cash) in your first retirement year. Each year after that, raise your take by the inflation rate. If you stick with that plan, your money should last for life. If you take more, you risk running out of money.

- Consider a visit to a financial planner who can run your finances through his or her computer and tell you where you stand. But not just any financial planner. Planners who sell products will find things for you to buy—and the commission makes them expensive. Look for a fee-only planner, who sells no products and charges only for the time spent. Two places to look: www.garrettplanningnetwork.com and www.napfa.org

5. Plan on Working!

The reality is that many would-be retirees haven't saved enough to support themselves for life. When considering whether you can quit, add together your annual pension, if any, your Social Security benefit, and 4 percent of your personal retirement savings (4 percent of the lump sum; don't count interest and dividends separately). If that's enough to live on (and you have health insurance), you're good to go. If your job has gone away, plan on working part time to fill the gap between your expenses and your income without having to dip into savings right away.

JANE BRYANT QUINN, the author of Smart and Simple Financial Strategies for Busy People, writes for Newsweek, Good Housekeeping, and Bloomberg News.

Keep Pace with Older Workers

Older employees—more than one-quarter of the workforce—bring experience to their jobs. Research proves they are as productive as youth. And by understanding aging, employers can make them even more productive.

ROBERT J. GROSSMAN

When Dan Smith, senior vice president of human resources at Borders Group in Ann Arbor, Mich., joined the company in 1995, the majority of Borders' workforce was under 30. As he looked to the future, he became concerned about unsettling labor forecasts, asking, "What will we do when the under-30 population starts to dry up?" His question led him to study the demographics of Borders' 30,000-strong empire, yielding an unanticipated revelation destined to dramatically alter Borders' employee mix and bottom line.

"Our stores with older workers had much lower turnover, did better financially, [and] all the workers were happier," Smith says. Looking at workers age 50 and over vs. those under 30, the comparison was startling as to loyalty and stability. "Older workers were more satisfied, were staying longer, and customer service seemed to be better in their stores. It became clear that we had to make these guys a bigger segment of our population."

Borders began to target people age 50 and over. Since then, the number of older workers at its stores has tripled. Eighteen percent of Borders' workers are over 50; two-thirds of those are between 50 and 60. The metrics they're delivering make Smith look like a genius: "In the retail book business, turnover is 100 percent to 120 percent," he says. "Ours is half that and trending down." Turnover is six times less for workers over 50 than for those under 30.

Borders' experience is no fluke. For managers concerned that older workers may wear out or falter, evidence proves clear: Blue- or white-collar, these folks remain loyal, reliable and as good as younger counterparts.

"There is no correlation between age and job performance," insists Richard Johnson, principal research associate at the Urban Institute in Washington, D.C., citing a statistically validated report that combines the results of many research studies of worker performance from ages 20 to 65.

One more thing: When many people think of older workers, they don't have 50- to 64-year-olds in mind.

Misconceptions

Opinions differ as to when workers cross the bridge from middle age. Professional football players grow old in their 30s; air traffic controllers face mandatory retirement at 56, pilots at 65 and federal law enforcement officers at 57. The Age Discrimination in Employment Act, applicable to employers with payrolls of at least 20, begins protecting workers at age 40.

AARP, seniors' formidable lobbying organization, clusters mature workers in one category: 55-plus. Company officials interviewed for this article—from Borders; Vanguard Group in Valley Forge, Pa.; and Bon Secours Richmond Hospital System in Richmond, Va.—use 50 as the tipping point. Labor economists and gerontologists voice preference for 50 as well.

Yet, when the term "older worker" is used, an image of a 50-year-old is not what comes up. More likely, it's a person in his 70s or older-alert, spry, with an inner drive that keeps him going while most peers play golf or canasta.

Take Hattie Davis, 86, a licensed practical nurse at Bon Secours. Davis has worked for many units at Bon Secours. With age, she found the physical aspects of her job—walking, lifting and standing patients—too demanding. Because Davis is a valued worker, HR officials moved her to the employee wellness program, where today she gives inoculations and performs other less strenuous duties.

Mature Workers: Myths and Realities

They cost more. Reality. Older workers ages 50 to 64 cost more, but not by much. The financial divide is not dramatic—only about 10 percent, according to Richard Johnson at the Urban Institute, who bases his estimate on compensation and health insurance costs.

If you're an economist, older workers are less productive because they may have higher salaries; if you're a psychologist, they're equally productive because they may have more experience, says Neil Charness, a professor of psychology at the Pepper Institute on Aging and Public Policy at Florida State University.

They're absent more. Myth. According to the U.S. Bureau of Labor Statistics, in 2007 full-time workers ages 25 to 54 were absent at a ratio of 3.2 per 100; workers age 55 and over were absent with greater frequency, but barely—3.6 per 100.

"We don't have any data that suggest older people are sick more," says Dan Smith, senior vice president of HR for Borders Group. If anything, they're more loyal and less likely to call in sick for false reasons. Borders finds that the opportunity to join a group for health care purposes is an enticement for older workers that costs the company little. "A lot of people come to us because we offer access; they pay the majority of the cost," Smith says.

Health costs are greater. Reality. There's a gradual increase in health care spending as workers age from 40 on. Any significant differential, however, does not occur until age 65 when chronic conditions tend to set in. In 2004, the difference in health care claims filed by workers ages 55 to 64 and employees ages 25 to 34 amounted to about $900 (see table at right). A Towers Perrin study of company-paid medical claim costs for AARP in 2005 found that employees ages 50 to 64 cost, on average, 1.4 to 2.2 times as much in health care costs as workers in their 30s and 40s.

In contrast, some companies, such as Vanguard Group, report that older workers actually cost them less for health care. "Our largest health costs come from preemie babies; it's not from things like high blood pressure," says Kathy Gubanich, managing director of HR.

Same for the Bon Secours Richmond Health System. "There's a false assumption that older workers cost more on your health plan," says Bonnie Shelor, senior vice president of human resources. "We have not found that to be true. That generation is more dependable and well than the younger generations. The population we have is very healthy [and] has a great attitude and work ethic."

They're harder to train. Myth and reality. Older workers generally require more help and hands-on practice. In response to a questionnaire from the Center on Aging and Work at Boston College in Chestnut Hill, Mass., 44 percent of HR managers said older workers are reluctant to try new technology. At Bon Secours, Shelor says some workers have been slower in catching on, but they come around when given more time.

Annual Private Health Insurance Claims

Median Cost by Age

Age	Claim Amount
20–24	$220
25–34	$278
35–44	$396
45–54	$715
55–64	$1,177

Source: Urban Institute.

Borders' application process ensures that candidates are comfortable with technology. "Our application process is entirely online—if they can get through the process, they can handle the technology," Smith says.

In a 2006 survey of more than 460 organizations, only 15 percent saw the technology gap as a potential downside to employing older workers.

They're coasting, waiting for retirement. Myth. In a national study of 600 organizations, when HR managers were asked to measure productivity of older workers, they reported no significant drop-off at older ages. The study also found older workers to be more committed to their careers than younger workers. "The myth is that they're just hanging on when they get close to retirement," says Marcie Pitt-Catsouphes, director of the Center on Aging and Work at Boston College. Though the study showed similarities in engagement, it also showed that significant percentages of workers in all age categories were coasting.

They require special treatment, causing intergenerational clashes. Myth and reality. At an intergenerational roundtable discussion in Portsmouth, N.H., last year, participants spoke freely about the generational divide. Baby boomers criticized younger colleagues for inappropriate dress, for spending too much time on cell phones and for being ill-mannered.

Younger workers countered by criticizing older workers for unwillingness to see the value of the energy and fresh thinking young people bring to collaboration and for failure of many to learn to use technology.

Still, the fear of intergenerational dissonance may be hype. "I've coached and counseled Borders' employees for years and have gotten in the middle of conflicts in our stores," Smith says. "If you have all employees between 20 and 25, there will be a lot of conflict; if you have a good mix, they tend to respect each other more. Maybe it's because there's a calming influence with older workers; there seems to be more respect."

—Robert J. Grossman

But Davis remains an outlier. There's a time warp between our image of older workers and reality. Instead, picture men and women in those Viagra commercials or the L'Oreal ads featuring 50-year-old movie star Andie MacDowell. Or Harrison Ford, 65, still doing his own stunts.

"We've gained almost 30 years of life expectancy in about 100 years—an enormous increase," says Neil Charness, a psychology professor at the Pepper Institute on Aging and Public Policy at Florida State University in Tallahassee. "Yet HR departments, like so many of our institutions, suffer from the fact that they're fairly slow-moving; they tend to follow policies and hold to attitudes driven by the near-distant past. When I was growing up and someone died at 65, it was considered a ripe old age. Today, you'd almost be horrified that someone died so young."

For more misconceptions, see the "Mature Workers: Myths and Realities" box.

Muffled Minority

Numbers tell the story. In 2007, according to the U.S. Bureau of Labor Statistics, of 146 million people working full time and part time in the United States, only 13 percent, or 5.6 million, were age 65 and over (see charts). And within that 13 percent, only about 20 percent, or 1.1 million, were still working full time. Undoubtedly, this number will increase in coming years as people choose to delay retirement for personal reasons or as a result of changes in government policy such as reductions in Social Security benefits. In the absence of an economic meltdown, these older workers will still be a small percentage of the workforce.

More significant are the 36.4 million predominantly full-time workers between the ages of 50 and 64—one-quarter of the U.S. workforce and growing. They're part of a huge muffled minority. Marilyn B. is an example.

A world-famous editor, Marilyn combines impeccable taste with an uncanny sense of what sells. She has spent more than two decades with the same global company working her way up the ladder. A top revenue producer, her books grace *The New York Times'* best-seller list.

> **"If you're productive, creative and making money for your employer, why should age be an issue? It's none of their business."**
>
> —Marilyn B.

Yet, like an undocumented worker, Marilyn won't give her real name or age. On the plus side of 60, she's wary about attracting the attention of colleagues and superiors

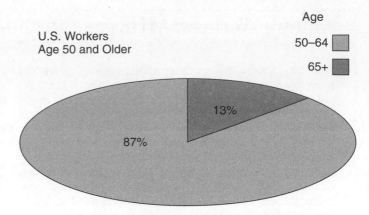

One in four U.S. workers has celebrated a 50th birthday. Of those, nearly 36.4 million range in age from 50 to 64 and 5.6 million are 65 or older, according to the U.S. Bureau of Labour Statistics in Washington, D.C. Of the former group, 50- to 54-year-olds number in the majority, as shown below.

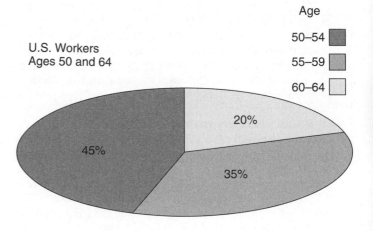

she fears may want to ease her off stage. "It makes me want to pop them in the nose," she says. "If you're productive, creative and making money for your employer, why should age be an issue? It's none of their business. I don't want to be judged by anything other than how competent I am."

Marilyn represents millions of workers critical to U.S. businesses whose fear of losing their jobs keeps them from telling employers the truth—that they're experiencing physical and mental changes that by their very nature influence how they do their work. As the Urban Institute research cited earlier proves, they're adapting, but at what cost? Could they do better? Employers, with some notable exceptions, seem content to let things slide.

"It's shortsighted," says Melissa Hardy, a professor and director of The Gerontology Center at Pennsylvania State University in University Park. Employers could do much to make work environments more hospitable to aging workers, but few organizations address these issues. "Workers won't raise them, and I suppose employers don't see how their failure to address them reflects on the bottom line," Hardy adds.

By understanding aging, employers can make mature workers even more productive.

By understanding aging, employers can make mature workers even more productive. Aging is a gradual process that sneaks up. "It's not like each day you notice a difference," Hardy says. "You think you're the same inside, but then something new comes up and it's a little harder to do." For more on how aging affects physical and mental processes, see the "Use It or Lose It" box.

Increasing the Odds

Yet people gain some, lose some. As physical and mental abilities decline, experience and determination help older workers compensate. For example, in workplaces where hearing or vision issues have not been addressed, older workers, often without realizing it, may concentrate more on compensating for their physical limitations. Workers with hearing problems may lip-read or rely on experience to discern spoken words they're really not hearing. This takes them away from focusing on higher-order decision-making and creativity.

The process "cascades," Charness says. "Hearing and seeing is no longer happening easily; you have to concentrate more at the expense of something else." It's a constant battle, and employers can help tip the scales the right way in several areas.

Adapting to change. If things aren't changing a lot, "crystallized" ability—the facility to access stored information such as verbal skill, vocabulary and knowledge of facts—carries you along. Where younger workers would have to problem-solve situations, mature workers already know what to do from experience.

But in some jobs—especially new ones or those that change—the balance shifts. Without experience to fall back on, older workers may have difficulty adapting.

This finding can present a dilemma for HR professionals because older workers frequently yearn for change and new opportunity. Unless the new job is tied to the worker's experience base, at the very least, more time to train and learn will probably be required. For example, adults in their 60s take roughly 50 percent to 100 percent longer than those in their 20s to learn and perform any new task, Charness says.

Targeting training. Experts say mature and younger workers do not respond the same way to training. They suggest that segmented approaches improve results. "Companies assume all people are the same; they choose to offer one-size-fits-all training, frequently online," says Alan Hedge, a biomedical and chemical engineering professor at Cornell University in Ithaca, N.Y., and Syracuse University in Syracuse, N.Y. "As a result, they see high drop-out rates. Even those who complete the training often don't retain well."

Training "300 workers with a PowerPoint presentation for three hours is not effective," Hardy says. "Hands-on training rather than lectures is better. When they age, people tend to learn visually and experientially at the same time. They also may feel pressure if the pace is too fast, a problem that can occur in mixed groups."

But older workers may not respond well to self-paced online learning because they may have trouble with the technology. While "Younger workers expect to interact through a computer screen, that's not how older workers interact, at least not as much," Hedge says. "The comfort level is not there. It's harder for older folks to read from the screen. That's why they print everything out; younger people don't do that."

Despite what experts say, most HR professionals show little inclination to single out mature workers for training. Borders offers the same training to all employees and reports no difficulties on the part of older workers. Vanguard also offers intergenerational training. Learning goes on between generations, says Kathy Gubanich, managing director of HR at Vanguard. "But our training is delivered in a variety of ways, geared to different learning styles," with e-learning and classroom components.

Older workers may not receive a proportionate allocation of training dollars. Some employers may suspect that it's more difficult to teach older people new skills or that their training funds can be spent more effectively on younger workers. In one survey, reported by AARP, only 51 percent of workers over 55 received formal training from employers during a 12-month period, compared with 79 percent of workers ages 25 to 34. Since studies show older workers' performance remains comparable to their younger counterparts', how, with less training, are they acquiring and maintaining their skills?

"In most organizations, training is informal—like sitting down and reading a manual on a procedure or on a software program," Johnson says. "Or people get together and learn one-on-one. Often, you figure it out yourself."

But research suggests that with appropriate formal training, workers across the board could be more productive. An "intensity index" designed by Hedge to measure how effectively a person performs certain tasks—some as basic as typing—suggests glaring gaps in performance that raise questions about training. "In many organizations, on a scale of one to 10, we're finding intensity scores in the four to five range," he says. "Loss of potential may in part

Use It or Lose It

What happens as we age? What do HR professionals need to know about the changes workers ages 50 to 64 go through? What can be done to help these workers be more productive?

Vision

People in their mid-40s—with women starting a year or two earlier—begin to suffer from presbyopia, a form of farsightedness. Their ability to see or read from a paper or computer screen becomes more difficult. When they perform close-up work, they may have headaches, eyestrain or fatigue. If they don't use glasses, they'll have to hold the newspaper farther and farther away or resort to surgery. An estimated 90 million people in the United States will have presbyopia by 2014.

Presbyopia is caused by loss of transparency in the lens of the eye, making it more difficult for light to come in. The contrast between what someone over 55 sees compared to younger workers is startling. To get the same visibility, you will need 10 times more light, says Alan Hedge, a biomedical and chemical engineering professor at Cornell and Syracuse universities.

Lighting can make a difference. Research by the Canadian Research Council in Ottawa shows that with properly adjusted light, people do 24 percent more work and are 42 percent more alert at the end of the day. Cornell University offers a "lighting visibility calculator" that measures the light a person needs in 10-year increments. (For a link to the calculator, see the online version of this article at www.shrm.org/hrmagazine)

How do you deal with workers requiring differing amounts of light? Companies such as Deutsche Bank install task lighting that enables each worker to self-select the amount of light he or she requires. In addition, illuminated keyboards make it easier for workers to transfer their gaze from monitor to keyboard.

Hearing

Age-related hearing loss, called presbycusis, usually begins in the 40s. Onset varies, depending on genetics, work setting, whether you've been exposed to a noisy environment at home and whether you use headphones to listen to music. Not everyone suffers from hearing loss, but many do. The number affected increases as people hit their 50s, 60s and beyond, with an estimated 50 percent of the population experiencing some hearing deficit.

As we age, the ability to hear higher pitches declines, affecting men earlier than women. The impact can be significant, cutting some people off—they miss what's going on, they're removed from the flow of conversation in the office—while others hear clearly.

Understanding the consonant sounds in speech depends on our ability to hear high pitches, says James K. Kane, Ph.D., an audiologist and scientific reviewer in the Federal Drug Administration's Office of Device Evaluation. "If one cannot hear the high-pitched sounds, speech becomes less intelligible."

Also, as we age, the decibel level required to fully comprehend speech tends to rise. And background noise that a younger person blocks out makes it harder to hear or concentrate. Noisy offices or factory floors can be tough. "You will disable a 55- or 60-year-old in a noisy environment," says Neil Charness, a professor of psychology at the Pepper Institute on Aging and Public Policy at Florida State University.

Employers can compensate for hearing loss by providing phones with higher volume controls. It's also advisable to remove unnecessary noise distractions from the work environment.

Dexterity and Flexibility

Thirty-one percent of jobs are primarily physical and require little cognitive ability. These are jobs that mature workers may have greater difficulty with. Workers lose speed, strength and dexterity as they age, beginning at age 40. They also tend to get heavier, gaining on average a pound a year, peaking in their 50s. It takes longer for them to do physical tasks—even tasks as basic as typing. "The older you get, the faster you lose it," Hedge says. "Muscles change; you can do strength training and it will help, but it doesn't create new muscle fibers; you're not creating new cells." Weight tends to level off in the 60s, then goes down as body cells are lost.

Still, you can slow the decline through exercise and practice. "Be a concert pianist well into your 70s and 80s and amaze people, but only if you practice every day. Play video games; you won't be good at it, but it helps train reaction time," Hedge says.

Overall, however, few people do much to maintain strength and dexterity, Hedge says. As a result, employers need to reorganize work so employees will have to remain active. Encourage people to stand and walk; support wellness activities. But inevitably, as strength and flexibility decline, employers need to look at job design, technology and ergonomics to help workers compensate.

Kathy Santini, vice president of surgical services at Bon Secours Richmond Health System, bears responsibility for more than 600 nurses in 57 operating rooms. With the average age of an OR nurse at 52, Santini has taken steps to reduce physical stress for the staff.

For lifting heavy equipment and patients, "We have lift teams on call. We've also [localized] supplies and meds so [the nurses] don't have to walk as far," she says.

Santini encourages ergonomic innovations that help curb carpal tunnel syndrome and reduce back problems, as discomfort may divert older workers' attention from their jobs.

Choosing the right chair, it seems, makes a difference. Snazzy mesh chairs may look good, but they don't offer enough padding for older workers, Hedge says. "Older people tend to need softer things to sit on."

Cognition

The number of jobs that require cognitive skills—reasoning, thinking, problem-solving and innovative solutions, for example—is increasing. Richard Johnson, principal research associate at the Urban Institute, estimates that 69 percent of jobs in the United States are in this category and that educated people ages 50 to 64 do them efficiently. "For most jobs that require cognitive skills, you won't see a cognitive decline through the worker's 60s," he says.

Such jobs require a combination of cognitive skills characterized either as "fluid abilities" or "crystallized abilities."

Fluid Abilities

Fluid abilities are "IQ items," such as abstract problem-solving and on-the-spot reasoning. They tend to decline with age. For example, numerical ability and capacity to master new material peaks at age 35. Then the skills begin to drop off and follow a line that slopes downward throughout life. The decline means it's ever harder for mature workers to learn new things. And when they learn, it takes longer, Johnson says. Still, he says practice can make a difference. Surgeons, dentists and musicians who maintain their skills at high levels do so through consistent, deliberate practice.

Short-term memory, another fluid ability, fades over time. People lose the ability to remember things that happened recently, or to repeat back a list of newly seen or heard items like an unfamiliar phone number. "Short-term memory loss is the tip-of-the tongue phenomenon; it happens to everyone," Hedge says. "You can't do much about it. People stress out about it, and that only makes it worse."

Long-term memory, in contrast, refers to knowledge acquired and stored throughout life. Your name, phone number and the alphabet are examples. Long-term memory stays with age.

Hedge says memory lapses occur when information you want to retain is not encoded into your long-term memory. You can train your brain to do this by engaging in cerebral pursuits outside of work. "The brain can shift neurons that run programs needed for doing activities like crossword puzzles, Sudoku, chess or bridge, and apply them to memory tasks," he says. Some companies encourage these activities during off-hours as part of wellness programs.

Self-organization can also help with short-term memory. "People attempt to remember too many things, and that's a prescription for failure," Hedge says. "Don't try to remember 10 things that you have to do. The magic number is seven, plus or minus two. You have a better chance of remembering five."

Crystallized Abilities

Crystallized abilities constitute the facility to access stored information—verbal skill, mastery of knowledge and facts. These skills, and the information acquired, accrete; they get better over time.

"Acquired knowledge, enhanced communication skills and sharper decision-making can offset age-related declines in mental efficiency," Charness says.

For example, older airline pilots taking flight simulation tests scored lower than younger counterparts on aspects of the test that required fluid ability. But their crystallized skills enabled them to earn overall higher safety scores.

Similarly, older lab workers studying specimens under microscopes were more efficient than younger workers because they knew what to look for. Mature hotel reservation clerks were more productive than younger associates, though they handled fewer calls, because their communication skills generated more bookings.

—Robert J. Grossman

---

be because companies are not focusing on training older workers." To learn more about the intensity index, visit www.prodyx.com.

Providing feedback. Most mature workers, contrary to common belief, are still interested in self-improvement and advancing their careers. They face disappointment in evaluations that give them short shrift. When appraised, especially by younger managers, feedback tends to be fleeting and flimsy, less geared to advice on how they could do their jobs better or extend their careers. "The signals that are subtly communicated are not encouraging," Hardy concludes, and his observations have been documented by AARP research.

Working at the Puzzle

In a 2006 survey of HR executives from more than 460 organizations, conducted by Buck Consultants of Houston, 88 percent identified integrating multiple generations of workers as the most significant business risk of employing older workers. One reason: They fear equity issues will arise among younger workers should they give older employees privileges such as flextime. Yet, a minority of companies that actively court older workers offers all employees special treatment—flextime, telecommuting, compressed and reduced schedules, and more. Further, companies that successfully integrate older workers into their workforces discover that other generations may have different priorities, but that the changes they put in place for their 55-to-64 cohort resonate with everyone.

One example: Gubanich estimates that almost 30 percent of Vanguard's full-time employees are over 50. Only 2 percent to 3 percent of Vanguard's 12,000 workers are part time. Because of U.S. Securities and Exchange Commission rules, the company doesn't offer telecommuting, but it does offer compressed schedules and other accommodations for all employees who require it.

True, flexibility makes HR's job tougher. For instance, in the Buck survey, 40 percent of the HR respondents identified "accommodating part-time and flexible schedules" as a significant business risk of employing mature workers.

But Bon Secour's Senior Vice President for Human Resources Bonnie Shelor says to attract and retain older workers in their prime, the risk is worth taking. When people have varying needs, "It's not as simple as setting one set of rules for everyone. It's like solving a complicated puzzle. We've proved that taking the time and energy to do it pays huge dividends in terms of morale, engagement and culture. Thirty percent of our 6,600 employees are over 50; they give us great critical thinking and wisdom. We couldn't exist without them."

ROBERT J. GROSSMAN, a contributing editor of *HR Magazine,* is a lawyer and a professor of management studies at Marist College in Poughkeepsie, N.Y.

From *HR Magazine,* May, 2008, pp. 39–46. Copyright © 2008 by Society for Human Resource Management. Reprinted by permission via the Copyright Clearance Center.

Color Me Confident

Why many Americans may be working when they retire.

PAUL MAGNUSSON

Despite everything, Susan Buer, a 46-year-old South Dakota homemaker, is confident that she'll have enough money to retire on. She's in the process of getting divorced, a situation that affects nearly half of all married couples, and one that usually leaves both partners worse off financially. She has less than $10,000 in savings. Credit card debt and a car loan cloud her future. She hasn't yet calculated how much she'll need to retire, although she's "very confident" she can do the math. "Eventually, I'll talk to a financial planner about all this, but I just haven't had the time yet," Buer says.

In her approach to retirement, Buer reflects the best and worst of many Americans—a can-do spirit and procrastination. According to a recent *AARP Bulletin* poll, many people are confident that they can meet their basic retirement expenses, yet have not done basic planning or calculated what funds they'll need. Many fear their employers will cut back on their health and pension benefits but have not begun to save adequately for the costs they'll face.

The poll, which surveyed 1,096 workers and 686 retirees age 40 and older, indicates that many Americans may not have adjusted to the new economic reality: that the responsibility for funding retirement is shifting from business and the federal government onto the shoulders of workers themselves.

This is happening gradually, as traditional "defined benefit" pensions, which are based on salary, are being replaced by more chancy "defined contribution" plans, such as a 401(k), that require employees to contribute a percentage of pay and bear much of the risk of investing the principal. In 1980, 83 percent of workers with pension plans were enrolled in a defined benefit plan. Today, that figure has shrunk to 21 percent, according to the U.S. Department of Labor.

A recent *Bulletin* poll indicates that many American workers may not have adjusted to the new economic reality: that responsibility for funding retirement is shifting from business and government onto workers themselves—and many have not begun to save for the costs they'll face.

Workers may not yet fully grasp their own increasing role in retirement planning or the implications of what Yale professor Jacob Hacker calls "the great risk shift." (see "Retirement Insecurity," *AARP Bulletin,* March). Although 68 percent of workers (or their spouses) said they've saved some money for retirement, 31 percent have not saved a dime. The most common reasons were "not enough income" and "high everyday expenses." Thirty percent also said that a lack of financial discipline was a contributing factor.

Just last month, the Center for Retirement Research at Boston College released a study that painted an equally gloomy picture of retirement, saying that 45 percent of working-age households are "at risk" of being unable to maintain their preretirement standard of living.

"Unless Americans change their ways, many will struggle in retirement," said CRR Director Alicia H. Munnell. "There is no silver bullet; the answer is saving more and working longer. Even relatively modest adjustments—working two extra years or saving 3 percent more—can substantially improve retirement security."

Rose-colored glasses seem to be particularly characteristic of the 75 percent of all workers who define themselves as "very confident" or "somewhat confident" about having enough money to live comfortably in their retirement years. Of that group, 48 percent haven't tried to calculate their retirement savings needs; 22 percent have saved no money so far for retirement; and 43 percent have less than $25,000 in savings and investments, excluding the value of their homes and defined benefit plans. Most worrisome, a third of them have no money in a 401(k), and 45 percent have no IRA savings.

However, when it comes to specifics like pensions, health care and debt, respondents express serious concerns. Among the findings:

Pensions. Forty percent of those who are employed—or whose spouses are employed—worry that their employers will reduce or eliminate pension or health care benefits before or during their retirement. In fact, some reported that such changes had already occurred in the last five years: elimination of a traditional defined benefit pension plan (10 percent) or the plan's benefits frozen or reduced (9 percent); traditional pension plan converted into a 401(k)-type defined contribution plan (15 percent); and health care benefits reduced (44 percent).

Social Security may help fill in the gaps. Thirty-nine percent of workers say they expect Social Security to be a major source of their retirement income—this compares with 58 percent of current retirees who report that Social Security is a major source of their income.

Health care. Twenty-eight percent of workers and 13 percent of retirees said they were concerned about not having enough money in retirement to pay for their medical expenses. And 40 percent of workers and 33 percent of retirees are worried about their ability to meet long-term care expenses.

Debt. Debt is a serious issue for both workers and retirees. More than half of workers see their (or their spouse's) current level of debt as a problem, compared with 30 percent of retirees. Workers are also more likely than retirees to carry a mortgage, credit card debt or a car loan, or even medical or dental debt.

So how much does it take to retire? There is no single answer. One rule of thumb is that workers should plan on replacing 60 to 70 percent of pretax employment income with savings and investments. Some may need less if all debts, mortgages and other loans are paid off and health care is covered.

And if there's a financial shortfall, continued employment may be a last resort. Two in 10 workers in the *Bulletin* poll say

---

86% of retirees and 75% of workers age 40-plus are at least somewhat confident they have or will have enough money for retirement.

31% of workers age 40 or older have not yet saved any money for their retirement.

28% of current retirees also acknowledge not saving any money for their retirement years before they retired.

58% of retirees report that Social Security is a major source of their income.

28% of workers and 13% of retirees are not confident they'll have enough money for retirement medical expenses.

40% of workers and 33% of retirees are not confident they can pay for long-term care.

53% of workers see their current level of debt as a problem, compared with 30% of retirees.

---

they plan to draw a major portion of their retirement income from a job. The back-to-work crew may just be the most realistic of all.

PAUL MAGNUSSON is a freelance writer in Washington.

Work/Retirement Choices and Lifestyle Patterns of Older Americans

HAROLD COX ET AL.

T his study examined the work, retirement, and lifestyle choices of a sample of older Indiana residents. The six lifestyles examined in this study were:

1. *to continue to work full-time;*
2. *to continue to work part-time;*
3. *retire from work and become engaged in a variety of volunteer activities;*
4. *to retire from work and become involved in a variety of recreational and leisure activities;*
5. *to retire from work and later return to work part-time; and*
6. *to retire from work and later return to work full-time*

These findings indicate that health was not a critical factor in the older person's retirement decision, and that those who retired and engaged in volunteer or recreational activities were significantly more satisfied with their lives than those who continue to work. Those who retired and engaged in volunteer or recreational activities scored significantly higher on life satisfaction than those who had returned to work full or part-time. There was no significant difference between those who had retired and those who had continued working in terms of how they were viewed by their peers. Of those who retired and then returned to work, the most satisfied with their lives were the ones who returned to work in order to feel productive. Those least satisfied with their lives were the ones that returned to work because they needed money.

Introduction

There are basically six different choices of lifestyles from which older Americans choose when they reach retirement age. They can (1) continue to work full-time, (2) reduce work commitments but continue to work part-time, (3) retire from work and become engaged in a variety of volunteer activities that provide needed services but for which they will receive no economic compensation or (4) retire from work and become involved in a variety of recreational and leisure activities, (5) retire from work and later return to work part-time, (6) retire from work and return to work full-time.

There are a multitude of life experiences and retirement patterns that may ultimately lead older persons to choose among the diverse ways of occupying themselves during their later years. Some enjoy their work as well as the income, status, privilege, and power that go with full-time employment and never intend to retire. Some retire intending to engage in recreational and leisure activities on a full-time basis only to find this lifestyle less satisfying than they imagined and ultimately return to work. The need to feel productive and actively involved in life is often a critical factor inducing some retirees to return to work. Some retirees who have become widowed, divorced, or never married find themselves too socially isolated in retirement. They return to work either full-time or part-time because their job brings them into contact with a variety of people, and therefore they are less isolated. Thus, there are a variety of reasons why older persons may continue to work or to become active volunteers during their later years. On the other hand, many persons retire, dedicate themselves to recreation and leisure activities, and are most satisfied doing so.

The purpose of this study was to determine which of these six groups were better off in terms of their health, life satisfaction, retirement adjustment and the respect they received from their peers.

A second factor, which will be examined in this study, is the advisability for both government and industry of encouraging older workers to remain in the labor force longer. Changes in Social Security regulations after the year 2000 are going to gradually increase the age of eligibility for Social Security payment from 62 to 64 for early retirement and from 65 to 67 for full retirement benefits. Will changes in the age of eligibility for retirement income derived from Social Security regulations be good or bad for older Americans?

Review of Literature
Work

The meanings of such diverse activities as work, leisure, and retirement to a member of a social system are often quite complex. Paradoxically, the relevance of work and leisure activities for an individual is often intertwined in his or her thinking.

Consequently, the concept of work or occupation has been difficult for sociologists to precisely define.

For some time sociologists have struggled to come up with an adequate definition of work. Dubin (1956), for example, defined work as continuous employment in the production of goods and services for remuneration. This definition ignores the fact that there are necessary tasks in society carried out by persons who receive no immediate pay. Mothers, fathers, housewives, and students do not receive pay for their valued activities.

Hall (1975) attempts to incorporate both the economic and social aspects of work in his definition: "An occupation is the social role performed by adult members of society that directly and/or indirectly yields social and financial consequences and that constitutes a major focus in the life of an adult." Similarly Bryant (1972) tries to include both the economic and social aspects of work life in his definition of labor: "Labor is any socially integrating activity which is connected with human subsistence." By *integrating activity* Bryant means sanctioned activity that presupposes, creates, and recreates social relationships. The last two definitions seem to take a broader view of work in the individual's total life. Moreover, they could include the work done by mothers, fathers, housewives, and students. The advantage of definitions that attach strong importance to the meaning and social aspects of a work role is that they recognize the importance of roles for which there is no, or very little, economic reward. The homemaker, while not receiving pay, may contribute considerably to a spouse's career and success. College students in the period of anticipatory socialization and preparation for an occupational role may not be receiving any economic benefits, but their efforts are crucial to their future career.

The most appropriate definitions of work, therefore, seem to be those that emphasize the social and role aspects of an occupation, which an individual reacts to and is shaped by, whether or not he or she is financially rewarded for assuming these roles. From the perspective of sociology, one's work life and the roles one assumes during the workday will, in time, shape one's self-concept, identity, and feelings about oneself, and therefore strongly affect one's personality and behavior. Moreover, from this perspective, the individual's choice of occupations is probably strongly affected by the desire to establish, maintain, and display a desired identity.

Individual Motivation to Work

Vroom (1964) has attempted to delineate the components of work motivation. The first component is wages and all the economic rewards associated with the fringe benefits of the job. People desire these rewards, which therefore serve as a strong incentive to work. Iams (1985), in a study of the post-retirement work patterns of women, found that unmarried women were very likely to work at least part-time after retirement if their monthly income was below $500. Hardy (1991) found that 80 percent of the retirees who later re-entered the labor force stated that money was the main reason they returned to work. The economic inducement to work is apparently a strong one.

A second inducement to work is the expenditure of physical and mental energy. People seem to need to expend energy

in some meaningful way, and work provides this opportunity. Vroom (1964) notes that animals will often engage in spontaneous activity as a consequence of activity deprivation.

A third motivation, according to Vroom, is the production of goods and services. This inducement is directly related to the intrinsic satisfaction the individual derives from successful manipulation of the environment.

A fourth motivation is social interaction. Most work roles involve interaction with customers, clients, or members of identifiable work groups as part of the expected behavior of their occupants.

The final motivation Vroom mentions is social status. An individual's occupation is perhaps the best single determinant of his or her status in the community.

These various motivations for work undoubtedly assume different configurations for different people and occupational groups. Social interaction may be the most important for some, while economic considerations may be most important for others. For still others the intrinsic satisfaction derived from the production of goods and services may be all-important. Thus, the research by industrial sociologists has indicated that there are diverse reasons why individuals are motivated to work.

The critical questions for gerontologists is whether the same psychological and social factors that thrust people into work patterns for the major part of their adult life can channel them into leisure activities during their retirement years. Can people find the same satisfaction, feeling of worth, and identity in leisure activities that they did in work-related activities? Streib and Schneider (1971) think they can. They argue that the husband, wife, grandmother, and grandfather's roles may expand and become more salient in the retirement years. Simultaneously, public service and community roles become possible because of the flexibility of the retiree's time. They believe that the changing activities and roles, which accompany retirement, need not lead to a loss of self-respect or active involvement in the mainstream of life.

Retirement Trends

Demographic and economic trends in American society have resulted in an ever-increasing number of retired Americans. Streib and Schneider (1971) observed that for retirement to become an institutionalized social pattern in any society, certain conditions must be met. There must be a large group of people who live long enough to retire, the economy must be sufficiently productive to support segments of the population that are not included in the work force, and there must be some well-established forms of pension or insurance programs to support people during their retirement years.

There has been a rapid growth in both the number and percentage of the American population 65 and above since 1900.

In 1900, there were 3.1 million Americans 65 and over, which constituted four percent of the population. Currently, approximately 31 million Americans are in this age category, which makes up 12.5 percent of the population. While the number and proportion of the population over 65 have been increasing steadily, the proportion of those who remain in the work force has decreased steadily. In 1900, nearly two thirds of those

Table 1 Civilian Labor Force Participation Rates: Actual and Projected*

	Men			Women		
Year	45–54	55–64	65 and Over	45–54	55–64	65 and Over
1950	95.8	86.9	45.8	37.9	27.0	9.7
1960	95.7	86.8	33.1	49.8	32.2	10.8
1970	94.2	83.0	26.8	54.4	43.0	9.7
1980	91.2	72.3	19.1	59.9	41.5	8.1
1986	91.0	67.3	16.0	65.9	42.3	7.4
1990*	90.7	65.1	14.1	69.0	42.8	7.0
2000*	90.1	63.2	9.9	75.4	45.8	5.4

Source: For the rates from 1950–1970: U.S. Department of Labor (1980:224). For the rates from 1980–2000: Bureau of Labor Statistics (unpublished data).
*Values are projections from the Bureau of Labor Statistics middle growth path.

65 worked. Sammartino (1979) reports that by 1947 this figure had declined to 47.8 percent. By 1987 only 16.5 percent of those 65 and older were still in the work force. In the past 20 years the decline in labor force participation in later years has extended into the 55–64 year old age group. Clark (1988) observed that between 1960 and 1970 the labor force participation of men (55–64) dropped from 86.8% to 83%. By 1990 the labor force participation rate of men in this age group (55–64) had dropped to 65.1% (see Table 1). Table 1 indicates that the labor force participation rates of women 55–64 rose from 27% to 43% from 1950 to 1970 but has remained relatively stable since 1970. Thus, while the labor force participation rate of 55-years and -older women has remained relatively stable since 1970, the labor force participation rate of women 45–54 has grown from 54.4% in 1970 to 69% in 1990. It would appear from these figures that, while younger women are in increasing numbers entering the labor force, women 55 and above are following the same path as their male counterparts and choosing to retire early.

Similarly, there appears to be a somewhat greater convergence in the work and retirement patterns of men and women when comparing 1900 with 1970. The earlier pattern of work histories seemed to be for men to enter the work force earlier and retire later; women tended to enter later and retire earlier. Current trends indicate that women are entering the work force earlier and working longer.

Men, on the other hand, enter the work force later and retire earlier. Thus, the work histories of men and women are becoming very similar, although men as a group still have longer work histories than women. Today, more women are both entering the labor force and also remaining in the labor force throughout their adult lives.

The trend for both men and women for the past 30 years has been for larger numbers to choose to claim Social Security benefits prior to age 65. Allen and Brotman (1981) point out that

in 1968, 48 percent of all new Social Security payment awards to men were to claimants under 65; by 1978 this figure had increased to 61 percent. In 1968, 65 percent of all new Social Security awards to women were to claimants under 65; in 1978, the figure was 72 percent.

Simultaneously, fewer persons are choosing to remain in the labor force beyond the age of 65. Soldo and Agree (1988) report that 62 percent of the men and 72 percent of the women who received Social Security benefits in 1986 had retired prior to age 65 and therefore were receiving reduced benefits. The General Accounting Office reports that almost two-thirds of those receiving private retirement benefits in 1985 stopped working prior to age 65. Of those who do remain in the labor force after age 65, Soldo and Agree (1988) report that 47 percent of the men and 59 percent of the women held part-time positions.

Quinn and Burkhauser (1990) report that probably the most critical factor in the decision to retire early is adequate retirement income. They found that between 1975 and 1990 the proportion of workers covered by two pension plans had risen from 21 percent to 40 percent. Moreover, Gall, Evans, and Howard (1997) report a number of studies that found that those with higher incomes, or at least adequate finances, were more satisfied with their life in retirement (Fillenbau, George, and Palmore 1985; Seccombe and Lee 1986; Crowley 1990; Dorfman 1992).

There is a multiplicity of problems confronting the individual at retirement: the lowering of income; the loss of status, privilege, and power associated with one's position in the occupational hierarchy; a major reorganization of life activities, since the nine-to-five workday becomes meaningless; a changing definition of self, since most individuals over time shape their identity and personality in line with the demands of their major occupational roles; considerable social isolation if new activities are not found to replace work-related activities; and a search for a new identity, new meaning, and new values in one's life. Obviously, the major reorganization of one's life that must take place at retirement is a potential source of adjustment problems. Critical to the adjustment is the degree to which one's identity and personality structure was attached to the work role. For those individuals whose work identity is central to their self-concept and gives them the greatest satisfaction, retirement will represent somewhat of a crisis. For others, retirement should not represent a serious problem.

Work and Retirement Patterns in Later Life

Beck (1983) identified three different work and retirement patterns of older persons which include:

1. the fully retired
2. the partially retired
3. the formerly retired

What could be added to Beck's pattern are "the never retired."

There are a number of different studies and authors who have attempted to identify the critical factor determining who will or will not work during their later years. Beck (1983) found that individuals with high job autonomy and high demand jobs were most likely to return to work after formal retirement. Those with the greatest financial need—service workers and laborers—were less likely to return to work despite financial limitations. Beck concludes that income was the critical factor in the motivation of workers who were very poor to return to work. Those in other income categories were less likely to return to work because of actual financial benefits as much as for other factors.

A number of other studies tended to support Beck's analysis of work and retirement patterns. Tillenbaum (1971) found that those with higher levels of education were more likely to continue working beyond age 65 or to return to work after retiring if they chose to do so. Quinn (1980) found the self-employed were much more likely to work beyond retirement age. Streib and Schneider (1971) found that white collar workers were significantly more likely than blue collar workers to return to work. They found no relationship between income and post-retirement work. Howell (1988) reports that those who formally retire and engage in no substantial work during the next three years are more likely to have been unemployed before retirement and to have lower incomes after retirement. They are also more likely to be nonwhite urban dwellers in poor health.

The past research has indicated then that those who either continue to work after retirement age or return to work after retiring are most likely to:

1. have stable employment patterns throughout their adult life;
2. be in white collar occupations;
3. have higher incomes;
4. have a higher number of years of education;
5. be self-employed.

Those least likely to either work after retirement age or return to work after retirement age:

1. those who experienced periods of unemployment throughout their adult life;
2. those in blue collar occupations;
3. those with low incomes;
4. those who have a lower number of years of education;
5. those who are of minority status (Tillenbaum 1971; Quinn 1980; Howell 1988).

These findings support the idea that many people who continue to work after retirement do so for other than financial reasons. If work was stable and both social and psychologically meaningful to the individual, he/she is much more likely to be found working during the retirement years.

As a rule, retirees do not return to jobs with low autonomy, poor working conditions, and difficult physical labor. Those who most need to continue working during the retirement years for financial reasons are least likely to be able to do so. This is most probably related to their inability to find gainful employment.

Volunteer Work in Retirement

Social integration refers to the individual being actively involved in a variety of groups and organization and thus integrated into the web of community activity. The active older person is likely to be involved in a variety of groups ranging from family to social clubs to church and community organizations. While work and career often place the individual in disparate groups and organizations throughout much of his/her adult life, active engagement in voluntary organizations is likely to keep the individual socially involved during their retirement years.

Moen, Dempster-McClain, and Williams (1992) report that studies as early as 1956 reporting that older persons participating in volunteer work on an intermittent basis and belonging to clubs and organizations were positively related to various measures of health. They concluded that occupying multiple roles in the community was positively related to good health.

A number of studies have found a positive relationship between social integration (in the form of multiple roles) and health in later life (Berkman and Breslow 1983; House, Landes, and Umberson 1988; Moen et al.; Williams 1992).

The researchers were unable to determine if multiple roles lead to improved health or if healthy people were more likely to engage in multiple roles. Moen et al. (1992), however, once again found that being a member of a club or organization appeared to be a critical factor in the current health of the individual, after previous health had been controlled. Paid work over the life course, while positively related to multiple roles in later life, was negatively related to measures of health. However, any volunteer activity at any time during adult life appears to promote multiple role occupancy, social integration, and health in later life.

Mobert (1983) observes that church affiliation itself was not considered a volunteer group or activity; however, membership in groups sponsored by the church such as choir, Old Timers, etc. was considered a volunteer activity. Moreover, church members generally remain active participants in church-related activities long after dropping participation from other voluntary associations (Gray and Moberg 1977). Markides (1983) and Ortega, Crutchfield, and Rusling (1983) argue that the church serves as a focal point for individual and community integration of the elderly and that this is crucial to their sense of well-being. Both of these studies found that church attendance was significantly correlated with life satisfaction.

Productivity in Later Life

Older workers who remain in the work force have been found to be just as productive as younger workers. An industrial survey conducted by Parker (1982) found that older workers were most often regarded as superior to younger workers. Adjectives used by employers to describe older workers were responsible, reliable, conscientious, tolerant, reasonable, and loyal. Older workers have greater stability, they miss work less frequently, change jobs less frequently, and are more dedicated and loyal to the employing organization. Welford (1988) found that performance on production jobs tends to increase with age. While this is true, employers generally offer incentive plans to encourage older workers to retire early. Older workers are generally higher on salary schedules, have accumulated more vacation time and fringe benefits. Thus, many employers see younger workers as cheaper. The fact that they are untested does not seem critical to the employer.

Fyock in discussing the early retirement policies of the 1970's states that:

Employers liked it because it enabled them to hire and promote younger, more recently trained and lower paid workers. The public liked it because it didn't appear to cost anything and because at age 62 or earlier they could expect to retire; older workers for obvious reasons loved it. (Fyock 1991:422)

Fyock (1991) warns however that we currently have an aging work force and that in the near future employers may find it to their advantage to encourage older workers to remain in the work force longer. She believes that employers often find that retirement appeals to their best, instead of the most expendable, employee.

Projected job growth coupled with a declining number of younger workers has raised concern about possible labor shortages. If these projections prove accurate and labor shortages do develop, the answer to the problem would seem to be the retention of older workers—the very workers employers are currently encouraging to retire. Dennis (1986), Sheppard (1990), and Fyock (1991) all argue that an aging labor force can be a source of opportunity for employers. The smart employers, they believe, will be the ones who know how to take advantage of the opportunity.

McShulski (1997) reports the need for a "soft landing" program which eases older workers out of the labor force on a very gradual basis. Encouraging retiring employees to work a reduced number of hours and handle more limited duties for less pay, helps both the company and the employee. Future retirees can impart relevant job information to their coworkers and teach less experienced employees about specific tasks and customer needs. Thus, working for reduced hours and more limited responsibilities results in a gradual transition to retirement, which is good for the company and the employee according to McShulski.

Retirement Policies and Older Workers

Industrialized societies traditionally have low fertility rates and long life expectancy, resulting in an ever-growing number and percentage of our population that is over 65. Thus, industrialized nations very early began to shift social welfare programs from younger persons to older persons. Many economists are questioning the willingness of society to continue to support an ever-growing number of older persons through public-funded retirement incomes.

Initially, in 1935 when Social Security was passed, both management and labor were anxious to get older persons out of the labor force. Management believed that older workers were

too expensive since they were high on salary schedules and had accumulated considerable fringe benefits. Labor unions believed that removing older workers would create jobs for younger workers. The public was happy since they were given economic help in support of their older family members and ultimately they looked forward to being able to retire themselves.

The post-WWII era saw major expansions in Social Security programs. Social Security was extended to cover nearly all wage earners and self-employed persons. The permissible retirement age was lowered to 62, and a national disability income program was added to Social Security. A legal interpretation of the Taft-Hartley Act resulted in private pension plans becoming legitimate items of collective bargaining. The result was that private pension plans have grown substantially from 1950 to present. As a result of these and related activities, a retirement norm has emerged in America. Most people now plan to retire and to live some part of their life out of the labor force.

Congress, with the passage of new Social Security legislation in 1983, began, for the first time, to question the desirability of removing seniors from the labor force. Concern about the financial solvency of the Social Security program led Congress and the President to increase Social Security taxes, to increase taxes on earned income of older persons, to tax Social Security benefits, and to raise the eligible age of Social Security benefits after the year 2000.

Retirement age will go up very gradually during the first quarter of the next century. Early retirement will be increased from 62 to 64 years of age. Full retirement will be increased from 65 to 67. Reduction in pension benefits for those who retire early will go up from 20% to 30% of their full retirement income. Those who stay at work after 65 will get a pension boost of 8% for each extra year of work instead of today's 3%.

The changes in Social Security benefits are clearly designed to encourage people to work longer and retire later. The question that remains, given the trend toward younger retirements, is will these changes really keep older workers in the work force longer or merely mean that more retirees will earn less and therefore more will fall below the poverty line.

Economists and labor planners have never been able to establish the fact that for every older worker who retires, a job is created for a younger worker. Changing technologies and the creation of new jobs have at different times created a greater or lesser demand for more workers. Morris (1986) states that:

If financial and social policy disincentives to employment could be reduced there is no prior reason to believe that the economy would be unable to expand gradually to accommodate more retired persons especially in part-time, self-employed, and service capacities (Morris 1986:291).

Morris (1986) argues that half of the Social Security recipients abruptly leave the labor force and the other half engage in some short-term labor force participation after they retire.

The critical question raised by Congress in changing Social Security benefits in 1983 is can government policies change the age at which people choose to retire. If the older person is to be encouraged to remain in the labor force longer, both the individual worker and the business/industrial community must be convinced of the advantages of keeping older persons in the labor force longer. There seems to be no question that older persons can be productive members of the labor force beyond the retirement age if they have the opportunity and choose to do so.

Hypothesis

1. Those working full-time or part-time will be in better health than those who have retired.
2. Those people who have retired will score higher on measures of life satisfaction than those working full or part-time.
3. Those retirees engaged in volunteer or leisure activities will score higher on measures of life satisfaction than those returning to work.
4. Those people working full-time or part-time during their later years will be more highly regarded by their peers.

Methodology

The questionnaire utilized in this study included the standard demographic variables, as well as measures of attitude toward retirement, the respondent's perceived state of health, life satisfaction, retirement adjustment, and his/her perceived status among friends.

The questionnaire was mailed to 597 members of the Older Hoosiers Federation and 200 Green Thumb workers in Indiana. The Older Hoosiers Federation is a volunteer groups of senior citizens who lobby for or against various state and federal legislation which they perceive would affect older Americans. They are primarily retired Americans over the age of 55. The Green Thumb workers are persons 55 and older who work on various parks, roads, and community projects. They are employed by the federal government in community service projects in order

to raise their income above the poverty level. A limitation of this study is that the sample was an available sample and not a random sample. It was the best available sample that the researchers could find at this time. There were 342 valid returns, which represented 42.91% of those surveyed.

Findings

The first hypothesis stated that those persons working full or part-time will be in better health than those who are retired. This hypothesis was not supported by the data. As Table 2 indicates, calculating the mean score on the subjects' perceived state of health for those working full-time, those working part-time, those retired and engaged in volunteer activities, and those retired and engaged in leisure activities and then performing a one-way analysis of variance resulted in a finding of no significant difference in the means of the four groups. While past studies of when people retire have indicated that perceived health and subjects' belief that they have adequate income to retire are often identified as the critical variables in the decision of when to retire, that would not appear to be the case with this sample. There were no significant differences in the perceived state of health for those subjects who were working in comparison to those subjects who were retired (Table 2).

Hypothesis Two stated that those persons who have retired will score higher on measures of life satisfaction than those who are working full or part-time. The mean scores on life satisfaction were calculated for those working full-time, those working part-time, those retired and engaged in volunteer activity, and those retired and engaged in leisure activity. The data indicated that those retired and engaged in volunteer activities and those retired and engaged in leisure activity scored significantly higher on measures of life satisfaction than those working either full or part-time (Table 3). The hypothesis was supported by the data (Table 3).

Hypothesis Three stated that those retirees engaged in volunteer or leisure activities will score higher on measures of life satisfaction than those who retired and then returned to work on a full-time or part-time basis. Mean life satisfaction scores

Table 2 One-Way Analysis of Variance: Mean Perceived Health Scores for Older Workers and Retirees

	Mean	N = 329
Work Full-Time	3.4706	51
Work Part-Time	3.2970	101
Retired/Engaged in Volunteer Activities	3.2867	143
Retired/Engaged Leisure Act.	3.2647	34

Source	D.F.	Sum of Squares	Mean Squares	F-Ratio	F-Probability
Between Groups	3	1.4682	.4891	.9956	.3951
Within Groups	325	159.6574	.4913		
Total	328	161.1246			

Table 3 One-Way Analysis of Variance: Mean Life Satisfaction Scores for Older Workers and Retirees

	Mean	N = 318
Work Full-Time	7.6372	49
Work Part-Time	7.1875	96
Retired/Engaged in Volunteer Activities	7.9928	139
Retired/Engaged in Leisure Activities	8.0000	34

Source	D.F.	Sum of Squares	Mean Squares	F-Ratio	F-Probability
Between Groups	3	40.4064	13.4688	8.2667	.0015
Within Groups	314	803.0056	2.5573		
Total	317	843.4119			

Table 4 One-Way Analysis of Variance: Mean Life Satisfaction Scores for Older Workers and Retirees

	Mean	N = 268
Returned to Work Full-Time	2.2000	5
Returned to Work Part-Time	2.0333	90
Retired/Engaged in Volunteer Activities	2.3885	139
Retired/Engaged in Leisure Activities	2.2941	34

Source	D.F.	Sum of Squares	Mean Squares	F-Ratio	F-Probability
Between Groups	3	6.9659	2.3220	5.9067	.0006
Within Groups	264	103.7804	.3931		
Total	267	110.7463			

were calculated for those who had retired and then returned to work full-time, those who had retired and then returned to work part-time, those who had retired and were engaged in volunteer activities, and those who had retired and were engaged in leisure activities. Those retired and engaged in volunteer or leisure activity scored significantly higher on life satisfaction than those who had retired and returned to work full or part-time. As Table 4 indicates there were only five people in this sample who had retired and returned to work full-time. Returning to work full-time was rare in this sample of people.

Hypothesis Four stated that those retirees who returned to work full or part-time will be more respected by their peers than those who have retired and engaged in volunteer or leisure activities.

In terms of their perceived respect by friends, those retired and returning to work full-time scored highest with a mean of 3.0. Those who retired and were engaged in volunteer activities scored second with a mean of 2.86. Those who retired and were engaged in leisure activities scored third with a mean of

2.76. Those who had retired and returned to work part-time perceived they were least respected by their friends with a score of 2.68. While the analysis of variance did not find significant differences in these means at the .05 level of significance, they were significant at the .07 level of significance. Since the .05 level of significance is the normal level of acceptance of the significance of difference between groups, this hypothesis was not supported by the data (Table 5).

In order to clarify how the retirees' decision to return to work would affect their life satisfaction, an additional calculation was done. One question asked those who had returned to work was why they had done so. The choices to this question were: I needed the money, I needed to do something that makes me feel productive, and I was lonely and bored and work gave me something interesting to do. Mean scores and measures of life satisfaction were calculated for each of these three groups (Table 6). The highest mean score was for the group who returned to work in order to feel productive, and their score was 8.27. The second highest mean score was for those who had returned to work because they were lonely and bored, and their score was 7.26.

Table 5 One Way Analysis of Variance: Mean Scores for Perceived Respect of Older Workers and Retirees by Their Peers

	Mean	N = 277
Returned to Work Full-Time	3.00006	4
Returned to Work Part-Time	2.6869	99
Retired/Engaged in Volunteer Activities	2.8643	140
Retired/Engaged in Leisure Activities	2.7647	34

Source	D.F.	Sum of Squares	Mean Squares	F-Ratio	F-Probability
Between Groups	3	2.0236	.6745	2.4254	.0657
Within Groups	272	75.8326	.2778		
Total	276	77.8556			

Table 6 One Way Analysis of Variance: Mean Scores on Life Satisfaction Based on the Reasons Individuals Returned to Work

	Mean	N = 130
Needed the money	6.7027	74
Wanted to feel productive	8.2703	37
Lonely & bored	7.2632	19

Source	D.F.	Sum of Squares	Mean Squares	F-Ratio	F-Probability
Between Groups	2	60.6360	30.3180	10.7420	.0000
Within Groups	127	358.4410	2.8224		
Total	129	419.0769			

The lowest mean score on life satisfaction was 6.7 for those who had been forced to return to work because they needed the money (Table 6). Thus, most of the people that returned to work did so because they needed the money, but they were the least satisfied with their lives.

Conclusion

The data from this study indicate that those who retire and engage in volunteer or recreational activities score higher on measures of life satisfaction than those that never retired. Of those that retired and then returned to work, those that did so because they wanted to feel productive scored highest on life satisfaction. Those that returned to work because they needed the money scored lowest on life satisfaction.

These findings would suggest that if the goal of the federal government is to keep older people in the labor force longer, some means must be found by which the older workers are kept at jobs in which they feel productive and needed. For the business community to continue, primarily for economic reasons, to encourage older workers to retire from highly skilled jobs in which they are more productive than younger workers does not seem desirable.

One possible solution to this problem might be for the federal government to give a tax incentive to businesses employing older workers so that the economic advantage business sees for retiring older workers and employing younger ones would diminish.

A major break in the cost of employing older workers in business would be for the federal government to develop a national health insurance program. One of the major costs to the employer of older workers is the amount of money they must put into health insurance for them. For the federal government to assume this cost would be a major reduction in the business cost of continuing to employ older workers.

Perhaps businesses could continue to utilize the talents of older workers by developing reduced and flexible work schedules which would pay them a lower salary but keep them involved in critical tasks for the industry, as suggested by McShulski (1997).

Since the trend of the last thirty years has been for an ever increasing number of workers to retire prior to age 65, perhaps the government's attempts to keep people in the workforce longer by increasing the age at which they can draw a Social Security check will not be successful. It is possible that through private savings, private investment programs, and pension programs financed by their employers, older workers will continue to retire prior to age 65.

On the other hand, improving technology may mean that business and industry will need fewer employees to produce the nations' goods and services, and therefore they will continue to encourage their workers to retire at younger ages.

The complexity and unpredictability of the factors involved makes predicting future employment and retirement patterns for older Americans at best hazardous and at worst impossible. Observing the results of economic and political pressures placed on both business and government by an ever increasing number of the baby boom generation arriving at retirement age in the next 25 years should prove interesting.

References

Allen, Carole and Herman Brotman. 1981. *Chartbook on Aging.* Washington, D. C.: Administration on Aging.

Beck, S. 1983. "Determinants of Returning to Work after Retirement." Final Report for Grant No. 1R23AG035:65–101, Kansas City, MO.

Berkman, Lisa F. and Lister Breslow. 1983. *Health and Ways of Living: The Alameda Country Study.* New York: Oxford University Press.

Clark, Robert. 1988. "The Future of Work and Retirement." *Research on Aging* 10:169–193.

Clifton, Bryant. 1972. *The Social Dimensions of Work.* Upper Saddle River, NJ: Prentice Hall.

Crowley, J. E. 1990. "Longitudinal Effects of Retirement on Men's Well-Being and Health." *Journal of Business and Psychology* 1:95–113.

Dennis, Helen. 1986. *Fourteen Steps to Managing an Aging Work Force,* edited by Helen Dennis, Lexington, MA: Lexington Books.

Dorfman, L. T. 1992. "Academics and the Transition to Retirement." *Educational Gerontology* 18:343–363.

Dubin, Robert. 1956. "Industrial Workers' Word: A Study of the Central Life Interests of Industrial Workers." *Social Problems* 3:131–142.

Fillenbau, G. G., L. K. George, and E. B. Palmore. 1985. "Determinants and Consequences of Retirement." *Journal of Gerontology* 39:364–371.

Fyock, Catherine. 1991. "American Work Force Is Coming of Age." *The Gerontologist* 31:422–425.

Gall, Terry, David Evans, and John Howard. May 1997. "The Retirement Adjustment Process; Changes in Well-Being of Male Retirees Across Time." *The Journal of Gerontology* 52B(3):110–117.

Gray, Robert M. and David O. Moberg. 1977. *The Church and the Older Person,* revised edition. Grand Rapids, MI: Ermanns.

Hall, Richard. 1975. *Occupations and the Social Structure.* Englewood Cliffs, NJ: Prentice Hall.

Hardy, Melissa. 1991. "Employment After Retirement." *Research on Aging* 13(3):267–288.

House, James S., Karl R. Landes, and Debra Umberson. 1988. "Social Relationships and Health." *Science* 241:540–545.

Howell, Nancy Morrow. 1988. "Life Span Determinants of Work in Retirement Years." *International Journal of Aging and Human Development* 27(2):125–140.

Iams, Howard M. 1985 "New Social Security Beneficiary Women." Correlates of work paper read at the 1985 meeting of the American Sociological Association.

Markides, Kyrakos S. 1983. "Aging, Religiosity and Adjustment: A Longitudinal Analysis." *Journal of Gerontology* 38:621–625.

McShulski, Elaine. 1997. "Ease Employer and Employee Retirement Adjustment with 'Soft Landing' Program." *HR Magazine,* Alexandria: 30–32.

Mobert, David D. 1983. "Compartmentalization and Parochialism in Religion and Voluntary Action Research." *Review of Religious Research* 22(4):318–321.

Moen, Phyllis, Donna Dempster-McClain, and Robin Williams. 1992. "Successful Aging: A Life Course Perspective on Women's Multiple Roles and Health." *American Journal of Sociology* 97(6):1612–1633.

Morris, Malcolm. 1986. "Work and Retirement in an Aging Society." *Daedalus* 115:269–293.

Ortega, Suzanne T., Robert D. Crutchfield, and William A. Rusling. 1983. "Race Differences in Elderly Personal Well-Being, Friendship, Family and Church." *Research on Aging* 5(1): 101–118.

Parker, Stanley. 1982. *Works and Retirement.* London: Allen & Unwin Publishers.

Quinn, Joseph and Richard Burkhauser. *1990 Handbook of Aging and the Social Sciences,* edited by Richard Beinstock and Linda K. Gorge. Academic Press.

Quinn, J. F. 1980. *Retirement Patterns of Self-Employed Workers in Retirement Policy on an Aging Society,* R. L. Clark ed., Durham, NC: Duke University Press.

Soldo, Beth J. and Emily M. Agree. 1988. *Population Bulletin* 43(3). Population Reference Bureau.

Sammartino, Frank. 1979. "Early Retirement." in *Monographs of Aging,* No. 1, Madison: Joyce MacBeth Institute on Aging and Adult Life, University of Wisconsin.

Seccombe, K. and G. R. Lee. 1986. "Gender Differences in Retirement Satisfaction and Its Antecedents." *Research on Aging* 8:426–440.

Sheppard, Harold. 1990. *The Future of Older Workers.* International Exchange Center on Gerontology, University of South Florida, Tampa. FL.

Streib, G. F. and C. J. Schneider. 1971. *Retirement in American Society.* Cornell University Press, Ithaca, NY.

Tillenbaum, G. C. 1971. "The Working Retired." *Journal of Gerontology* 26:1:82–89. U. S. Department of Labor, Civilian Labor Force Participation Rates: Actual and Projected 1980.

Vroom, Victor. 1964. *Work & Motivation.* New York: John Wiley.

Welford, A. T. 1988. "Preventing Adverse Changes of Work with Age." *American Journal of Aging and Human Development* 4:283–291.

UNIT 6

The Experience of Dying

Unit Selections

Key Points to Consider

- What could be done to improve the quality of palliative care in the United States?

- What are the steps a person goes through in the grieving process?

- What are the end-of-life preferences of the terminally ill?

- Should dying patients be told the truth about their impending death, or should the information be withheld? Defend your answer.

- What are the six mind frames toward death that a person might adopt after being informed of their impending death?

Student Website
www.mhhe.com/cls

Internet References

Agency for Health Care Policy and Research
   http://www.ahcpr.gov
Growth House, Inc.
   http://www.growthhouse.org
Hospice Foundation of America
   http://www.HospiceFoundation.org

Modern science has allowed individuals to have some control over the conception of their children and has provided people with the ability to prolong life. However, life and death still defy scientific explanation or reason. The world can be divided into two categories: sacred and secular. The sacred (that which is usually embodied in the religion of a culture) is used to explain all the forces of nature and the environment that can neither be understood nor controlled. On the other hand, the secular (defined as "of or relating to the world") is used to explain all the aspects of the world that can be understood or controlled. Through scientific invention, more and more of the natural world can be controlled. It still seems highly doubtful, however, that science will ever be able to provide an acceptable explanation of the meaning of death. In this domain, religion may always prevail. Death is universally feared. Sometimes, it is more bearable for those who believe in a life after death. Here, religion offers a solution to this dilemma. In the words of anthropologist Bronislaw Malinowski (1884–1942):

Religion steps in, selecting the positive creed, the comforting view, the culturally valuable belief in immortality, in the spirit of the body, and in the continuance of life after death. (Bronislaw Malinowski, *Magic, Science and Religion and Other Essays,* Glencoe, IL: Free Press, 1948)

The fear of death leads people to develop defense mechanisms in order to insulate themselves psychologically from the reality of their own death. The individual knows that someday he or she must die, but this event is nearly always thought to be likely to occur in the far distant future. The individual does not think of himself or herself as dying tomorrow or the next day, but rather years from now. In this way, people are able to control their anxiety about death.

Losing a close friend or relative brings people dangerously close to the reality of death. Individuals come face to face with the fact that there is always an end to life. Latent fears surface. During times of mourning, people grieve not only for the dead, but also for themselves and for the finiteness of life.

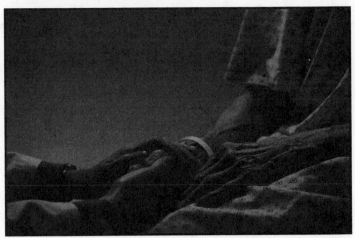

© Comstock/PunchStock

The readings in this section address bereavement, grief, and adjustments to the stages of dying. Stephen Connor, in "Development of Hospice and Palliative Care in the United States," points out the things that need to be done and the changes that need to be made to improve the quality of palliative care in this country. In "The Grieving Process," the authors list and describe the stages of grief that the individual will experience following the death of a loved one.

The authors of "End-of-Life Preferences: A Theory-Driven Inventory" point out the conditions which people with a known terminal illness would prefer to end their lives with compared with what life ending conditions the general public would prefer. In "Mind Frames towards Dying and Factors Motivating Their Adoption by Terminally Ill Elders," Tracy Schroepfer describes the six different mind frames people can hold regarding their own death once they recognize that they are terminally ill.

Development of Hospice and Palliative Care in the United States

Stephen R. Connor

Introduction

More than 30 years have passed since palliative care was introduced in the United States, and what began as a small rebellion has evolved into a fairly large health care industry. Although the palliative care movement has considerably improved the care given to those at the end of life, many challenges remain for palliative care providers in the United States. Some of these challenges have arisen out of the seeds planted in the early years of the U.S. hospice movement.

Early U.S. Hospice History

Palliative care began in the United States through an effort to transplant hospice care from the United Kingdom to the United States. In 1963, Florence Wald, then Dean of the School of Nursing at Yale, invited Dr. Cicely Saunders from London to give a series of lectures on hospice care. Cicely Saunders, matriarch of the worldwide hospice movement, had developed approaches to managing pain and the total needs of the dying patients based on the philosophy of using a team to treat the whole person. Cicely's visit eventually led to the formation of the first U.S. hospice in Branford, Connecticut, which began serving patients at home in 1973.

It is significant that in the United States great emphasis was placed on care in the home, in contrast to the United Kingdom, where hospice care began primarily in inpatient settings. This reflected a number of U.S. factors including a desire for independence, a distrust of medical institutions, and a lack of resources for non-profit hospices operating outside mainstream medicine.

Although some have said that hospice began in the United States as an anti-physician movement, this is not precisely accurate. There was certainly, from the beginning, a strong involvement in hospice from nurses, chaplains, and psychosocial professionals. However, early pioneers in hospice care also included many physicians who, like their other professional colleagues, shared a concern for how the health care system was caring—or more accurately, not caring—for the dying.

Much has been written about the institutionalization of the U.S. health care system—the pervasive attitude of denial and the view of death as the enemy. What was happening in the middle 1970s in the United States as the nescient hospice movement was beginning, reflected the U.S. society as a whole. A consumer movement was underway to take back control of various social institutions, including churches, community services, and health care, from birth to death.

Another significant feature of hospice's development in the United States was the involvement of volunteers. In the beginning everyone was essentially a volunteer, either lay or professional. As hospice has progressed in the United States, lay volunteers have continued to play an important role and have been fundamental in establishing hospice. Today, approximately 400,000 volunteers work in U.S. hospices.

To nurture those in the hospice field, a series of national meetings were convened in Connecticut in 1975, in Boonton, New Jersey in early 1977, and in Marin County in early 1978. These meetings led to the formation of the National Hospice Organization (NHO) in 1978. The first large national NHO conference was held in Washington, D.C. in October 1978 and the first Standards of a Hospice Program of Care were published by NHO in 1979. In 1999, NHO changed its name to the National Hospice and Palliative Care Organization to reflect the melding of traditional hospice care with palliative care in the United States.

Even at this early stage of development, hospice leaders were working with key legislative leaders to develop a system to reimburse hospice care in the United States. Before reimbursement could occur, however, data had to be collected to demonstrate what hospice actually did and what costs were involved. The Health Care Finance Administration (now Center for Medicaid and Medicare Services) conducted a national demonstration project involving 26 hospices throughout the United States to study the effect of reimbursed hospice care. The results of this demonstration project enabled government and hospice representatives to develop a model for how hospice care could be organized and funded, and a bill was introduced to Congress creating a new Medicare entitlement for hospice care.

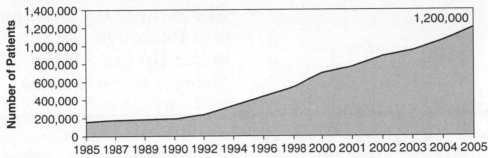

Figure 1 Hospice patients served 1985–2005.

Medicare Hospice Benefit

The Hospice Medicare Benefit (MHB), which was established in 1982 through amendments to the Social Security Act, was included in the Tax Equity and Fiscal Responsibility Act (TEFRA). It was the only new benefit added to Medicare under President Ronald Reagan's administration, and included a three-year sunset provision requiring a report back to Congress on hospice's impact and reauthorization before becoming a permanent benefit in 1985.

The MHB was a unique addition to the U.S. health care system. Prior to implementation of the MHB, the government "reimbursed" providers for their cost in delivering care. With the MHB, a provider was paid a set amount under a prospective reimbursement system. By creating a set payment for hospice care, the government was sharing the risks with a provider. If a patient's cost exceeded the MHB payment, the hospice lost money or had to find other sources of payment. If the MHB payment exceeded a patient's cost, the hospice was allowed to keep the gain even though all hospices originally were not-for-profit organizations.

The set MHB payments were based on the cost of care in the original hospice demonstration project and assumed that each hospice was in compliance with all the standards of hospice care at the time. These standards were changed into Medicare *Conditions of Participation* or regulations that had to be met for a provider to receive payment. Key provisions of the *Conditions of Participation* required hospices to:

- admit eligible patients with a terminal illness with a prognosis of six months or less who chose not to continue curative treatment and agree to hospice care;
- re-certify surviving patients as being terminally ill at specified intervals;
- meet administrative requirements including a governing body, an interdisciplinary team, a plan of care for each patient, a medical record for each patient, a medical director, regular training, quality assurance, use of volunteers, and maintenance of professional management of the program; and
- provide core services by hospice employees including a physician, nurse, counselor, and medical social worker; and provide other non-core services including physical, occupational, and speech therapy, home health aides/homemakers, medical equipment and supplies, medications, and short term inpatient care for symptom management and respite.

MHB payment is made for each day of hospice care on a per diem basis at one of four rates: routine home care; continuous home care for crisis periods in lieu of hospitalization; general inpatient care for severe symptom management; and inpatient respite care to give up to five days break for caregivers.

Growth of Hospice and Palliative Care in the United States

Over the last 25 years, since the enactment of the MHB, hospice has grown considerably and is now the fastest growing benefit in the Medicare program. Even with that, it still represents less than 3% of Medicare expenditures. For the first 10 years following implementation of the benefit, there was slow growth as community-based hospices learned to adapt to meeting regulatory requirements. However, growth in the 1990s and through 2005 was enormous (see Figure 1) and in 2005 more than 1.2 million people received hospice care in the United States. That same year NHPCO estimates that at least one of every three deaths, of all causes, in the United States was under hospice care.

There have been a number of significant changes to the hospice population over the last 25 years. Initially, more than 90% of hospice patients had a primary diagnosis of malignancy. In 2005, the percent of hospice admissions with a cancer diagnosis had dropped to less than 50%. Also, length of service in hospice dropped from an average of around 70 days to less than 50 days. More concerning is that the median time in hospice dropped to around 20 days, with more than 30% of patients receiving service for seven days or less. These lengths of service have improved slightly in the last few years (see Figure 2), but are still historically low.

The number of sites where hospice care is delivered has grown significantly in recent years (see Figure 3). Over a 20-year period, from 1985 to 2005, the number of hospice sites has increased from around 1,500 to more than 4,000. This growth has been fueled both by the MHB and by increased acceptance of hospice in the U.S. health care system. Also contributing to the growth of hospice has been the growth of for-profit hospices, with over a third of U.S. hospice organizations being for-profit corporations today.

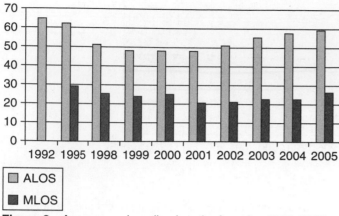

Figure 2 Average and median length of service 1992–2005.

Challenges for Hospice and Palliative Care in the United States

Changes to the Hospice Medicare Benefit

Medicare reimbursement has been the driving force behind hospice's tremendous success in reaching people at the end-of-life in the United States. At the same time, however, regulatory requirements of the MHB have limited the provision of palliative care primarily to those near death. Palliative care services can be provided to patients under existing general Medicare requirements but do not facilitate interdisciplinary care that is essential to palliative care. Physicians and physician surrogates can bill for evaluation and management, licensed psychologists and social workers can bill for some psychological services, and home health agencies can provide general home care, but only under hospice is interdisciplinary care reimbursed as a package.

Some have called for the creation of a specific palliative care benefit in the United States that is separate from hospice. There is concern that creating a parallel palliative care benefit in the United States could result in competition between hospice and palliative care providers. What is needed most are payment provisions that reinforce provisions of good palliative care at various points in the continuum of care for patients with life-threatening illnesses.

Hospice and palliative care leaders in the United States acknowledge that a change is needed in the payment system for palliative care. There is also an understanding that changes to health care reimbursement will occur incrementally and not all at once. What seems to be needed is careful study of the impact of changes and additions to the payment system so that unintended negative consequences can be mitigated.

There is, for instance, a growing consensus that the current restriction on "curative" treatment is not helpful and is the primary cause of late referral to hospice. This treatment restriction was imposed on hospice providers by the director of the Reagan administration's budget office, out of fear that giving patients palliative care and allowing them to continue chemotherapies and other treatments would be too expensive.

While hospice providers at the time did not want to encourage patients to continue treatments that would make their symptom management more difficult and their quality of life poor, patient autonomy and each patient's right to make their own personal decisions about treatment was respected. In fact, the first National Hospice Organization standard for hospice programs of care in 1979 stated that hospice care was "appropriate" care and went on to define appropriate care as a combination of palliative and curative therapies.

A number of studies conducted through the Robert Wood Johnson Foundation's Promoting Excellence in End-of-Life Care program have demonstrated in various settings that removing the curative treatment restriction under the MHB would not in fact be more expensive to the Medicare program (see http://www.promotingexcellence.org/i4a/pages/index.cfm?pageid=1).

In the last 10 years, there has been considerable growth in programs that deliver palliative care in hospitals and in the community. These programs mostly developed outside of hospices and were the result mainly of limitations on hospice eligibility and the need to provide palliative care more broadly to those who had symptom control problems and serious illness but who were not yet terminally ill. A study of end-of-life care in teaching hospitals in the United States (SUPPORT, 1995) revealed that hospitalized patients often had unmet needs for pain control and that treatment wishes were often unknown or ignored, even when useful information was readily accessible to physicians and specially trained nurses were available for patients and families.

The growth in specialist palliative care in the United States has been dramatic. The Center to Advance Palliative Care reports that the number of palliative care programs increased from 632 (15% of hospitals) in 2000 to 1,240 (30% of hospitals) in 2006—a 96% increase in only five years. Also, NHPCO reports that 64.6% of hospice providers now report the provision of some palliative care outside their hospice program.

A number of additional new developments have shown that palliative care, including hospice, is becoming more accepted in the U.S. health care system. Recently, the American Board of Medical Specialties approved hospice and palliative medicine as a recognized sub-specialty. So far, 10 specialties have indicated their interest in allowing their members to sub-specialize in this field, including: Psychiatry and Neurology, Internal Medicine, Family Medicine, Radiology, Surgery, Anesthesiology, Physical Medicine & Rehabilitation, Obstetrics/Gynecology, Pediatrics, and Emergency Medicine.

Also, the Accreditation Council for Graduate Medical Education has begun to accredit fellowship programs in palliative medicine and the Hospice and Palliative Nurses Association offers certification for advanced practice nurses, registered nurses, and nursing assistants. The American Academy for Hospice and Palliative Medicine is growing into a professional society for physicians and the Center to Advance Palliative Care has initiated a National Palliative Care Research Center. While these developments indicate that hospice and palliative care are coming of age in the United States, there remain many challenges and inequities.

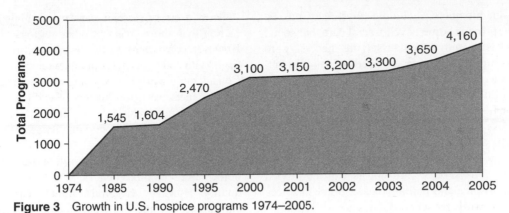

Figure 3   Growth in U.S. hospice programs 1974–2005.

Current hospice providers have a considerable amount of flexibility in how they define curative and palliative treatments. Under Medicare regulations each hospice team determines whether a treatment is curative or not. Very few of the newer treatments available to cancer patients and others with life-threatening conditions can be viewed as curative. A growing number of hospices are implementing "open access" policies wherein all patients with limited prognoses are admitted without regard to their current treatment choices. The hospice then works with the patient and treating physicians to decide which are appropriate to continue based on the patient's goals for care. This approach usually results in earlier hospice referral and enough increased reimbursement to cover the added treatment costs.

Another significant regulatory barrier is the requirement that hospice patients have a prognosis of six months or less if the disease runs its normal course. This requirement is a barrier to timely hospice palliative care. However, to eliminate the six-month prognosis requirement necessitates replacing it with "something else" and that "something else" should not be more onerous than the original requirement.

This problem can be placed on a continuum, with one end being complete reliance on the use of physician judgment and the other end being the use of objective measurable criteria with no judgment involved. There are problems with either of these approaches. Physician judgment has been shown to be notably inaccurate (Christakis, 1999) and many problems are associated with the use of rigid criteria, notably with the application of home health skilled need or homebound criteria and rigid application of local coverage determinations by the Medicare fiscal intermediaries on who is eligible for hospice care.

Some have suggested expanding the six-month criteria to 12 months. This could make it easier for patients to acknowledge the possibility of their approaching death and physicians might find it easier to agree to making such a prognosis, much like the surprise question of "would you be surprised if this patient were alive a year from now?" However, expanding the prognostic criteria doesn't fundamentally change the issue of having to make a determination that death is approaching. Moreover, the federal government has indicated that such a change would be scored as a potential doubling of the cost of hospice care. Therefore, this approach is not likely to occur.

What is needed then is an expansion of hospice benefits to include reimbursement for interdisciplinary consults at an earlier stage of the illness and for care management services prior to admission to a formal hospice service. Such consults and services could be tied to the existence of a life-threatening diagnosis, rather than requiring a prognosis and would require a referral. Such consults are being done now on a limited basis in hospitals, nursing facilities, and residences. Care management programs are emerging; however, to be most effective, the provider needs to have the capacity to do more than just talk on the phone and give advice. To prevent hospitalization, it is sometimes necessary to go to the patient even if it is 2 A.M. Currently, hospices have the most well developed after-hour service delivery capacities.

Workforce Issues

Such an expansion of palliative care will require a substantial increase in a competent workforce. Now that hospice and palliative medicine has been accepted as a recognized sub-specialty, there may be increased incentive for new and existing physicians to enter the field. However, as seen in the sub-specialty of geriatrics, which has not grown in spite of a growing and recognized need, there need to be adequate incentives to attract competent physicians to the field.

Similarly for nursing, which will soon confront a much more significant shortage than has been reported due to large scale retirements, palliative care needs to attract caring and competent professional nurses and skilled nursing assistants. Certification by the National Board for Certification of Hospice and Palliative Nurses is growing and helping to ensure basic competency for nursing professionals. There are currently no recognized certification programs in hospice and palliative care for psychosocial professionals, chaplains, or hospice administrators.

Social workers have been providing the bulk of psychosocial services in hospice programs. This is due to the fact that social work is a required core hospice service and that social workers, if adequately trained in mental health, can also meet the hospice's required need for counseling services. However, there is growing concern that hospices and palliative care programs are not devoting adequate resources to psychosocial services, which are thought to be one of the defining characteristics of the field.

Certainly all team members, including physicians, nurses, and volunteers, can provide some psychosocial care, but social workers, psychologists, and psychiatrists are necessary to address the often complex dynamics and needs of families facing a death. Also, there has been much new knowledge in the field of mental health that may not be adequately applied to the dying and their families. Just providing active listening or providing "supportive" care is not enough. Opportunities for healing relationships and promoting growth at the end of life are major outcomes of good hospice care.

Spiritual and religious services are not as well developed as they could be in hospice and palliative care. Some hospices employ staff chaplains while most coordinate care with community clergy. Most clergy report that their seminarian training was wholly inadequate to prepare them to minister to the dying. Few clergy have undertaken chaplaincy training and when ministering to patients and families are at risk of doing as much harm as good; for example, when patients are left feeling their illness is punishment for misdeeds or lack of faith. Still, spiritual support is generally better in hospice care than in the general health care system and opportunities to help patients find meaning are among the most important of hospice interventions.

If current projections are correct, then more than twice as many hospice professionals and volunteers will be needed in the next 20 years to meet the unmet need for palliative care and the growing numbers of older people in our society. Already, hospices do not have enough physicians to provide optimal care and could use many more to enhance the quality of services.

Access and Quality

The challenge for hospice and palliative care providers can be boiled down to achieving unfettered access to quality palliative care for all who need it. Initially, hospice care in the United States was limited to mainly white suburban cancer patients. Over the past 30 years access has improved considerably and is close to but not yet at parity with population needs. A recent report (Connor et al., in press) demonstrates that blacks are now 7% less likely to receive hospice care than whites. Data for other minority groups is difficult to analyze and the U.S. society is growing increasingly multi-racial.

Significant improvement has been made in improving access to hospice for patients with non-cancer diagnoses, and hospice is now caring for about 60% of all patients who die from cancer. However, access to hospice for patients with solid organ failure, dementia, and frailty still has a long way to go and is limited by current regulatory requirements and prognostic uncertainties. Determining prognosis in non-cancer populations remains a challenge, though recent efforts to improve NHO's original prognostic guidelines are underway.

There remains considerable geographic disparity in access to hospice care (Connor et al., under review), with rates of hospice use ranging from 11% of all deaths in Alaska to 49% of all deaths in Arizona in 2002. Access to hospice and palliative care in very rural areas is a considerable concern.

Most users of hospice care report higher ratings of satisfaction than those dying in other settings (Teno et al., 2004). However, consumer expectations for end-of-life care are low to begin with and there is a general tendency toward leniency bias. Considerable work is now being done to develop sensitive and specific measures for providers of end-of-life care. As hospice and palliative care have grown in the United States, there has not been as much attention to quality as in the rest of the health care system.

Initial focus was on improving the quality of nursing home care, which has generated the most concern about poor quality. However, hospitals, home health agencies, physician practices, and other Medicare providers have now had to develop accountability measures, many of which are now publicly reported on websites such as Home Health Compare and Nursing Home Compare. Hospice will join their ranks before long.

Most current efforts to measure quality in hospice and palliative care are aimed at drawing out from patients and families feedback about their perception and evaluation of the care they have received. This is only fair as these are important outcomes that we can't risk manage and are inherently important to consumers. We also need to look beyond this feedback to look at how our organizations are functioning, how our workforce is improving, and how we measure changes in the patient's condition in an increasingly electronic world of medical records.

In summary, the hospice and palliative care experiment in the United States is continuing to evolve and grow. While we were wrong to believe that the need for specialized palliative care would be eliminated by now, we can hope that in another 20 years we may see a health care system that provides easy access to palliative care throughout the continuum of care for all those with life-threatening illnesses and, in Cicely's words, is provided by people who can give with both their minds and hearts.

References

Christakis, N. (1999). *Death foretold: Prophecy and prognosis in medical care.* Chicago: University of Chicago Press.

Connor, S., Elwert, F., Spence, C., & Christakis, N. (under review). Racial disparity in hospice use in the United States in 2002. *Social Science and Medicine.*

Connor, S., Elwert, F., Spence, C., & Christakis, N. (in press). Geographic variation in hospice use in the United States in 2002. *Journal of Pain and Symptom Management.*

SUPPORT Investigators. (1995). A controlled trial to improve care for seriously ill patients. *Journal of the American Medical Association, 274*(20), 1591–1598.

Teno, J., Clarridge, B., Casey, V., Welch, L., Wetle, T., Sheild, R., & Mor, V. (2004). Family perspectives on end of life care at the last place of care. *Journal of the American Medical Association, 291*(1), 88–93.

The Grieving Process

Michael R. Leming and George E. Dickinson

Grief is a very powerful emotion that is often triggered or stimulated by death. Thomas Attig makes an important distinction between grief and the grieving process. Although grief is an emotion that engenders feelings of helplessness and passivity, the process of grieving is a more complex coping process that presents challenges and opportunities for the griever and requires energy to be invested, tasks to be undertaken, and choices to be made (Attig, 1991, p. 387).

Most people believe that grieving is a diseaselike and debilitating process that renders the individual passive and helpless. According to Attig (1991, p. 389):

It is misleading and dangerous to mistake grief for the whole of the experience of the bereaved. It is misleading because the experience is far more complex, entailing diverse emotional, physical, intellectual, spiritual, and social impacts. It is dangerous because it is precisely this aspect of the experience of the bereaved that is potentially the most frustrating and debilitating.

Death ascribes to the griever a passive social position in the bereavement role. Grief is an emotion over which the individual has no control. However, understanding that grieving is an active coping process can restore to the griever a sense of autonomy in which the process is permeated with choice and there are many areas over which the griever does have some control. . . .

Coping with Grief

The grieving process, like the dying process, is essentially a series of behaviors and attitudes related to coping with the stressful situation of changing the status of a relationship. . . . Many have attempted to understand coping with dying as a series of universal, mutually exclusive, and linear stages. However, because most will acknowledge that not all people will progress through the stages in the same manner, we will list a number of coping strategies used as people attempt to resolve the pain caused by the loss of a significant relationship.

Robert Kavanaugh (1972) identifies the following seven behaviors and feelings as part of the coping process: shock and denial, disorganization, volatile emotions, guilt, loss and loneliness, relief, and reestablishment. It is not difficult to see similarities between these behaviors and Kübler-Ross's five stages (denial, anger, bargaining, depression, and acceptance) of the dying process. According to Kavanaugh (1972, p. 23), "these seven stages do not subscribe to the logic of the head as much as to the irrational tugs of the heart—the logic of need and permission."

Shock and Denial

Even when a significant other is expected to die, at the time of death there is often a sense in which the death is not real. For most of us our first response is, "No, this can't be true." With time our experience of shock diminishes, but we find new ways to deny the reality of death.

Some believe that denial is dysfunctional behavior for those in bereavement. However, denial not only is a common experience among the newly bereaved, but also serves positive functions in the process of adaptation. The main function of denial is to provide the bereaved with a "temporary safe place" from the ugly realities of a social world that offers only loneliness and pain.

With time the meaning of loss tends to expand, and it may be impossible for one to deal with all of the social meanings of death at once. For example, if my wife dies, not only do I lose my spouse, but also I lose my best friend, my sexual partner, the mother of my children, a source of income, the person who writes the Christmas cards, and so on. Denial can protect me from some of the magnitude of this social loss, which may be unbearable at one point in time. With denial, I can work through different aspects of my loss over time.

Disorganization

Disorganization is that stage in the bereavement process in which one may feel totally out of touch with the reality of everyday life. Some go through the 3-day time period just prior to the funeral as if on "automatic pilot" or "in a daze." Nothing normal "makes sense," and they may feel that life has no inherent meaning. For some, death is perceived as preferable to life, which appears to be devoid of meaning.

This emotional response is also a normal experience for the newly bereaved. Confusion is normal for those whose social world has been disorganized through death. When my father died, my mother lost not only all of those things that one loses with a death of a spouse, but also her caregiving role—a social role and master status that had defined her identity in the 5 years that my father lived with cancer. It is only natural to experience confusion and social disorganization when one's social identity has been destroyed.

Volatile Reactions

Whenever one's identity and social order face the possibility of destruction, there is a natural tendency to feel angry, frustrated, helpless, and/or hurt. The volatile reactions of terror, hatred, resentment, and jealousy are often experienced as emotional manifestations of these feelings. Grieving humans are sometimes more successful at masking their feelings in socially acceptable behaviors than other animals, whose instincts cause them to go into a fit of rage when their order is threatened by external forces. However apparently dissimilar, the internal emotional experience is similar.

In working with bereaved persons over the past 15 years, I have observed that the following become objects of volatile grief reactions: God, medical personnel, funeral directors, other family members, in-laws, friends who have not experienced death in their families, and/or even the person who has died. I have always found it interesting to watch mild-mannered individuals transformed into raging and resentful persons when grieving. Some of these people have experienced physical symptoms such as migraine headaches, ulcers, neuropathy, and colitis as a result of living with these intense emotions.

Guilt

Guilt is similar to the emotional reactions discussed earlier. Guilt is anger and resentment turned in on oneself and often results in self-deprecation and depression. It typically manifests itself in statements like "If only I had . . . ," "I should have . . . ," "I could have done it differently . . . ," and "Maybe I did the wrong thing." Guilt is a normal part of the bereavement process.

From a sociological perspective, guilt can become a social mechanism to resolve the **dissonance** that people feel when unable to explain why someone else's loved one has died. Rather than view death as something that can happen at any time to any one, people can **blame the victim** of bereavement and believe that the victim of bereavement was in some way responsible for the death—"If he had been a better parent, the child might not have been hit by the car," or "If I had been married to him I might also have committed suicide," or "No wonder he died of a heart attack, her cooking would give anyone high cholesterol." Therefore, bereaved persons are sometimes encouraged to feel guilt because they are subtly sanctioned by others' reactions.

Loss and Loneliness

As we discussed earlier, loss and loneliness are the other side of denial. Their full sense never becomes obvious at once; rather, each day without the deceased helps us to recognize how much we needed and depended upon those persons. Social situations in which we expected them always to be present seem different now that they are gone. Holiday celebrations are also diminished by their absence. In fact, for some, most of life takes on a "something's missing" feeling. This feeling was captured in the 1960s love song "End of the World."

Why does the world go on turning?
Why must the sea rush to shore?
Don't they know it's the end of the world
'Cause you don't love me anymore?

Loss and loneliness are often transformed into depression and sadness fed by feelings of self-pity. According to Kavanaugh (1972, p. 118), this effect is magnified by the fact that the dead loved one grows out of focus in memory—"an elf becomes a giant, a sinner becomes a saint because the grieving heart needs giants and saints to fill an expanding void." Even a formerly undesirable spouse, such as an alcoholic, is missed in a way that few can understand unless their own hearts are involved. This is a time in the grieving process when anybody is better than nobody and being alone only adds to the curse of loss and loneliness (Kavanaugh, 1972, p. 118).

Those who try to escape this experience will either turn to denial in an attempt to reject their feelings of loss or try to find surrogates—new friends at a bar, a quick remarriage, or a new pet. This escape can never be permanent, however, because loss and loneliness are a necessary part of the bereavement experience. According to Kavanaugh (1972, p. 119),the "ultimate goal in conquering loneliness" is to build a new independence or to find a new and equally viable relationship.

Relief

The experience of relief in the midst of the bereavement process may seem odd for some and add to their feelings of guilt. My mother found relief in the fact that my father's battle with cancer had ended, even though this end provided her with new problems. I have observed a friend's relief 6 months after her husband died. This older friend of mine was the wife of a minister, and her whole life before he died was his ministry. With time, as she built a new world of social involvements and relationships of which he was not a part, she discovered a new independent person in herself whom she perceived was a better person than she had ever been.

Although relief can give rise to feelings of guilt, like denial, it can also be experienced as a "safe place" from the pain, loss, and loneliness that are endured when one is grieving. According to Kavanaugh (1972, p. 121):

> The feeling of relief does not imply any criticism for the love we lost. Instead, it is a reflection of our need for ever deeper love, our quest for someone or something always better, our search for the infinite, that best and perfect love religious people name as God.

Reestablishment

As one moves toward reestablishment of a life without the deceased, it is obvious that the process involves extensive adjustment and time, especially if the relationship was meaningful. It is likely that one may have feelings of loneliness, guilt, and disorganization at the same time and that just when one may experience a sense of relief something will happen to trigger a denial of the death. What facilitates bereavement and adjustment is fully experiencing each of these feelings as normal and realizing that it is hope (holding the grieving person together in fantasy at first) that will provide the promise of a new life filled with order, purpose, and meaning.

Reestablishment never occurs all at once. Rather, it is a goal that one realizes has been achieved long after it has occurred. In some ways it is similar to Dorothy's realization at the end of *The Wizard of Oz*—she had always possessed the magic that could return her to Kansas. And, like Dorothy, we have to experience our loss before we really appreciate the joy of investing our lives again in new relationships.

The Four Tasks of Mourning

In 1982 J. William Worden published *Grief Counseling and Grief Therapy*, which summarized the research conclusions of a National Institutes of Health study called the Omega Project (occasionally referred to as the Harvard Bereavement Study). Two of the more significant findings of this research, displaying the active nature of the grieving process, are that mourning is necessary for all persons who have experienced a loss through death and that four tasks of mourning must be accomplished before mourning can be completed and reestablishment can take place.

According to Worden (1982, p. 10), unfinished grief tasks can impair further growth and development of the individual. Furthermore, the necessity of these tasks suggests that those in bereavement must attend to "grief work" because successful grief resolution is not automatic, as Kavanaugh's (1972) stages might imply. Each bereaved person must accomplish four necessary tasks: (a) accept the reality of the loss, (b) experience the pain of grief (c) adjust to an environment in which the deceased is missing, and (d) withdraw emotional energy and reinvest it in another relationship (Worden, 1982).

Accept the Reality of the Loss

Especially in situations when death is unexpected and/or the deceased lived far away, it is difficult to conceptualize the reality of the loss. The first task of mourning is to overcome the natural denial response and realize that the person is dead and will not return.

Bereaved persons can facilitate the actualization of death in many ways. The traditional ways are to view the body, attend the funeral and committal services, and visit the place of final disposition. The following is a partial list of additional activities that can assist in making death real for grieving persons.

1. View the body at the place of death before preparation by the funeral director.
2. Talk about the deceased and the circumstances surrounding the death.
3. View photographs and personal effects of the deceased.
4. Distribute the possessions of the deceased among relatives and friends.

Experience the Pain of Grief

Part of coming to grips with the reality of death is experiencing the emotional and physical pain caused by the loss. Many people in the denial stage of grieving attempt to avoid pain by choosing to reject the emotions and feelings that they are experiencing. Some do this by avoiding places and circumstances that remind them of the deceased. I know of one widow who quit playing golf and quit eating at a particular restaurant because these were activities that she had enjoyed with her husband. Another widow found it extremely painful to be with her dead husband's twin, even though he and her sister-in-law were her most supportive friends.

J. William Worden (1982, pp. 13–14) cites the following case study to illustrate the performance of this task of mourning:

> One young woman minimized her loss by believing her brother was out of his dark place and into a better place after his suicide. This might have been true, but it kept her from feeling her intense anger at him for leaving her. In treatment, when she first allowed herself to feel anger, she said, "I'm angry with his behavior and not him!" Finally she was able to acknowledge this anger directly.

The problem with the avoidance strategy is that people cannot escape the pain associated with mourning. According to Bowlby (cited by Worden, 1982, p. 14), "Sooner or later, some of those who avoid all conscious grieving, break down—usually with some form of depression." Tears can afford cleansing for wounds created by loss, and fully experiencing the pain ultimately provides wonderful relief to those who suffer while eliminating long-term chronic grief.

Adjust to an Environment in which the Deceased is Missing

The third task, practical in nature, requires the griever to take on some of the social roles performed by the deceased, or to find others who will. According to Worden (1982, p. 15), to abort this task is to become helpless by refusing to develop the skills necessary in daily living and by ultimately withdrawing from life.

I knew a woman who refused to adjust to the social environment in which she found herself after the death of her husband. He was her business partner, as well as her best and only friend. After 30 years of marriage, they had no children, and she had no close relatives. She had never learned to drive a car. Her entire social world had been controlled by her former husband. Three weeks after his funeral she went into the basement and committed suicide.

The alternative to withdrawing is assuming new social roles by taking on additional responsibilities. Extended families who always gathered at Grandma's house for Thanksgiving will be tempted to have a number of small Thanksgiving dinners after her death. The members of this family may believe that "no one can take Grandma's place." Although this may be true, members of the extended family will grieve better if someone else is willing to do Grandma's work, enabling the entire family to come together for Thanksgiving. Not to do so will cause double pain—the family will not gather, and Grandma will still be missed.

The final task of mourning is a difficult one for many because they feel disloyal or unfaithful in withdrawing emotional energy from their dead loved one. One of my family members once said that she could never love another man after her husband died. My twice-widowed aunt responded, "I once felt like that, but I now consider myself to be fortunate to have been married to two of the best men in the world."

Other people find themselves unable to reinvest in new relationships because they are unwilling to experience again the pain caused by loss. [A] quotation from John Brantner . . . provides perspective on this problem: "Only people who avoid love can avoid grief. The point is to learn from it and remain vulnerable to love."

However, those who are able to withdraw emotional energy and reinvest it in other relationships find the possibility of a newly established social life. Kavanaugh (1972, pp. 122–123) depicts this situation well with the following description.

> At this point fantasies fade into constructive efforts to reach out and build anew. The phone is answered more quickly, the door as well, and meetings seem important, invitations are treasured and any social gathering becomes an opportunity rather than a curse. Mementos of the past are put away for occasional family gatherings. New clothes and new places promise dreams instead of only fears. Old friends are important for encouragement and permission to rebuild one's life. New friends can offer realistic opportunities for coming out from under the grieving mantle. With newly acquired friends, one is not a widow, widower, or survivor—just a person. Life begins again at the point of new friendships. All the rest is of yesterday, buried, unimportant to the now and tomorrow.

End-of-Life Preferences
*A Theory-Driven Inventory**

The study aimed at making a theory-driven inventory of end-of-life preferences. Participants were asked about a variety of preferences representing all eight motivational states described in Apter's Metamotivational Theory (AMT; Apter, 2001). Data from a convenience sample of 965 community participants and a convenience sample of 81 persons suffering from a terminal illness were examined using exploratory and confirmatory factor analysis. Ten factors were evidenced; they were easily interpretable in the AMT framework. In decreasing order of importance, people would, at the time of their death, like to have an understanding doctor, to be at peace with themselves, to remain autonomous, to keep a sense of humor, to remain able to oppose any decision taken without their consent, to remain an object of love, to remain a reference for others, to have resolved conflicts with others, to leave their businesses in good order, and to find themselves at peace with God.

SYLVIE BONIN-SCAON ET AL.

Dying persons often have to face pain, dependence, and loss of dignity. Their plight is distressing to them and to everyone around them (Kapo, Morrison, & Liao, 2007; Plonk & Arnold, 2005). Previous studies of end-of-life preferences, using qualitative or quantitative approaches, have shown that a great diversity of end-of-life issues are considered important by people in general, by people who are in the process of dying, and by caregivers. Among the issues most frequently mentioned, one can quote:

a. maintaining professional and personal role functions in the context of ongoing treatment (Volker, Kahn, & Penticuff, 2004), completing meaningful goals (Rankin, Donahue, Davis, Katseres, Wedig, Johnson, et al., 1998), and having one's financial affairs in order (Steinhauser, Christakis, Clipp, McNeilly, McIntyre, & Tulsky, 2000a; Steinhauser, Clipp, McNeilly, Christakis, McIntyre, & Tulsky, 2000b);

b. maintaining one's sense of humor (Kuhl, 2002; Steinhauser et al., 2000a, 2000b);

c. remembering one's personal accomplishments (Kuhl, 2002; Steinhauser et al., 2000a, 2000b), discussing spiritual experiences and concerns (Vig, Davenport, & Pearlman, 2002), and expressing readiness for death, (Rankin et al., 1998);

d. avoiding inappropriate prolongation of dying (Singer, Martin, & Kelner, 1999), and opposing the use of heroic measures (Duffy, Ronis, Fowler, Myers Schim, & Jackson, 2006);

e. maintaining physical independence, maintaining personal hygiene, controlling treatment choices, choosing food and drink intake (Rankin et al., 1998), being kept clean, knowing what to expect about one's condition, maintaining one's dignity, and being free of shortness of breath, naming a surrogate decision-maker, and having left treatment preferences in writing (Chochinov, Hack, Hassard, Kristjanson, McClement, & Harlos, 2002; Steinhauser et al., 2000a, 2000b; Volker et al., 2004);

f. having a nurse with whom one feels comfortable, having someone who will listen, trusting one's physician, having a physician with whom one can discuss fears (Ferris, von Gunten, & Emanuel, 2003; Kuhl, 2002; Steinhauser et al., 2000a, 2000b; von Gunten, 2005;), appearing calm and tranquil, being free of pain and anxiety, and expressing symptom control (Jayawardena & Liao, 2006; Pierson, Curtis, & Patrick, 2002; Rankin et al., 1998; Singer, Martin, & Kelner, 1999; Vig et al., 2002; Volker et al., 2004; West, Engelberg, Weinrich, & Curtis, 2005);

* This work was supported by the Ethics and Work laboratory (Institute for Advanced Studies), and the "Université de Toulouse" (CLLE-LTC, UTM, CNRS, EPHE).

g. resolving unfinished business with family or friends (Kuhl, 2002), having a physician who knows one as a whole person (Steinhauser et al., 2000a, 2000b), and disengaging gradually from significant others (Rankin et al., 1998);

h. exchanging affection with others (Kuhl, 2002; Rankin et al., 1998), saying goodbye to important people, sharing time with close friends, and believing the family is prepared for one's death (Pierson et al., 2002; Steinhauser et al., 2000a, 2000b; Vig et al., 2002; Volker et al., 2004).

Most of these issues have also been mentioned by patients in studies about what motivates terminally ill persons to consider (or not consider) a hastened death (Schroepfer, 2006).

The first objective of the present set of studies was to make a systematic, theory-driven inventory of these preferences. The second objective was to structure them into a number of intelligible factors. The third objective was to relate them to several broad characteristics of the participants: age, gender, education, and religious involvement. These three objectives were pursued in Study 1. The fourth objective was to compare the preferences expressed by people in general with those expressed by persons who are highly concerned about their own impending death; that is, by people whose doctors have told them they have a terminal condition. This objective was pursued in Study 2. In view of the diversity of these preferences, which has been illustrated in the previous point, the theoretical framework chosen was a broad one. Michael Apter's Metamotivational Theory (AMT; Apter, 2001, 2007).

This theory posits that the fundamental psychological motives, and the values they represent, consist of four pairs of opposites. The first pair of contrasting motives are telic and paratelic. The basic value of the telic motive is that of achievement, or progress toward important goals in the future, and it can be characterized as serious in style. Examples of possible telic-type preferences are "Being able to manage one's finances until the last moment," and "Having enough time to finish an important project." Both wishes are serious ones. As already shown by Steinhauser et al. (2000a, 2000b), even if, at the time of death, the future may appear limited, considerations as regards the future may not be absent from the preferences people are willing to express.

The telic motive contrasts with the paratelic motive. The basic value here is that of immediate enjoyment, with an orientation toward the present moment and toward ongoing activities and experiences in themselves. This motive may be said to display a playful style. Examples of possible paratelic-type preferences are "Being able to enjoy life until the last moments" and "Keeping a sense of humor." Although these wishes may appear at variance with the fact of dying, Steinhauser et al. (2000a, 2000b) found that "maintaining one's sense of humor" was considered a priority by most patients.

The next pair of motives is composed of the conformist and negativistic motives. The conformist motive has the basic value of fitting in (or, more strongly, of duty) and a compliant style that accepts the need for rules and welcomes the structure they provide. Examples of possible conformist-type preferences are "Being at peace with oneself" and "Having the sense of a personal accomplishment." These wishes express the feeling of having behaved in life in a correct, moral way; in other words, the feeling of having accomplished one's duty. Among religious persons, these wishes may have an additional religious tonality: "Feeling at peace with one's God" and "Being able to receive the sacraments." Rankin et al. (1998) have already suggested that recalling lifetime memories, reviewing life's accomplishments, and discussing spiritual experiences and concerns were indicators for dignified dying. Pierson, Curtis, and Patrick (2002) showed that for some patients spiritual aspects of dying were necessary components of a "good" death.

In contrast, the negativistic motive represents the basic value of freedom and a challenging style that experiences rules of all kinds as limitations and constraints and feels the need to break free from them. Examples of possible negativist-type preferences are "Being able to oppose certain decisions taken for oneself by the family or by the doctors" and "Being able to be alone from time to time." Duffy, Ronis, Fowler, Myers Schim, & Jackson (2006) have already highlighted the importance of opposing the use of heroic measures for patients.

The mastery motive has the basic value of power and control, whether over people, objects, or situations. Here the style is a competitive one that aims to dominate or at least to command respect. This contrasts with the sympathy motive, with the basic value of love and a caring style that allows the expression of intimacy and tenderness. Finally, the autic motive has the basic value of individuality and a self-oriented style in which the outcomes of actions are evaluated by the individual in terms of how they affect that individual personally. In contrast, the alloic motive has the basic value of transcendence of one's own condition and an other-oriented style involving identification with others (individuals, groups, causes) and genuine unselfishness in the sense of wanting to do things for the sake of the other rather than oneself.

In many cases, the mastery-sympathy motives and the autic-alloic motives combine to form four different pairs of motives: autic mastery, autic sympathy, alloic mastery, and alloic sympathy (Apter, 2001; Cottencin, Mullet, & Sorum, 2006; Makris & Mullet, 2009). Examples of possible autic mastery-type preferences are: "Being able autonomously to feed oneself" and "Not being connected to a machine." In both examples, the basic idea is remaining, as far as possible, an autonomous person, that is, a person with sufficient mastery of oneself. In Apter's framework this type of preferences more precisely refers to what is called intra-autic mastery. As already shown by Steinhauser et al. (2000a, 2000b), being kept clean, knowing what to expect about one's condition, and maintaining one's dignity were considered important by most patients.

Other examples of possible autic-mastery-type preferences are "Having been able to express all grievances one wanted to express to others before dying" and "Remaining a reference for the others until the last moment." In both cases, these preferences express the need for maintaining the self, at least at a symbolic level, in a controlling position. In Apter's framework, this type of preference more precisely refers to what is called auto-centric mastery. Rankin et al. (1998) have already suggested that resolving important issues and concerns and disengaging gradually from significant others were indicators of dignified dying.

Autic sympathy-type preferences derive from the need to keep love relationships intact: "Being accompanied by a close member of the family until the last moment," "Not dying alone." These relationships are usually with family. Kuhl (2002) has suggested that to take someone's hand at the last moment may be a priceless opportunity. They may also involve the care personnel because dying may frequently be dying in a hospital, or because nurses and doctors are sometimes the only persons available. In this later case, autic sympathy-type preferences refer directly to the quality of the caring relationship. Examples of possible autic sympathy-type preferences involving the care personnel are "Having a competent and understanding doctor" and "Receiving adequate pain relief treatment." Volker et al. (2004) have already showed that control of pain and other symptoms associated with disease was among the more important patient concerns.

Alloic mastery-type preferences refers to the ability to find one's place into hierarchies, to obey orders, to respect and honor the persons who are in charge of the community, and to act as a responsible citizen. Examples of possible alloic mastery-type preferences is "Remaining a good citizen (a patriot) until the last moment" and "Remaining able to show respect for the doctors and the nurses."

Finally, examples of possible alloic sympathy-type preferences are "Being granted forgiveness by the persons one has hurt during one's life" and "Knowing that one's death will not have dramatic consequences for the family." As already shown by Volker et al. (2004), managing the impact of one's death on family is an important patient concern.

Study 1

In Study 1, a group of adults judged to what extent a list of end-of-life conditions and situations were important. Four hypotheses were formulated.

The first hypothesis was that a complex structure (see Kuhl, 2002), comprised of factors consistent with AMT, would be able to satisfactorily account for the data. At least eight factors are expected: Telic (leaving one's affairs in order), Paratelic (keeping a sense of humor), Conformist (being at peace with oneself or with God), Negativist (being able to oppose unwanted treatments), Autic Mastery (keeping enough autonomy and being respected), Autic Sympathy (keeping close to the family), Alloic Mastery (remaining able to show respect and consideration to people), and Alloic Sympathy (being at peace with significant others).

The second hypothesis was that gender would have a positive impact on autic sympathy and alloic sympathy scores. Females are expected to be more other-oriented than males (e.g., Heilman & Chen, 2005). As a result, females might consider that being in the company of the family (not being left alone) and resolving past conflicts with others before dying are more important at the moment of dying than do males.

The third hypothesis was that educational level would have a positive impact on telic and negativist scores. It was assumed that more educated persons would be more concerned about completing an important project or achieving something significant before dying than less educated persons. Also, it was assumed that more educated persons would better understand the type of treatments they were offered and, as a result, would feel themselves in a better position to accept or refuse them than less educated persons.

The fourth hypothesis was that religious involvement would have a positive impact on conformist scores. Religious persons were expected to be more concerned than non-religious persons with the ideas of feeling at peace not only with their God but also with other persons.

Method
Participants

The sample was composed of 965 non-paid, voluntary participants (658 females and 307 males). They were aged 18 to 99 with a mean age of 43.76 years ($SD = 20.58$). Two hundred twenty-four participants were 18–24 years old, 273 were 25–39 years old, 230 were 40–59 years old, and 238 participants were older than 60. All the older participants were autonomous and lived at home.

Two hundred sixty-five participants had not completed secondary education, 106 had completed secondary education, 410 had also obtained a 2–3 year college degree, and 184 had gone on to obtain a master's or doctoral degree. Five hundred and thirty participants were married or lived with a regular partner, 51 were divorced, 75 were widowed, and 309 were single. Three hundred forty-six declared they did not believe in God, 330 believed in God but did not attend church on a regular basis, and 289 did attend church on a regular basis. Two hundred seventy-one participants reported that their life had already been put in danger. Five hundred forty-one had already lost at least one very close relative (mother, father, or sibling).

Participants were contacted during daylight hours on campus and in the streets of several small, medium, or big towns located in the west and in the south of France. The six investigators solicited every third passerby until they had contacted 1500 individuals. The potential participants were told that our research team was conducting a survey on the conditions in which people in general would prefer to be at the time of death, and they were given either some examples of the questions or shown the first page of the questionnaire. The acceptance rate was moderately high: 64% of the people contacted agreed to participate in the study. The main reason for refusing to participate was lack of time; it took approximately 30 minutes to fill out the questionnaire.

Material

The questionnaire had the following introduction:

> In the last moments of life, a certain number of factors become very important. Not to be all alone, to be kept clean, to have effective pain treatment are generally considered as important factors in the hour of death. We need

your help to make the most complete inventory possible of these factors. It is for this reason that we ask you to rate the importance of the factors that we present in this questionnaire. Circle each time the expression (from of little importance to extremely important) that best corresponds to your current opinion. Of course, there is neither a good, nor a bad reply. It is your opinion, and your opinion only, that interests us.

The questionnaire itself was composed of 120 items that covered the eight domains suggested in AMT (Apter, 2001). This list was composed of 42 items borrowed from Steinhauser et al. (2000a), 15 items inspired by Pierson, Curtis, and Patrick (2002), and 63 new items inspired by Reversal Theory (see Table 1 for an overview of the items). Responses were given on a 7-point scale ranging from "of little importance" to "extremely important." The intermediate levels were "not very important," "somewhat important," "important," "very important," and "very, very important." Additional questions asked for demographic information.

Procedure

Each participant responded individually. After the participant agreed to participate in the study and gave written consent, the investigator either administered the survey right away at the participant's home or made an appointment to meet later at the participant's home or office or in a room at the university. In all cases, the participant worked in a familiar, calm setting. Four hundred eighty-three participants were presented the items in one order and 482 in the reverse order. No time limit was imposed.

Results

Each rating by each participant was converted to a numerical value expressing the distance (the number of points, from 1 to 7) between the chosen point on the response scale and the left anchor, serving as the reference. These numerical values were then subjected to graphical and statistical analyses.

Exploratory Factor Analysis

The sample was randomly divided in two equivalent sub-samples. A first exploratory factor analysis was conducted on the first sub-sample ($N = 482$) of participants. Using the scree test to determine the number of factors arising from this analysis, 10 factors with eigenvalues higher than 1 emerged. This 10-factor solution was retained and subjected to VARIMAX rotation. Examination of the results allowed the researchers to select a sub-sample of 60 items with loadings higher than .30 on at least one of the 10 factors. A second factor analysis was conducted on these 60 items on the same participants sub-sample. A 10-factor solution was found again. Eigenvalues ranged from 1.25 to 14.52. Results are shown in Table 1.

The first factor, which explained 8% of the variance, was called *Keeping close to loved ones* since it loaded positively on items expressing the need for another's affection and love and the desire to die in a familiar place (e.g., not dying alone and being able to decide where to die). The mean values for the

items loading on this factor (loading > .40) ranged from 5.27 to 5.61; that is, they were intermediate between the "very important" and "very, very important" levels of the response scale.

The second factor, which explained 6% of the variance, was named *Keeping enough autonomy* since it loaded positively on items expressing a will to remain autonomous and in complete control of oneself (e.g., being able to feed oneself autonomously, not being connected to machines). The mean values for the items loading on this factor ranged from 4.92 to 5.80; that is, they also corresponded to "very important."

The third factor, which explained 5% of the variance, was called *Feeling at peace with God* since it loaded positively on items expressing the need to be at peace with God (e.g., receiving sacraments), and, interestingly, hostility toward assisted suicide. The mean values for the items loading on this factor ranged from 3.57 to 4.42; that is, they were intermediate between the "somewhat important" and "important" levels of the response scale.

The fourth factor, which explained 7% of the variance, was labeled *Inspiring respect* since it loaded positively on items expressing the need to retain some personal control over others until the last moment (e.g., being able to formulate the grievances one has toward others before dying, remaining a reference for others). The mean values for the items loading on this factor ranged from 4.19 to 4.62; that is, they corresponded to "important."

The fifth factor, which explained 6% of the variance, was called *Enjoying life until the last moment* since it loaded positively on items expressing the need to enjoy, as far as possible, the last moment in life (e.g., keeping a sense of humor, spending time with good friends). The mean values for the items loading on this factor ranged from 4.17 to 4.85; that is, they corresponded to the "important" level of the response scale.

The sixth factor, which explained 4% of the variance, was named *Feeling of accomplishment* since it loaded positively on items expressing the satisfaction of having accomplished one's duty in life (e.g., being at peace with oneself, having a sense of personal accomplishment). The mean values for the items loading on this factor ranged from 5.02 to 5.85; that is, they were intermediate between "very important" and "very, very important."

The seventh factor, which explained 5% of the variance, was called *Leaving one's affairs in order* since it loaded positively on items expressing the need to put one's affairs into good order before dying (e.g., being able to manage one's finances until the last moment, being an example of responsibility until the last moment). The mean values for the items loading on this factor ranged from 3.64 to 4.52; that is, they corresponded to the "important" level of the response scale.

The eighth factor, which explained 6% of the variance, was labeled *Remaining able to oppose unwanted treatments* since it loaded positively on items expressing a will to resist unwanted family decisions or undesired medical treatments (e.g., being able to oppose any undesired invasive treatment, being still able to express anger when necessary). The mean values for the items loading on this factor ranged from 3.55 to 4.34; that is, they corresponded to "important."

Table 1 Results of the Exploratory Factor Analysis Conducted on the 60 Items (Study 1, First Sub-Sample). Results of the Confirmatory Factor Analysis Conducted on the 30 Items (Study 1, Second Sub-Sample). Results of the Confirmatory Factor Analysis Conducted on the 24 Items (Study 2).

Items	Exploratory Factor Analysis (60 items)										CFA (30 items)	CFA (24 items)
	I	II	III	IV	V	VI	VII	VIII	IX	X		
Keeping close to loved ones												
To not die alone*	.76	.09	.06	.04	.05	.09	−.05	−.02	.17	.16	.88	1.00
To know you will be able to take someone's hand at the last moment*	.69	.11	.07	.07	.09	.08	−.10	.02	.24	.22	.77	.95
To have a family member or someone close to you (a spouse, a friend) present at the bedside until the end*	.73	.06	.09	.12	.13	.06	−.01	.08	.24	.28	.88	.90
To have someone who can stay close to you	.70	.00	.08	.12	.14	.12	−.05	.04	.25	.33		
To decide on the place where you will die*	.69	.09	−.08	−.03	.06	.04	.18	.32	.10	.05		
To be able to die at home*	.66	.03	.19	.00	−.07	.09	.16	.21	.03	−.04		
To have around you certain personal objects of symbolic importance (photos)	.42	.09	.11	−.09	.11	.12	.11	.26	.11	.21		
Keeping enough autonomy												
To not be kept alive by artificial means	.12	.79	−.06	.03	−.04	.09	−.04	.18	.04	.00	.59	
To be able to feed yourself	.03	.74	−.06	.31	.09	−.01	.09	.26	.02	.07	.96	
To not find yourself connected to a machine*	.10	.70	.02	.05	.15	.03	.12	.13	−.04	.00	.75	
To not be a heavy burden on your family*	−.05	.62	−.02	.09	.15	.06	.22	−.13	.11	.12		
To be able to go to the bathroom with dignity	.07	.61	.01	.23	.12	−.05	.26	.16	.06	.21		
To not be an object of pity and tearful demonstrations	.15	.58	−.08	.16	.20	.12	.00	.07	.12	.15		
Feeling at peace with God												
To be able to receive communion	.13	−.04	.86	.04	.00	−.03	.12	−.02	.11	.07	.81	.94
To feel at peace with your God*	.06	.00	.82	.08	−.01	.09	.07	−.02	.19	.12	.93	.94
To be in a condition to pray or to attend church*	.24	−.04	.81	.02	.01	−.01	.12	.01	.12	.05	.82	.99
To be visited regularly by a religious authority*	.00	.02	.55	.35	.09	−.01	.08	.01	.50	−.07		
To be able to have recourse, if need be, to physician-assisted suicide	.13	.32	−.49	.10	.07	−.11	.00	.27	−.08	−.02		
Inspiring respect												
To remain useful to others until the end*	.00	.13	−.14	.54	.06	.03	.29	.41	−.01	.09	.72	.80
To know you will leave positive signs of your existence (writings, actions, creations, accomplishments)*	.15	.12	.24	.69	.01	.12	.00	.06	.17	.17	.67	.52
To remain until the end a point of reference for others	−.12	.15	.06	.62	.23	.05	.21	.02	.06	−.08	.61	.90

To get everything off your chest before dying	.13	.05	−.09	.64	.22	.01	.11	−.10	−.07	.04	
To have known how to obtain forgiveness from those you have recently wronged	.10	.10	.12	.67	.01	.09	−.04	.34	.16	.10	
To be able to forgive all the persons who recently wronged you	.02	.33	.09	.56	−.05	.08	−.11	.34	.11	.00	.95
To be able to keep a smile around others until the very end	.06	.16	.00	.52	.34	.15	.12	−.01	.05	.32	.79
To not become a heavy burden on society*	−.11	.38	−.08	.50	.07	−.12	.25	−.11	−.07	.19	.87
Enjoying life until the least moment											
To keep a sense of humor*	−.16	.24	.04	.11	.68	.08	.06	.02	−.06	.02	.74
To have a physician and care takers who have a sense of humor	−.05	.18	.08	.06	.70	.02	.05	.09	.00	.28	.63
To be able still to laugh a little	.18	.07	−.17	.07	.63	.15	.10	.17	−.13	.16	.64
To be able to say a final warm goodbye to the persons you have known well	.25	−.02	−.02	.30	.58	.14	.06	.07	.12	.12	
Feeling personal accomplishment											
To be able to have some good moments with your friends*	.24	.02	−.06	.09	.53	.18	.00	.13	.22	.19	.85
To be able to reminisce with those close to you about past good times	.37	.09	.05	.09	.46	.02	.13	.08	.27	.18	.85
To be able to say a final goodbye to all the persons you love*	.36	.08	−.02	.04	.49	.19	−.04	.02	.33	.24	.59
To be at peace with yourself	.07	.13	.18	.04	.05	.70	−.04	.10	.37	.09	.85
To know you have done your duty	.08	.16	.13	.07	.10	.70	.02	.15	.34	.10	.73
To be able still to experience some personal fulfillment	.20	.03	−.08	.03	.23	.68	.11	.16	−.07	.10	.67
To have a feeling of personal accomplishment*	.17	−.06	−.03	.18	.13	.69	.08	.19	.16	−.03	
Leaving one's affairs in order											
To be able to manage your financial affairs until the end*	.01	.09	.02	.11	−.11	.16	.78	−.01	−.14	.09	.95
To leave your affairs in order	.01	.26	.10	.01	.01	.08	.71	−.07	.02	.15	.84
To be able to designate a proxy*	−.04	.18	.15	.13	.15	−.10	.48	.07	.22	−.01	.85
To remain until the end an example for others	.10	.03	.22	.16	.30	−.18	.60	.07	.20	−.09	
To be able to finish an important project	.12	.09	.09	.18	.25	.06	.76	.17	.22	.06	
Remaining able to oppose oneself											
To be able to decide yourself about stopping treatment	.22	.06	−.12	.25	.18	.14	.05	.62	.20	.24	.62
To be able to oppose every attempt at invasive treatment	.16	.28	−.04	.02	.06	.13	−.06	.65	.17	.23	.75
To have the possibility of indicating firmly your treatment preferences*	.25	.10	−.06	.22	−.01	.06	.06	.60	.12	.34	.74
To be able to be alone from time to time	.03	.17	.09	−.05	.22	.23	−.03	.60	.05	.16	
To be able still to get angry if you are mistreated in any way	.29	.06	−.14	.14	.06	.28	.15	.56	.04	.26	
Always to have very clear information about your condition*	.12	.23	−.07	.09	.22	.05	.10	.41	.18	.34	.60
Being at peace with significant others											
To have resolved all conflicts with those close to you*	.18	.05	.06	.24	.06	.21	.02	−.06	.70	.19	.81

(continued)

Table 1 Results of the Exploratory Factor Analysis Conducted on the 60 Items (Study 1, First Sub-Sample). Results of the Confirmatory Factor Analysis Conducted on the 30 Items (Study 1, Second Sub-Sample). Results of the Confirmatory Factor Analysis Conducted on the 24 Items (Study 2) (continued)

Items	Exploratory Factor Analysis (60 items)										CFA (30 items)	CFA (24 items)
	I	II	III	IV	V	VI	VII	VIII	IX	X		
To have been forgiven by persons whom you might have wronged during your life	.10	−.07	.14	.24	−.03	.14	.04	.21	.57	−.05	.76	.93
To be able to forgive all the persons who wronged you during your life	.20	.09	.20	−.12	.05	.07	.03	.16	.70	.22	.88	.90
To know that your death will not result in big problems for your descendants	.16	.10	.14	−.05	.07	.07	.07	.12	.79	.12		
To be able to talk to a physician about your fears and anxieties*	.21	.03	.12	−.11	.06	.05	.07	.12	.77	.21		
To have been able to have a positive discussion with persons with whom you had been in conflict	.16	.01	.07	.22	.04	.18	.04	.05	.72	.04		
Benefiting appropriate care												
To be able to obtain adequate pain treatment*	.20	.19	−.11	.19	.12	.20	−.01	.16	.11	.49	.81	.31
To have a physician who knows how to listen to you*	.15	.05	.08	.14	.14	.00	.08	.16	.21	.76	.77	.86
To have a competent physician*	.18	.02	.02	.21	.12	.07	.09	.16	.11	.78	.71	.97
To have a physician to whom you can say anything*	.14	.27	.13	.05	.17	−.13	.10	.11	.14	.55		
To be able to oppose any attempt to perform euthanasia without your request	.26	.09	.19	−.02	.13	.14	−.03	.26	.08	.62		
To have caregivers you trust*	.21	.04	.04	−.08	.25	.10	.07	.25	.10	.67		
Explained variance	4.73	3.84	3.25	3.92	3.60	2.65	2.92	3.43	4.51	4.08		
Percent of explained variance	.08	.06	.05	.07	.06	.04	.05	.06	.08	.07		

*Items that were borrowed or directly inspired from Steinhauser et al. (2000a).

108

The ninth factor, which explained 8% of the variance, was named *Being at peace with significant others* since it loaded positively on items expressing the wish that one's death would not be too dramatic for others and the wish to reconcile with estranged others before dying (e.g., being able to solve all remaining conflicts with others). The mean values for the items loading on this factor ranged from 3.58 to 4.74; that is, they corresponded to the "important" level.

Finally, the tenth factor, which explained 7% of the variance, was called *Benefiting from appropriate medical care* since it loaded positively on items expressing concerns about good medical care and trust in the caring personnel (e.g., having an understanding doctor, obtaining adequate pain relief). The mean values for the items loading on this factor ranged from 5.23 to 6.17; that is, they were intermediate between "very important" and "very, very important."

Confirmatory Factor Analyses

A confirmatory analysis was then conducted on the second half of the sample ($N = 483$). The model tested was a correlated 10-factor model. Owing to the great number of factors, only three items for each factor, the ones with the highest loadings in the exploratory analysis and with clearly different meaning, were introduced in the model. All the path coefficients were significant. The indices of fit were judged satisfactory: CFI = .91, RMR = .06, RMSEA = .061 [.057 – .065], $Chi^2/df = 1018/361 = 2.81$.

Analyses of Variance

For each of the 10 factors, an overall score was computed by averaging the scores of the corresponding three items retained in the model. These overall scores, computed over the entire sample, ranged from 3.44 to 5.43, evidencing differences in level of importance as a function of the type of end of life preference considered, $F(9,8676) = 300.09, p < .001$.

A MANOVA with an Age × Gender, 4 × 2 design was conducted on the 10 series of scores. In view of the great number of analyses done in Study 1, the significance threshold was set at .001. The effect of age was significant, $R(30,2783) = 10.85$, $p < .001$. The effect of gender was also significant, $R(10,948) = 19.13, p < .001$. Subsequently, a series of ANOVAs with an Age × Gender, 4 × 2 design were conducted, one for each series of scores.

As we wanted to examine the effect of educational level, independently of age and gender, a MANCOVA with an Educational level, 4 design, was conducted on the 10 series of scores. Covariates were age and gender. The effect of educational level was significant, $R(30,2789) = 4.64, p < .001$. Subsequently, a series of 10 ANCOVAs with an Educational level, 4 design, were conducted, one for each series of scores. Covariates were age and gender.

As we also wanted to examine the effect of religious involvement, independently of age and gender, a MANCOVA with a Religious involvement, 3 design, was conducted on the 10 series of scores. Covariates were age and gender. The effect of religious involvement was significant, $R(20,1902) = 35.96$, $p < .001$. Subsequently, a series of 10 ANCOVAs with a

Religious involvement, 3 design, were conducted, one for each series of scores. Covariates were age and gender.

As regards the *Leaving one's affairs in order* factor, the effect of age was significant, $F(3,957) = 18.75, p < .001$. The older the participant, the higher the *Leaving one's affairs in order* score (from 3.58 to 4.43). The effect of educational level was also significant, $F(3,959) = 5.86, p < .001$. The higher the educational level, the lower the *Leaving one's affairs in order* score (from 3.64 to 4.31).

As regards the *Feeling at peace with God* factor, the effect of age was significant, $F(3,957) = 18.70, p < .001$: the older the participant, the higher the *Feeling at peace with God* score (from 3.17 to 4.24). The effect of gender was also significant, $F(1,957) = 27.77, p < .001$. The females' score (3.78) was higher than the males' (3.08). The effect of religious involvement was also significant, $F(2,960) = 325.66, p < .001$. The higher the religious involvement, the higher the *Feeling at peace with God* score (from 2.20 to 5.26).

As regards the *Feeling of accomplishment* factor, the effect of age was significant, $F(3,957) = 22.77, p < .001$. The older the participant, the lower the *Feeling of accomplishment* score (from 5.77 to 4.99). The effect of educational level was also significant, $F(3,959) = 8.82, p < .001$. The higher the educational level, the higher the *Feeling of accomplishment* score (from 5.06 to 5.66).

As regards the *Remaining able to oppose unwanted treatments* factor, the effect of age was significant, $F(3,957) = 17.73$, $p < .001$. The older the participant, the lower the *Remaining able to oppose unwanted treatments* score (from 5.26 to 4.59). The effect of gender was also significant, $F(1,957) = 83.45$, $p < .001$. The females' score (5.40) was higher than the males' (4.68). The effect of religious involvement was also significant, $F(2,960) = 27.74, p < .001$. The higher the religious involvement, the lower the *Remaining able to oppose unwanted treatments* score (from 5.49 to 4.70).

As regards the *Keeping close to loved ones* factor, the effect of age was significant, $F(3,957) = 7.60, p < .001$. The older the participant, the lower the *Keeping close to loved ones* (from 5.42 to 4.87). The effect of gender was also significant, $F(1,957) = 100.21, p < .001$: the females' score (5.73) was higher than the males' (4.76). The age × gender interaction was significant, $F(3,957) = 7.23, p < .001$. The male-female difference was higher among younger participants than it was among older participants.

As regards the *Benefiting from appropriate medical care* factor, the effect of gender was significant, $F(1,957) = 76.09$, $p < .001$. The females' score (5.64) was higher than the males' (4.97). Finally, as regards the *Being at peace with significant others* factor, the effect of gender was significant, $F(1,957) = 21.75, p < .001$. The females' score (4.53) was higher than the males' (4.01).

Discussion

Study 1 was aimed at structuring the many conditions and situations people in general would like to find at the moment of their own death. The first hypothesis, based on AMT (Apter, 2001, 2007) and on previous work by Steinhauser et al. (2000a) and

Kuhl (2002), was that a complex structure should be evidenced, and that this structure should be comprised of factors consistent with AMT. This is what was found, except that only seven of the hypothesized factors were evidenced, and that several of these factors—conformist, autic sympathy, and autic mastery—were found in different versions. One version of the conformist factor had a strong religious orientation. It mainly involved being at peace with God. The other version of the conformist factor had no religious orientation. It mainly involved being at peace with oneself for having accomplished one's duty in life. One version of the autic sympathy factor involved the immediate family, and the other version involved the care giving personnel (doctors and nurses). One version of the autic mastery factor involved the level of personal autonomy and the other version involved respect from others and dignity.

In view of the very particular situation studied here, these results make sense. Some people are very religious and other people are not. The emergence of two different conformist factors (feeling personal accomplishment and being at peace with God) expresses this differentiation between participants. Also, in the hospital the nursing personnel assume some of the functions the family assumed before the hospitalization. The emergence of two different autic sympathy factors (keeping close to loved ones and benefiting appropriate care) expresses this differentiation in roles. As for the autic mastery-type factors, at the time of dying, the person's attention is logically centered on the body, hence the occurrence of two autic mastery factor, one that refers to the body (keeping enough autonomy) and the other that refers to the environment (inspiring respect). In addition, it was shown through confirmatory factor analysis that this factor structure, although more complex than expected, was robust.

Practically all these factors of conditions and situations were considered as important ones. Except for religious conformity, the mean score was located between "important" and "extremely important." In decreasing order of importance, people in general would, at the moment of their death, like: to have a competent and understanding doctor, able to free them from pain; to be at peace with themselves; to remain conscious and autonomous; to keep a sense of humor; to remain able to oppose any decision taken without their consent; to remain an object of love until the last moment; to remain a reference for others until the last moment; to have resolved past conflicts with others; to leave their businesses and finances in good order; and to find themselves at peace with God.

The second hypothesis was that gender would positively impact autic sympathy and alloic sympathy scores. This is what was observed. Among females, being in the company of family members was considered as "very, very important" and having resolved past conflicts was considered as intermediate between "important" and "very important." Among males theses conditions were considered as "very important" and "important," respectively. In addition, as regards the keeping close to loved ones scores, gender differences were considerably reduced among older persons. No significant difference between males and females was observed in being at peace with oneself scores. Unexpectedly, however, females were more negativist (opposing others' decisions) than males; it is possible that, in general,

women find it more difficult than do men to get their family and caretakers to comply with their wishes.

The third hypothesis was that educational level would positively impact telic and negativism scores. This was not observed. In fact, the more educated persons were less concerned about leaving their affairs in order than the less educated persons. Possibly they had been more able to foresee their end and had time already to put their affairs in order. On the other hand, a positive relationship was observed between educational level and being at peace with oneself scores. The most educated considered being at peace with oneself as intermediate between "very important" and "very, very important."

The fourth hypothesis was that religious involvement would have a positive impact on conformity scores. The results supported this hypothesis. Among the more religious persons, being at peace with one's God was considered as slightly more than "very important." Among the less religious persons, this was considered as "not very important." In addition an effect of religious involvement was also found on negativist scores. Among the more religious persons, being able to oppose any decision taken without one's consent was considered as intermediate between "important" and "very important." Among the less religious persons, this was considered as "very, very important."

Several differences linked with age also deserve comments. Age positively impacted being at peace with God scores. Among the older group, being at peace with one's God was considered as intermediate between "important" and "very important." For being at peace with oneself scores, however, the observed impact was in the reverse direction, even though, among the older group, being at peace with oneself was still considered as "very important." Unexpectedly, age had a positive impact on leaving one's business in order scores, and a negative impact on remaining able to oppose unwanted treatment scores, and keeping close to loved ones scores. The latter is consistent with findings showing that older persons are more willing than younger persons to defer health care decisions to the experts (e.g., Ligneau-Hervé, Mullet, & Sorum, 2004) and with the fact that, as people age, their circle of close relatives and friends tends to become more and more reduced.

Study 2

Study 2 was aimed at testing the robustness of the model found in Study 1 and at comparing the responses given by people in general and by persons whose doctors had told them their condition was terminal. A reduced questionnaire of 24 items was devised, drawn from the items used in Study 1. For the sake of brevity and in deference to those with terminal conditions, only eight factors were retained, and each factor was represented by only three items. The keeping enough autonomy factor was not included because its items (e.g., being connected to a machine) where, after discussion with the nursing staff, judged as potentially upsetting to patients who knew their life was really at an end. Also, to shorten the questionnaire further, the conformity questions were restricted to those about religious conformity.

Method

Participants

The sample was composed of 81 non-paid participants (39 females and 42 males) recruited on a voluntary basis. They were aged 24 to 97. Their mean age was 65.51 years ($SD = 16.94$). They were all hospital patients. Forty-six participants had not completed secondary education and 35 had completed at least secondary education. Thirty-three participants were married or living with a regular partner, 10 were divorced, 25 were widowed, and the others were single or did not answer. Twenty-two participants declared they did not believe in God, 37 believed in God but did not attend church on a regular basis, and 22 did attend church on a regular basis.

Participants were contacted in the hospital through sessions of information about cares, treatments, and cancer. The investigator was a licensed psychologist who was also a registered nurse. She solicited 107 patients, telling them that the research team was conducting a survey on the conditions in which people would like be at the time of death. She showed them either some sample questions or the first page of the questionnaire. Seventy-six percent of the people contacted agreed to participate in the study. The main reasons for refusing to participate were tiredness and the fear to meet with a psychologist.

Material

The questionnaire was composed of 24 items that covered the eight domains that were selected. As in Study 1, responses were given on a 7-point scale ranging from not important to extremely important. Additional questions concerned demographical data.

Procedure

Each participant responded individually. After they agreed to participate in the study and gave written informed consent, the investigator immediately conducted the survey. Forty-three participants were presented the items in one order and 38 participants were presented the items in the reverse order. No time limit was imposed.

Results

As in Study 1, each rating by each participant was converted to a numerical value expressing the distance between the chosen point on the response scale and the left anchor. These numerical values were then subjected to graphical and statistical analyses.

Confirmatory Factor Analyses

A confirmatory analysis was conducted on the whole sample. The model tested was the correlated 8-factor model that is shown in Table 1 (right column). All the path coefficients were significant. The indices of fit were judged satisfactory: CFI = .92, RMR = .08, RMSEA = .069 [.050 – .088], $Chi^2/df = 364/224 = 1.62$.

Analyses of Variance

For each of the eight factors, an overall score was computed by averaging the scores of the corresponding three items in the model. These overall scores, computed over the entire sample, ranged from 2.60 to 4.88, evidencing differences in level of importance as a function of the kind of need considered, $F(7,560) = 22.13$, $p < .001$.

As we wanted to examine the effect associated with the current health status of the participants, independently of the effect of age, gender, educational level, and religious involvement, a MANCOVA with Sample (Study 1 versus Study 2) as the independent factor was conducted on the eight series of scores. The whole sample considered in Study 1 was used. Covariates were age, gender, educational level, and religious involvement. In view of the great number of analyses, the significance threshold was set at .001. The effect of Sample was significant, $R(8,1030) = 58.22$, $p < .001$. Subsequently, a series of eight ANCOVAs with Sample (Study 1 versus Study 2) as the independent factor was conducted on each of the eight series of scores. Covariates were age, gender, educational level, and religious involvement. Results are shown in Table 2.

For two factors—*Remaining able to oppose unwanted treatment* and *Being at peace with significant others*—scores were significantly higher among participants who knew their death was temporally close than among the other participants, $F(1,1040) = 34.48$ and 21.36, respectively, $p < .001$. Among those who knew their death was temporally close, being able to oppose any unwanted treatment was judged as "very important" (4.82), and being able to resolve all past conflicts with others was judged as intermediate between "important" and "very important." Among the other participants, they were judged as only "important."

For two other factors—*Keeping close to loved ones* and *Inspiring respect*—there was no differences between the two groups; that is, knowing their life was in danger did not change the importance given to remaining an object of love until the last moment or remaining a reference for others as long as possible.

For the four remaining factors—*Leaving one's affairs in order, Enjoying life until the last moment, Being at peace with God,* and *Benefiting appropriate medical care*—scores were significantly lower among participants who knew their death was temporally close than among the other participants, $F(1,1040) = 108.44, 109.95, 59.16,$ and 45.88 respectively, $p < .001$. Among the participants who knew their death was temporally close, leaving one's affairs in order, keeping a sense of humor, and being at peace with one's God were judged as intermediate between "not very important" and "somewhat important." Having competent and understanding caregivers was judged as intermediate between "important" and "very important."

Discussion

The conditions in which people with a known terminal disease would prefer to end their lives represent the same wide assortment of motivations regarding the conditions they want in place when they die as found in people in general. In decreasing order of importance, people suffering from a terminal illness would, at the moment of their death, like to:

a. keep close to loved ones and to remain an object of love until the last moment;

b. remain able to oppose any decision taken without their consent, any unwanted treatment;

Table 2 Differences in Mean Score between Healthy Adults and Terminally Ill Patients for the Eight Preference Factors (from Table 1)

Factor	Motivational Type	Sample Type		$F(1,1040)$	p
		Adults	Dying Patients		
Leaving one's affairs in order	Telic	4.15	2.73	108.44	.001
Enjoying life until the last moment	Paratelic	4.62	2.82	109.95	.001
Feeling at peace with God	Religious conformity	4.00	2.59	59.16	.001
Remaining able to oppose unwanted treatment	Negativism	4.06	4.82	34.48	.001
Keeping close to loved ones	Autocentric sympathy	5.45	4.88	0.10	ns
Benefiting appropriate care	Autocentric sympathy	5.67	4.58	45.88	.001
Inspiring respect	Autocentric mastery	4.35	4.33	0.38	ns
Being at peace with significant others	Allocentric sympathy	4.03	4.51	21.36	.001

c. have a competent and understanding doctor, able to free them from pain;

d. to have resolved past conflicts with others;

e. to keep inspiring respect and remain a reference for others until the last moment;

f. to keep a sense of humor;

g. to leave their businesses and finances in good order; and

h. to find themselves at peace with God.

Practically all these end of life conditions were considered as important, which is consistent with the findings of previous studies (e.g., Kuhl, 2002; Steinhauser et al., 2000a, 2000b).

Differences were, however, found between Study 1 and Study 2 as regards the importance of each type of motivation. In particular, people who know they are dying are more concerned than others in keeping control of their manner of dying, namely by preventing unwanted treatments. They are more concerned also to make sure their past conflicts with others are resolved; they appear to want to set their corner of the world right before they die.

General Discussion

These two studies demonstrated: that people have a wide range of ideas about how they would want to die; that the relative importance of these ideas differs in an interpretable way according to age, gender, educational level, and religiosity; and that the relative importance of these ideas is different for people with terminal illnesses. The greater understanding of what constitutes a "good death" provided by our findings—and by the ways in which the groups differ—are of importance to clinicians, to those close to dying people, and to policy makers.

What then is added by organizing the responses to the questions into factors and by categorizing the factors in accordance

with AMT? First, the discovery through the factor analysis of 10 factors that can be described coherently by the psychological categories proposed by the theory supports the view that the viewpoints on end of life preferences corresponding to these factors are largely independent. In other words, when considering the importance for a dying person of, for example, leaving one's affairs in order, feeling at peace with significant others, and inspiring respect, we are not considering three times the same aspect of end of life preferences in different guises but are really considering three different, empirically separable aspects. In other words, the taxonomy that is offered is not redundant. Second, the appearance of most of Apter's categories support the view that most (if not all) important factors regarding end of life preferences have been considered. In addition, the complexity of this motivational structure is consistent with Schroepfer's (2006) suggestion that motivating factors that may, at first glance, appear as unitary factors (such as the family), must be considered under different perspectives: the family as a provider of love and psychological support (keeping close to loved ones) and the family as a receiver of love and psychological support (being at peace with significant others).

Third, this taxonomy may be useful for the family and for the care giving personnel in their daily contacts with dying persons, as well as for the persons in charge of the hospital in their effort to provide the best possible environment to their patients. This complete and non-redundant taxonomy may serve as a basis for checking whether all important factors of end of life preferences have been considered. Accordingly, each person approaching a dying person may want to ask herself a limited but comprehensive set of questions, such as the following. As a close relative of this person, have I done everything possible to allow this person to finish any project considered as important or to reassure her that the project will be pursued by somebody else? Have I done everything possible to allow this person to enjoy her last moments in life (e.g., through conversations, lectures, or good TV programs); to oppose unwanted decisions or unwanted encounters; to make her will known and respected by her care givers; to feel loved despite her present health state and her possible changes in appearance; to feel that she has been important for her various relatives, friends, and colleagues and that she is still a point of reference for others? Have I done everything possible to resolve my own personal conflicts with this person and to help her to feel forgiven by the persons she may have hurt in the past? As a member of the care giving staff, have I done everything possible to give this person some privacy; to allow her to meet with a pastor or a priest and with other people of importance to her; to know and respect her will concerning care and treatment; and to alleviate her suffering?

Directors of hospitals and long-term care facilities can use this taxonomy to create an environment and a care giving staff that are responsive to all their dying patients' preferences. Researchers can use it to create an instrument for measuring the extent to which terminally ill people are satisfied with their care and environment from the different viewpoints evidenced in the present study (see Schroepfer, 2006). They can also use this instrument to compare the effectiveness of different medical settings in satisfying the needs and desires of terminally ill patients, to compare the effects of different programs, and to assess the needs of different groups of people (Duffy et al., 2006, Higginson, 2005; McFarland & Rhoades, 2006; Steinhauser, 2005).

References

Apter, M. J. (Ed.). (2001). *Motivational styles in everyday life: A guide to reversal theory.* Washington, DC: American Psychological Association.

Apter, M. J. (2007). *Reversal theory: The dynamic of motivation, emotion and personality.* Oxford: Oneworld Publications.

Chochinov, H. M., Hack, T., Hassard, T., Kristjanson, L. J., McClement, S., & Harlos, M. (2002). Dignity in the terminally ill: A cross-sectional, cohort study. *Lancet, 360,* 2026–2030.

Cottencin, A., Mullet, E., & Sorum, P. C. (2006). Consulting an alternative practitioner: A systematic inventory of motives. *Journal of Alternative and Complementary Medicine, 12,* 791–798.

Duffy, S. A., Ronis, D., Fowler, K., Myers Schim, S., & Jackson, F. C. (2006). Differences in veterans' and nonveterans' end-of-life preferences: A pilot study. *Journal of Palliative Medicine, 9,* 1099–1105.

Ferris, F. D., von Gunten, C. F., & Emanuel, L. L. (2003). Competency in end-of-life care: Last hours of life. *Journal of Palliative Medicine, 6,* 605–613.

Heilman, M. E., & Chen, J. J. (2005). Same behavior, different consequences: Reactions to men's and women's altruistic citizenship behavior. *Journal of Applied Psychology, 90,* 431–441.

Higginson, I. J. (2005). End-of-life care: Lessons from other nations. *Journal of Palliative Medicine, 8,* s161–s173.

Jayawardena, K. M., & Liao, S. (2006). Elder abuse at end of life. *Journal of Palliative Medicine, 9,* 127–136.

Kapo, J., Morrison, L. J., & Liao, S. (2007). Palliative care for the older adult. *Journal of Palliative Medicine, 10,* 185–209.

Kuhl, D. (2002). *What dying people want: Practical wisdom for the end of life.* Toronto: PublicAffairs.

Ligneau-Hervé, C., Mullet, E., & Sorum, P. C. (2004). Age and medication acceptance. *Experimental Aging Research, 30,* 253–273.

Makris, I., & Mullet, E. (2009). A systematic inventory of motives for becoming an orchestra conductor: A preliminary study. *Psychology of Music.*

McFarland, K. F., & Rhoades, D. R. (2006). End-of-life care: A retreat format for residents. *Journal of Palliative Medicine, 9,* 82–89.

Pierson, C. M., Curtis, J. R., & Patrick, D. L. (2002). A good death: A qualitative study of patients with advanced AIDS. *AIDS Care, 14,* 587–598.

Plonk, W. M., & Arnold, R. M. (2005). Terminal care: The last weeks of life. *Journal of Palliative Medicine, 8,* 1042–1054.

Rankin, M. A., Donahue, M. P., Davis, K., Katseres, J. L., Wedig, J. A., Johnson, M., et al. (1998). Dignified dying as a nursing outcome. *Outcomes Management for Nursing Practice, 2,* 105–110.

Schroepfer, T. A. (2006). Mind frames towards dying and factors motivating their adoption by terminally ill elders. *Journal of Gerontology: Social Sciences, 61B,* S129–S139.

Singer, P. A., Martin, D. K., & Kelner, M. (1999). Quality end-of-life: Patients' perspectives. *Journal of the American Medical Association, 281,* 163–168.

Steinhauser, K. E., Christakis, N. A., Clipp, E. C., McNeilly, M., McIntyre, L., & Tulsky, J. A. (2000a). Factors considered important at the end of life by patients, family, physicians and other care providers. *Journal of the American Medical Association, 284,* 2476–2482.

Steinhauser, K. E., Clipp, E. C., McNeilly, M., Christakis, N. A., McIntyre, L., & Tulsky, J. A. (2000b). In search of a good death: Observations of patients, families and providers. *Annals of Internal Medicine, 132,* 825–831.

Steinhauser, K. E. (2005). Measuring end-of-life outcomes prospectively. *Journal of Palliative Medicine, 8,* s30–s41.

Vig, E. K., Davenport, N. A., & Pearlman, R. A. (2002). Good deaths, bad deaths, and preferences for the need of life: A qualitative study of geriatric outpatients. *Journal of the American Geriatric Society, 50,* 1541–1548.

Volker, D. L., Kahn, D., & Penticuff, J. H. (2004). Patient control and end-of-life care Part II: The patient perspective. *Oncology Nursing Forum, 31,* 954–960.

von Gunten, C. F. (2005). Interventions to manage symptoms at the end of life. *Journal of Palliative Medicine, 8,* s88–s94.

West, H. F., Engelberg, R. A., Wenrich, M. D., & Curtis, J. R. (2005). Expressions of nonabandonment during the intensive care unit family conference. *Journal of Palliative Medicine, 8,* 797–807.

Mind Frames towards Dying and Factors Motivating Their Adoption by Terminally Ill Elders

Objectives. This study was designed to advance the understanding of the physical and psychosocial factors that motivate terminally ill elders not only to consider a hastened death but also *not* to consider such a death.

Methods. I conducted face-to-face in-depth qualitative interviews with 96 terminally ill elders. An inductive approach was taken to locating themes and patterns regarding factors motivating terminally ill elders to consider or not to consider hastening death.

Results. Six mind frames towards dying emerged: (a) neither ready nor accepting; (b) not ready but accepting; (c) ready and accepting; (d) ready, accepting, and wishing death would come; (e) considering a hastened death but having no specific plan; and (f) considering a hastened death with a specific plan. From the data emerged approaches towards dying and accompanying emotions characterizing each mind frame, as well as factors motivating their adoption by elders. The results showed that psychosocial factors served more often than physical factors as motivators.

Discussion. The results demonstrate the importance of assessing the mind frame adopted by a terminally ill elder and his or her level of satisfaction with it. Terminally ill elders may experience a higher quality dying process when a traditional medical care approach is replaced by a holistic approach that addresses physical, spiritual, emotional, and social needs.

TRACY A. SCHROEPFER

A national mandate has been put forth to improve the comfort or palliative care provided to terminally ill individuals. This mandate is particularly relevant to Americans older than age 65, whose numbers have tripled in the 20th century and who have experienced a significant increase in their life expectancy (Hetzel & Smith, 2001). Elders now experience the greatest number of deaths in the United States (Arias, 2003), deaths that are often of poor quality. Research has shown that American elders experience severe pain in their dying process (Bernabei et al., 1998; SUPPORT Investigators, 1997), are undermedicated for their pain (Bernabei et al.; Cleeland et al., 1994), receive health care at odds with their end-of-life preferences (SUPPORT Investigators), experience psychosocial suffering (Chochinov et al., 2002; Pessin, Rosenfeld, & Breitbart, 2002), and experience existential suffering (Black & Rubinstein, 2004). These poor-quality dying experiences have contributed to the demand for the legalization of physician-assisted death, a demand that has raised ethical concerns and has led to research on the number of individuals requesting this option and the factors motivating them to do so. Knowledge of these factors serves to inform and guide health care practitioners in their quest to improve palliative care. It can also be argued, however, that knowledge of the factors that contribute to a quality dying process such that terminally ill individuals are motivated *not* to consider a hastened death is also essential to providing quality palliative care. This latter avenue of research has received little, if any, attention. The purpose of this article is to advance the understanding of physical and psychosocial factors that motivate terminally ill elders not only to consider a hastened death but also not to consider such a death.

Current Findings Regarding the Consideration to Hasten Death

Two types of studies emerge from a review of the literature on the consideration to hasten death: retrospective and prospective. Retrospective studies ask physicians, nurses, social workers, or survivors of the deceased to write case studies or answer surveys concerning the motivating factors cited by now-deceased patients who had considered or requested physician-assisted death prior to their death. Prospective studies interview a mix of individuals with a terminal illness (an illness likely to result in death) and people who have been defined as terminally ill (having fewer than six months to live) and ask whether they have considered hastening their death and, if so, their reasons for doing so.

Retrospective case study results have found that psychosocial factors play a more significant role than physical factors as motivators of a hastened death. Health care professionals have reported psychosocial factors that include a decreased ability to participate in activities that made life enjoyable (Chin, Hedberg, Higginson, & Fleming, 1999; Oregon Department of Human Services [ODHS], 2000, 2001, 2002, 2003), fear of future pain (Chin et al.; ODHS, 2000, 2001, 2002, 2003; Volker, 2001) or of uncontrollable symptoms, loss of meaning in life (Meier et al., 1998), the feeling that one is a burden (Back, Wallace, Starks, & Pearlman, 1996; Meier et al.; ODHS, 2001, 2002, 2003), loss of dignity (Back et al.; Meier et al.), loss of autonomy (Chin et al.; ODHS, 2000, 2001, 2002, 2003), loss of control over bodily functions (Back et al.; Chin et al.; ODHS, 2000, 2001, 2002, 2003) and over manner of death (ODHS, 2000; Volker), and loss of control in general (Back et al.). These studies reported neither depression nor religiosity, factors often discussed in relation to hastening death, as significant factors. Only two studies (Back et al.; Meier et al.) reported evidence of pain as a motivator.

Two retrospective studies that employed a quantitative approach also found that psychosocial factors were key motivators of the consideration to hasten death; they did not find pain to be a significant factor (Ganzini et al., 2002; Jacobson et al., 1995). Hospice nurses and social workers reported that a desire to control the circumstances of death, the wish to die at home, the feeling that living was pointless, and a loss of dignity were most often discussed by patients desiring a hastened death (Ganzini et al.).

Quantitative prospective studies support the importance of psychosocial factors and provide evidence of the role physical factors play in the consideration to hasten death. These studies found that patients with a terminal illness or who were terminally ill were not likely to attend church (Breitbart et al., 1996) or to be religious (Breitbart et al.; Emanuel, Fairclough, Daniels, & Clarridge, 1996), had few social supports (Breitbart et al.), experienced a low quality of social support (Arnold, 2004; Breitbartet al., 1996; Chochinov et al., 1995), and perceived their caregiving needs as high (Emanuel, Fairclough, & Emanuel, 2000). Emotionally, these patients reported a higher level of anxiety, a lower level of hope (Arnold) and a higher level of depression (Arnold; Breitbart et al.; Chochinov et al., 1995; Emanuel et al.) than did those individuals not considering a hastened death. Results regarding the role of pain were mixed. Three studies found that pain was not significantly related to the consideration to hasten death (Breitbart et al.; Chochinov et al., 1995; Emanuel et al., 1996), but two later studies found it to be a significant predictor (Arnold; Emanuel et al., 2000). These prospective studies did not measure loss of control.

The only qualitative study on the consideration to hasten death that could be located was conducted by Lavery, Boyle, Dickens, Maclean, and Singer (2001) on patients with HIV-1 or AIDS. According to this study, two major themes developed from discussions with participants considering a hastened death. The first theme involved a sense of disintegration, which resulted from the multiple symptoms and loss of bodily functions that eventually led participants to a dependency on others and a loss of dignity. The second theme, loss of community, reflected the lack of contact these individuals had with others. Participants also reported that the result of experiencing disintegration and loss of community was a perceived loss of self.

Much can be learned from these studies that can be used to guide health care practitioners in their quest to improve end-of-life care. Loss of self, dignity, and autonomy; loss of control over bodily functions and manner of death; lack of enjoyment and meaning in life; lower quantity and quality of social support; lack of hope; and higher levels of anxiety and depression are all key psychosocial factors that motivate some terminally ill individuals to consider hastening their death. Although pain was a significant predictor of hastening death in only two studies, fear of future pain or uncontrollable suffering surfaced as a key factor in most studies. Clearly, some individuals who are not suffering in the present fear they will be suffering at some point in the future.

Addressing Current Limitations

Although current empirical evidence regarding the factors that motivate terminally ill individuals to consider hastening their death has provided insight into this issue, three major limitations exist that need to be addressed. First, the considerable research on hastening death described in the preceding section was conducted retrospectively (either with physicians or survivors) or prospectively (with patients who had a terminal illness). Studies conducted with physicians or survivors result in second-hand information that may not provide an accurate record of patients' motivating factors. Although prospective studies do provide firsthand information, they too are problematic. Some patients with a terminal illness may be in the early stages of their illness and so are being asked to speculate about whether they would consider hastening death before death becomes imminent; in the later stages of their illness, their feelings may change. Prospective studies that include only terminally ill individuals are the most likely to provide the information necessary to understand the motivating factors for considering a hastened death.

Second, the main approach taken in research on considering a hastened death has been to measure quantitatively factors presumed to be key motivators, such as pain and depression. This approach has provided important information and should be continued. However, due to the current lack of information on the motivating factors for considering a hastened death, it may also be useful to step back and take a more open-ended approach to this research. The qualitative method is not constrained by what has been hypothesized; it allows for the exploration of the individual's reasoning regarding his or her consideration to hasten or not to hasten death, and it allows one to discover the unknown. As evidenced in the literature review above, this method has rarely been used. Continuing to limit research in this manner may result in crucial factors remaining undetected, unaddressed, and not well understood.

Third, the lack of attention given to studying the factors that motivate terminally ill individuals not to consider hastening their death may limit the understanding of factors key to a quality dying experience. The current approach of focusing on the factors motivating the consideration to hasten death assumes that such information provides all the knowledge necessary for improving palliative care. Extending this approach to include asking individuals what it is about their dying process that keeps them from considering a hastened death can also serve to inform palliative care.

The current study addresses each of these three limitations. I used a prospective qualitative approach, sampled only elders who had fewer than six months to live, and examined the factors motivating the consideration not to hasten death in addition to factors motivating the consideration to hasten death.

Methods
Sample
The selection criteria for the study were threefold. Respondents had to (a) be 50 years of age or older; (b) be deemed mentally competent by their physician, nurse, or social worker; and (c) have been given a prognosis by a physician of 6 months or less to live. I initially set the age selection criterion at 60 years or older in order to coincide with typical age definitions of elders. Six months into the study, however, I lowered the criterion to 50 years or older in order to obtain a sufficient number of male participants so that I could examine gender differences.

I used purposive sampling. I contacted hospices, hospital-based inpatient palliative care programs, and hospital-based outpatient clinics caring for the terminally ill throughout Michigan in hopes of obtaining a population that varied with regard to race, education, and occupation. Of the 17 programs contacted, 10 agreed to participate: 2 palliative care programs, 2 hospital outpatient clinics, and 6 hospices. Ninety-six terminally ill elders were approached by either a social worker or a nurse regarding the study, and all agreed to participate.

Participating elders ranged in age from 51 to 98 ($M = 73.5$). The majority of elders were White (84.4%), 15.6% were Black, and a little more than half were married (52.1%). Elders were quite varied in their religious preferences: Catholic (19.8%), Methodist (14.6%), Baptist (15.6%), other Protestant religions (35.4%), Jewish (2.1%), and no religious preference (12.5%). Most elders had some form of cancer (49.0%); others were diagnosed with end-stage renal disease (26.0%) or heart disease (15.6%). A small percentage (9.4%) of elders was dying of respiratory, neurological, or other diseases.

Data Collection
In face-to-face interviews, I asked respondents if they had given serious thought to hastening their death since finding out they had a serious illness that may shorten their life. If they answered no, I asked about their reasons for not considering a hastened death. If they answered yes, I asked how they were considering hastening their death and whether they were still thinking about doing so. If they were no longer considering doing so, I asked about their reasons for having once considered hastening their death, and their reasons for no longer thinking this way. If they were still considering a hastened death, I asked their reasons for thinking about doing so. All interviews were audiotaped and transcribed.

When answering these questions, respondents did not appear to construct their reality as they went along or to do so within the boundaries of hastening or not hastening death. Most respondents raised the topic on their own and began describing their mind frame towards dying prior to being asked questions regarding considering a hastened death. Although some respondents did not raise the topic and, when asked, dismissed any thought of hastening their death, their responses regarding why they would not do so were immediate and very indepth. I had the sense that they had already given the issue much thought and were simply sharing those thoughts with me.

Data Analysis
I analyzed the content of answers for themes regarding respondents' reasons for considering or not considering a hastened death: Content analysis involved "identifying" and "categorizing" the main themes and patterns found in the data (Patton, 1990, p. 381). I took an inductive method in locating these themes and patterns. That is, I did not determine the themes and patterns prior to the analysis; rather, they emerged from repeated readings of the transcripts (Patton). I used this approach to identify respondents who were considering a hastened death and those who were not considering one, as well as the psychosocial and physical factors motivating their considerations. As a reliability check, a hospice social worker independently coded the thematic areas identified, and we reached complete agreement.

Results
As was previously discussed, studies on the consideration to hasten death have traditionally assumed that terminally ill individuals face their dying in one of two ways: not considering a hastened death or considering a hastened death. I initially approached the present study operating under these same assumptions. Content analysis of the qualitative data revealed, however, that this dichotomous approach is an over-simplification of an elder's potential mind frame towards dying. No label in the death and dying literature appeared adequate to describe what evolved in the qualitative analyses, and so I chose the term *mind frame* to refer to the overall attitude or orientation an elder had adopted towards his or her dying. Six distinct mind frames towards dying emerged: (a) neither ready nor accepting; (b) not ready but accepting; (c) ready and accepting; (d) ready, accepting, and wishing death would come; (e) considering a hastened death but having no specific plan; and (f) considering a hastened death with a specific plan. Figure 1 illustrates how these six mind frames fall within the two traditional categories. Table 1 provides descriptive information regarding the elders who adopted each mind frame. I did not gather information regarding the approach or mind frame respondents had taken to previous life crises or whether past experiences influenced their current mind frame towards dying.

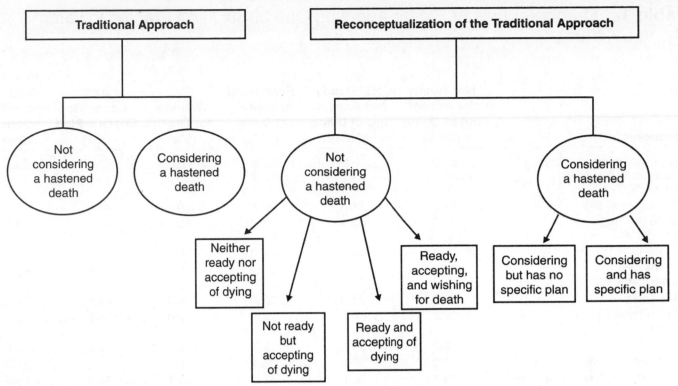

Figure 1   Traditional approach to research on considering a hastened death and a new conceptualization.

Approach Towards Dying, Accompanying Emotions, and Motivating Factors

Each mind frame towards dying that emerged from the interviews was distinguished by an approach towards dying, personal characteristics, accompanying emotions, and factors motivating the elder to adopt a particular mind frame. Motivating factors emerged from responses to the questions about the elders' reasons for either not considering or considering a hastened death. The approaches, personal characteristics, emotions, and motivating factors characterizing each mind frame are summarized in the following sections.

It is important to note that respondents did not appear to shift from one mind frame to another during their interviews. Although 15 respondents spoke of having transitioned earlier in their dying process from another mind frame (this topic will be discussed in another article), neither they nor the other respondents appeared to shift from one mind frame to another during the interview. I did not determine the reasons for this consistency; however, one could speculate that the factors motivating their adoption of a mind frame did not change during the interview process and so neither did the mind frame itself.

Mind Frame 1: Neither Ready Nor Accepting

Approach towards dying. Thirty-three elders (34%) spoke strongly about not being ready to die or willing to accept that death was imminent. Two approaches towards dying characterized this mind frame: fighting to live, and hoping or believing science would find a cure.

The predominant approach that emerged among these elders was that of fighting to live and not giving in to the disease. One 74-year-old divorced woman stated adamantly, "And I'm not ready, and I'll tell you why. They can say four months; I'm going to live longer than that." A 51-year-old man who stated emphatically, "I figure, I don't really have to die if I don't want to and I'm not going to," talked about his wife's determination and how he had adopted her attitude.

The second approach towards dying centered on the belief and hope that science would find a cure and that the elders would survive their illness. A 63-year-old elder said, "They're going to find a cure for everything I've got, and I'm going to be able to live a lot longer." This woman spoke with quiet resolve throughout the interview, as did the other respondents who spoke of a cure being found for their illness.

Personal characteristics. Respondents adopting this mind frame towards dying had a mean age of 69 and had, on average, less than a high school education. They were predominantly women (52%), White (79%), married (67%), and of the Protestant faith (70%).

Accompanying emotions. Elders who had adopted this mind frame spoke adamantly about their feelings and appeared to possess a strong will to live. They were dismissive of any questions or thoughts regarding dying. When discussing the issue of dying, they were not tearful; rather, they often showed anger or derisive humor. These elders did not view any aspect of dying as positive.

Factors motivating lack of readiness regarding dying. Elders discussed being with family, enjoying life, and

117

Table 1   Demographics of Elders Adopting One of Six Mind Frames towards Dying (N = 96)

Demographic	Not-Ready nor Accepting of Dying (34%)	Not Ready but Accepting of Dying (25%)	Ready and Accepting of Dying (16%)	Wishing for Death (6%)	Hasten Death, No Specific Plan (9%)	Hasten Death, Specific Plan (9%)
Age, in years (M)	69.3	71.9	81.3	83.2	73.8	74.0
Education, in years (M)	11.6	11.5	12.3	11.5	13.6	14.4
Gender (%)						
Female (n = 54)	51.5	58.3	66.7	50.0	44.4	66.7
Male (n = 42)	48.5	41.7	33.3	50.0	55.6	33.3
Race (%)						
Black (n = 15)	21.2	20.8	6.7	0.0	11.1	11.1
White (n = 81)	78.8	79.2	93.3	100.0	88.9	88.9
Marital status (%)						
Married (n = 50)	66.7	45.8	26.7	50.0	44.4	66.7
Not married (n = 46)	33.3	54.2	73.3	50.0	55.6	33.3
Religion (%)						
None (n = 12)	15.2	12.5	13.3	16.7	0.0	11.1
Catholic (n = 19)	15.2	25.0	33.3	16.7	11.1	11.1
Protestant (n = 63)	69.7	62.5	53.3	66.7	88.9	55.6
Jewish (n = 2)	0.0	0.0	0.0	0.0	0.0	22.0
Primary diagnosis (%)						
Cancer (n = 47)	54.5	54.2	46.7	16.7	55.6	33.3
End-stage renal disease (n = 25)	36.4	25.0	20.0	16.7	0.0	33.3
Heart disease (n = 15)	6.1	16.7	26.7	66.7	11.1	0.0
Other diseases (n = 9)	3.0	4.2	6.7	0.0	33.3	33.3

having unfinished business as the factors motivating their lack of readiness regarding dying. Family was the factor discussed most often, and many elders became tearful when talking about leaving family behind. They enjoyed being with their family and watching their children and grandchildren grow up. Some elders felt their family members still needed their help and so wanted to stay alive. Lack of acceptance by some elders who were also not ready to die was motivated by their religious beliefs or a fear of death. Most of the women and only a few men, regardless of age or race, believed that God wanted them to fight to live as long as possible: "See, I believe the good Lord is healing me . . . I'm going through a healing process now, and He's healing me every day. And as long as I feel good and have a positive attitude, that's the way it's going to be. And I really believe that I will be healed sooner or later."

Several men and one woman spoke of fearing the unknown, being alone in the grave, and being afraid that loved ones would forget them after they die. An 81-year-old widower depicted these fears clearly: "There's no future in dying. And, uh, you have to stay all alone in the grave and everything . . . If you die, uh, isn't nobody going to care anyway. They're going to forget you in less than two months." The future pictured by these elders at the time of the interview did not include their death.

Mind Frame 2: Not Ready but Accepting
Approach towards dying. Of the 96 persons interviewed, 24 elders (25%) indicated they were not ready to die but that they had accepted the fact that they were dying. The main approach

towards dying expressed by these 24 elders was the recognition that death is natural. Although they spoke of not being ready for death, they did accept death as a natural part of life and were matter-of-fact in their approach. One 73-year-old married woman stated, "Like I say, I don't want to die, but when that time comes, if that's it, that's it." A 74-year-old never-married man took a similar approach: "Oh, I don't think much about it [dying]. I just don't, uh, dwell on that too much. It's, oh, it's just something that, it happens to everybody. It's inevitable."

Personal characteristics. Respondents who had adopted this mind frame had a mean age of 72 and had slightly less than a high school education. Almost two thirds were women (58%), slightly more than half were not married (54%), 79% were White, and 63% were Protestant.

Accompanying emotions. Elders who had adopted Mind Frame 2 appeared less adamant about their approach towards dying than did elders who had adopted Mind Frame 1. They were calm when talking about their approaching death and did not appear to be in a hurry to move on to other topics.

Factors motivating lack of readiness regarding dying. As with elders who had adopted Mind Frame 1, family and unfinished business were mentioned as motivators for lack of readiness on the part of elders who had adopted Mind Frame 2. Most elders reported that they did not want to hasten their death because they were enjoying their life. This enjoyment of life included being with family and still having the ability to take an active role in their lives.

When elders who had adopted Mind Frame 2 spoke of families, the nature of the family ties differed from those of elders who had adopted Mind Frame 1. Only a few elders discussed how their loved ones still needed them. Instead, most spoke of how the instrumental and emotional support received from family members served as a motivator not to hasten the time they had left. A 73-year-old married man stated, "They [family] care about me and will, will walk that extra mile for me." In addition, these elders were concerned about how emotionally difficult their death would be on their families. A 71-year-old married woman stated with sadness, "I guess it's going to be harder on them than on me because I won't be here . . . They've got all the mourning to do and everything."

Unfinished business, a factor reported by elders who had adopted Mind Frame 1, was also reported by elders who had adopted Mind Frame 2. The difference, however, was that unfinished business was discussed in terms of a sense of purpose or responsibility. As one 74-year-old never-married man noted, "I have taken it upon myself to decorate the graves on Memorial Day. And that's quite a job, by the way. Somebody has to decorate the family graves, and I've sort of assumed that responsibility for myself."

Factors motivating acceptance of dying. Religious beliefs, which motivated elders who had adopted Mind Frame 1 not to be accepting of their dying, were a factor cited by elders who had adopted Mind Frame 2 regarding their acceptance of dying. The beliefs of both groups of elders centered on God's will regarding their acceptance of dying, but the two groups differed in their view of what was God's will. Elders who were neither ready nor accepting of their dying defined God's will as for them to fight death. Elders who were not ready but who had accepted their dying reported that it was in God's power to decide the time of death. Although they did not feel ready to die, this latter group of elders accepted that time of death was God's will, not their decision to make, as expressed in the following statement made by a 71-year-old widow: "So I said, well, Lord, I'm just not ready to go, but if it's Your will, I will go."

Elders who had adopted Mind Frames 1 and 2 viewed death differently regarding the non-acceptance or acceptance of dying. Elders who were not accepting of their dying espoused a negative view of death that included fear of the unknown. In comparison, elders who were accepting of their dying took a matter-of-fact approach towards dying. They viewed death as inevitable and either reported not being fearful or spoke of their fear in a matter-of-fact way:

> Everybody's scared of dying, I think. It's the inescapable fact. We don't . . . everybody wants to see the sun come up. There is a certain amount of fear attached, I think. You know, even though we know that death is inevitable and it's going to happen to each and every one of us, we fear the unknown. Yeah. We fear the unknown.

Unlike elders who had adopted Mind Frame 1, the future these elders pictured did include their death.

Mind Frame 3: Ready and Accepting

Approach towards dying. Fifteen elders (16%) indicated a readiness and acceptance regarding dying. Not only did these elders talk about not being afraid to die, many saw death as the avenue to a better place than they were in at the present. One 92-year-old widow said simply, "I'm not scared to die. I know there is a better place for me." Others spoke of their belief in the goodness of God and of reunions with deceased loved ones.

The majority of these elders viewed death as a natural part of life. Some talked about how happy they would be when death finally arrived and that they were simply waiting: "I'm going to be happy when I leave this earth. I guess it's kind of a selfish attitude, but I'll be out of my misery . . . All I'm doing is just passing time. I'm just waiting for the day."

Personal characteristics. Respondents who had adopted this mind frame had a mean age of 81 and had, on average, a high school education. Two thirds of these respondents were women, three fourths were not married, 93% were White, and slightly more than half were Protestant.

Accompanying emotions. Elders with this mind frame revealed two predominant emotions towards life and death. Some elders had found peace and were enjoying the time they had left. Others had not found peace, nor were they enjoying the time they had left. These individuals were simply waiting for death to come as they no longer felt they could justify their existence.

Factors motivating readiness for dying. Enjoying life was reported by several elders when describing their readiness to die. Because it was measured in relation to the limited time the elders had remaining before dying, enjoyment of life differed between elders who had adopted Mind Frame 2 and those who had adopted Mind Frame 3. A 92-year-old widow who was ready and accepting of death stated with a smile, "Whatever God gives me, I'm willing to take."

Several elders talked about no longer enjoying life; that their lives were full of sadness; and that they felt useless, dependent, and burdensome to others. These individuals were simply waiting for death to come, as evidenced by the following 75-year-old widow's statement:

> And, uh, so I'm ready to go any time. It's hard on the family, and I'm really not living. Even here [her son's house] with my family. I get up, and they're wonderful to me, and I'm so thankful I have a place to be. But, uh, they're trying too hard, and it's putting them out . . . They say it isn't, but you know it is. But like I say, I'm ready to cash in my chips.

A few elders discussed the openness they shared with family regarding their impending death and the loving manner in which their family responded to this openness. This openness appeared to allow them to ready themselves for death by being able to make plans and express feelings they needed to express before they died. For example, an 84-year-old widow stated, "Well, they [her sons] asked me . . . what kind of funeral do I want . . . We've always talked about death very openly, because we all know it's going to happen some day to one of us. So you might as well . . . be ready."

Other elders' readiness for death was explained in terms of their age. They had lived what they felt was a long time and so were taking their impending death in stride. One widow stated, "I just figure I'm 70 years old, and you kind of expect you got to die sometime, and you got to have some kind of a disease. You know, so I just kind of put it in my stride."

Factors motivating acceptance of dying. Three motivating factors were discussed by elders who were accepting of their impending death: (a) the belief that one's time of death was God's decision and not their decision, (b) having no fear of death, and (c) the belief that dying may be better than living: The first two factors were also cited by elders who had adopted Mind Frame 2. In addition, elders who had adopted Mind Frame 3 reported being motivated by their belief that death would be better than their current state of living. One 80-year-old married woman said, "I feel, uh, that I've accepted it [dying], know what I'm saying? So, and there's worse things. Oh, yeah. There's worse things than dying. Sometimes it's worse living." Although her statement could be interpreted as a wish for death to come, when directly asked, she denied ever wishing for death.

Mind Frame 4: Ready, Accepting, and Wishing for Death

Approach towards dying. When asked if they had seriously considered hastening death, six elders (6%) were adamant that they would not consider taking any action but that they did wish death would come soon. These individuals were similar to those who had adopted Mind Frame 3 except they explicitly spoke of wishing daily for death to come. Even though each talked about how difficult life was for them, all six elders were steadfast regarding not considering a hastened death. One 93-year-old widow stated, "I wish I could go to a better place, but I will not take my own life."

Personal characteristics. Respondents who had adopted this mind frame had a mean age of 83 and had, on average, less than a high school education. Fifty percent of these respondents were women, 50% were married, 100% were White, and two thirds were Protestant.

Accompanying emotions. Elders who had adopted Mind Frame 4 demonstrated different emotions than elders who had adopted Mind Frame 3. Elders who were ready and accepting appeared peaceful or were simply waiting for death to come. Elders who were also wishing for death, however, displayed conflicting emotions regarding living and dying. At times, they laughed nervously about their situation, and at other times they spoke with great sadness, often crying. Elders who had adopted Mind Frames 3 and 4 did share feelings of uselessness and a sense that they could no longer justify their existence.

Factors motivating wish for death. Half of these elders spoke only of psychosocial reasons for wishing death to come

soon. Several elders were no longer enjoying life, and one 87-year-old woman reported feeling useless: "It's just the way I feel like it, you know, like I might as well go. What good am I anymore, you know."

Other elders also discussed physical motivators, including exhaustion and daily pain. A 90-year-old widow noted, "Sometimes I feel so rotten that I don't care anymore." Others, like this 93-year-old widow, expressed a fear of future suffering as a reason for wishing death to come: "My first husband, he suffered a long time. He had on those machines, and I used to say, 'God,' I said, 'don't let me go under those machines.' "

Factors motivating against the consideration to hasten death. When these elders were asked why they had never moved beyond wishing for death to considering hastening it, two factors emerged. The first was the belief that the time of one's death was God's decision, as demonstrated by a married 84-year-old man's statement: "I leave that [dying] up to the good Lord, and He'll take you when He wants you." The other factor was family. Elders talked about the love and support of their family and friends, as well as wanting to protect them from the pain that their suicide would bring.

Mind Frame 5: Considering a Hastened Death but Having No Specific Plan

Approach towards dying. The approach nine elders (9%) took towards dying was to consider hastening their death. However, although they were considering hastening their death, they had not developed a specific plan to actually do so.

Personal characteristics. Respondents who had adopted this mind frame had a mean age of 74 and had, on average, some college education. Men outnumbered women, a slightly higher percentage were not married (57%), 90% were White, and the majority was Protestant (89%).

Accompanying emotions. These elders demonstrated conflicting emotions regarding their desire to hasten death and their taking the next step to develop a specific plan to carry out that desire. Their voices resonated with the emotional pain involved in considering hastening their death and taking the necessary actions to make it happen. As was the case with individuals who had adopted Mind Frames 3 and 4, individuals who had adopted Mind Frame 5 felt they could not justify their existence.

Factors motivating the serious consideration of a hastened death. The factors motivating these elders to consider a hastened death were mostly psychosocial in nature, as they were for those elders who had adopted Mind Frame 4. Eight of the nine elders who had adopted Mind Frame 5 reported psychosocial factors that included loneliness, not enjoying life, lack of hope, boredom, uselessness, and being a burden. One 92-year-old man aptly expressed his lack of enjoyment in life: "I, if I could do away with myself, I would . . . I had to give up everything . . . golfing and bowling, sex life, riding my bike."

Physical factors served as motivators for four of the nine elders. Two of these individuals were suffering pain at the time of the interview. One 53-year-old married woman reported despondently, "I'm tired. I'm tired of the struggle and the fighting and the pain and all of that." A 75-year-old married man, who was one of two elders not currently experiencing pain but fearful of future suffering, stated sadly, "I, I fear some of the, uh, some of the physical stress that may come in the course of my dying. Nobody chooses to die little by little. At least, I can't visualize that."

Factors motivating the lack of a specific plan to hasten death. All nine elders who had adopted this mind frame were suffering emotionally and/or physically such that death was preferable to living, yet they had not developed a specific plan for hastening death. Although only a few elders stated this preference specifically, others echoed this sentiment but used different words. For example, one 72-year-old widower stated in a voice full of despair, "I just want to get it over with . . . Tomorrow is the same thing, the same thing." Discussions with these individuals revealed the physical limitations and psychosocial reasons preventing them from actually developing a plan to hasten their death.

Three elders were physically unable to hasten their death due to the limitations placed on them by their disease. For example, one man had multiple system atrophy and could only move his lips. These individuals would have required assistance to carry out any plan but either lacked family or friends who might have provided such assistance or, out of love and a sense of responsibility, would not ask them to do so.

The six elders who possessed the physical ability to carry out a plan without assistance had yet to develop one because of their family and friends. For example, two individuals were suffering from respiratory diseases that made breathing difficult, painful, and exhausting. One woman, who was presented at the interview, stated that she knew her terminally ill husband wanted to hasten his death but was vehemently opposed because she felt unable to cope without him. The other elder's spouse, who was not present at the interview, was unaware of his wife's desire to hasten death. The wife, however, knew that her husband was dependent on her emotionally and financially; this dependence kept her from developing a plan. Faced with the love and support they both gave to, and received from, others, these two elders could not make a plan.

Only one elder cited religious beliefs as her reason for not developing a specific plan. Although this 87-year-old widow felt that "there doesn't seem to be any hope for anything," and she refused to explain what her religious beliefs were, she felt strongly that these beliefs would not permit her to take the next step towards hastening her death.

Except for the respondent who felt that her religious beliefs would not allow her to make a specific plan to hasten her death, I felt the others would make a plan in the future should their circumstances change. The physical and psychosocial anguish expressed by these elders was very real. If someone had volunteered to assist them, or if their spouses had changed their mind regarding not wanting them to leave, I believe these elders would have sought the opportunity to develop a plan.

Mind Frame 6: Considering a Hastened Death with a Specific Plan

Approach towards dying. The remaining nine elders (9%) were seriously considering hastening their death and had a specific plan of action. One 55-year-old married man had developed a suicide plan he could carry out on his own were his suffering to intensify. Three elderly women (aged 65, 70, and 79), two of whom were married, all had end-stage renal disease and planned to go off dialysis. They had discussed with their physicians stopping their dialysis treatment and their physicians told them they would support their decision and provide the necessary assistance. A 75-year-old married woman had contacted the Hemlock Society and had received their support. Two elderly women and two elderly men (aged 75, 91, 69, and 76, respectively) were considering physician-assisted death and had received verbal support from their physician, with whom they had a close relationship. One of the women stated, "I have considered, I do like this physician-assisted suicide. With the assistance of a doctor, so you won't have a, a, messy death . . . and they [doctors] have said that any time I'm going to want to, it's up to me. That's right. I'm very glad about it. Yeah."

Personal characteristics. Respondents who had adopted this mind frame had a mean age of 74 and had, on average, some college education. Two thirds were women, two thirds were married, and 90% were White. Although more than half of these respondents were Protestants, all respondents of Jewish faith ($n = 2$) were in this category.

Accompanying emotions. Some of these individuals were very emotional when speaking of hastening their death, whereas others had a matter-of-fact approach to the topic. Elders who had family or friends felt conflicting feelings when they spoke of the impact their plan might have on loved ones. Elders who had adopted Mind Frames 3, 4, 5, and 6 all shared feelings of uselessness and the sense that their existence could no longer be justified.

Factors motivating the serious consideration of a hastened death. All nine elders reported psychosocial factors as playing a crucial role in their desire for a hastened death. Eight of the nine elders expressed feeling useless. The frustration of feeling useless was evident in a 70-year-old widow's inability to do the normal tasks of daily living: "I just can't do what I used to. Urn, I can't go out, I can't go to the store . . . I can't write a check for nothing. I, it's just a lot of things . . . Oh, I hate it." A 91-year-old widow talked about how she no longer felt useful to others: "There's not any good reason for me to go on living. Nobody really needs me . . . I'm really not serving any purpose. If you don't, aren't needed by anybody, you kind of have a different feeling about life."

Six elders felt life no longer brought any enjoyment. Each day was filled with the limitations of their illness and the misery it wrought on their lives. One 76-year-old man had reached the point in his illness where he had lost the ability to move his body or speak. He had always loved to socialize, travel, and work—all things he was no longer able to do. Not being able to communicate with others or get around like he used to had a profound negative impact on him.

In addition to expressing psychosocial factors as motivators, two elders who were currently only experiencing mild physical discomfort feared they would suffer terribly as death drew near. One elder had heard on television and read in the newspaper about how painful dying had been for other Americans and feared the same fate. The other elder had witnessed his mother's suffering and was reminded daily of her terrible experiences.

The desire to hasten death was strong for the nine elders, and they all noted how having a plan provided a sense of control in case living became too unbearable. One 91-year-old widow was fueled by her desire for control over her body: "I just feel sometimes as though cancer is, uh, an opponent. And, it seems to me, it says to itself, 'I am in control of this body. This is mine, I will do whatever I want to with it.'" She spoke with her long-time doctor about physician-assisted death, and he promised his support when she was ready. She felt that although the cancer now had the upper hand, she had the ultimate control through physician-assisted death.

Factors motivating against implementation of plan to hasten death. Although all nine elders possessed a plan for hastening their death, they had not yet set an exact time for putting their plan into action. For some, physical limitations prevented them from carrying out their plan alone. For others, life was still bearable and they felt the need to protect their family from the taint and pain their suicide would bring. At that moment, the factors motivating elders not to move forward with their plan were proving stronger than the motivators for hastening death.

For some elders, physical limitations resulted in their not being able to carry out specific suicide plans. They had waited too long to put them into action and now were physically unable to do so. The anger and frustration felt by these individuals was expressed clearly by a 69-year-old married man who was suffering with amyotrophic lateral sclerosis: ". . . I can't pull the trigger. Too weak. I'd have to make a fixture and fasten it and have a string and pull my arm."

Although some elders had family who could assist and were supportive of their plan to hasten death, they could not bring themselves to accept their family's assistance. They did not want to place loved ones in this position and were hoping to find others who would do so; they also did not feel comfortable about approaching their physician.

For the elders who were physically able to carry out their plan, family also played a role in their not yet having executed the plan. These individuals talked about the emotional pain a hastened death would bring their loved ones. Feelings of protecting family members from this emotional pain were uppermost in their minds. One 55-year-old married man, whose son

had killed himself, his wife, and his children, was reluctant to put his wife through his own suicide if possible:

> And basically for one reason. Yeah, I'll tell you. We lost our son and his family back in '91 . . . It was to do with drugs. And we don't know . . . what happened, but supposedly he, he shot and killed his wife and the two-year-old son. And then himself, and they had a five-month-old baby that was suffocated . . . We found them, which made it ten times worse. And because of that, I would never do that to my wife. I wouldn't do that.

For the other elders who also could go through with their plan without any assistance, life was still bearable. However, should the time come when they could no longer tolerate their lives, they indicated that their plan would be put into action.

All nine elders were experiencing critical junctures in their dying process. Either life had become unbearable due to their illness, or they feared it would be so in the future. The only solution they saw to address their physical and emotional pain was to hasten their death, and they were strong in their conviction to do so, if it became necessary.

Discussion

Prior studies on factors motivating terminally ill individuals to consider a hastened death assumed that they faced their dying by either considering or not considering a hastened death. This dichotomy was originally proposed for the present study; however, as the respondents' stories unfolded, it quickly became clear that these 96 terminally ill elders had mind frames towards dying that were much more complex. Instead of the simple consideration to hasten or not to hasten death, six mind frames towards dying emerged. Furthermore, elders with differing mind frames were struggling with various issues related to their dying. Elders not considering a hastened death reported grappling with issues of readiness and acceptance, whereas elders wishing for or considering a hastened death reported grappling with whether to take action.

Researchers can draw no conclusion from the data regarding whether elders' six mind frames fall along a continuum from neither ready nor accepting of dying to having a specific plan by which to hasten death. To consider these mind frames as a continuum implies that (a) these mind frames are stages terminally ill elders move through, and (b) one stage progresses to the next. The data support neither implication. Fifteen elders reported moving from one mind frame to another during their dying process, whereas others reported only having experienced one mind frame (this topic will be discussed in another article). Elders who reported changing their mind frame did not necessarily move sequentially consistent with the mind frames being a continuum or a series of stages. Although the cross-sectional data do not provide information on the issue of progression, they do provide insights into personal characteristics, approaches towards dying, and accompanying emotions that characterize each mind frame, as well as the factors that motivate its adoption by the elder.

Personal Characteristics

The elders who participated in this study did not enter into their dying process with a blank slate; rather, each brought with them values, beliefs, and experiences based on their age, education, gender, race, marital status, and religion (see Table 1). It was noted earlier that information was not gathered regarding the mind frame respondents had adopted in previous life crises, or whether past experiences influenced their current mind frame. Respondents' personal characteristics, however, serve to provide some of this information.

Age and race showed some patterns in relation to respondents' readiness for death. Respondents who were not ready to die, regardless of whether they did or did not accept death, were younger (71 and 69 years old, respectively), on average, than respondents who were ready and accepting (81 years old) or wishing for death (83 years old). It could be that age may reflect the timing of the death; that is, younger elders may feel that death is coming sooner than they had anticipated and so they are less ready for it. Race also revealed an important pattern, in that few Black respondents reported a readiness to die, and none wished for death. It is unclear why Black respondents might lack readiness, but it could be related to their spiritual beliefs.

Education, gender, marital status, and religion revealed some noteworthy patterns with regard to respondents who were considering a hastened death. Regardless of whether they did or did not have a specific plan, respondents who were considering a hastened death reported having at least some college education (14 and 13 years, respectively), whereas respondents who had adopted other mind frames reported having a high school education or less. Education may provide knowledge of end-of-life options as well as access to resources necessary to hasten one's death. It is also important to note that a higher percentage of women than men reported having a specific plan to hasten their death, although the reason for this pattern is not clear. For the most part, respondents who were married and who were considering a hastened death had a specific plan, whereas unmarried respondents who were considering a hastened death did not. Having a partner to assist with hastening death may make it easier to develop a specific plan and act on it. Finally, although Catholics reported a high level of acceptance of dying regardless of their level of readiness, both Jewish respondents possessed a specific plan to hasten death. Again, it is difficult to speculate about the reasons for this difference.

The patterns noted above provide support for delving more deeply into the role that a respondent's personal characteristics may play in the adoption of his or her mind frame. A mixed-method research approach would help gather information not only on which characteristics play a role in the adoption of mind frames but also on how they do so.

Importance of the Psychosocial Aspects of Dying

Family relationships; unfinished business; enjoying life; fear of dying; having lived a long time already; not enjoying life; feeling bored, lonely, useless, dependent, and burdensome to others; lack of hope; lack of control; religious beliefs; fear of future suffering; and physical suffering were all factors that motivated the elders interviewed for this study to adopt one of six mind frames. Many of these factors reflect what has been found in previous studies; however, the current study provides rich information on how the factors motivate the adoption of different mind frames towards dying. It is important to note that in the present study, as well as in the studies reviewed earlier in this article, psychosocial factors were mentioned as motivating factors more often than were physical factors. Physical suffering, however, is not a factor that can be ignored. In the current study, physical suffering was a motivating factor for 3 of the 6 respondents who were wishing for death to come and for 2 of the 9 respondents who were considering a hastened death but had no specific plan on how to bring it about. Although elders discussed psychosocial issues more often than physical ones, it may be that some of these issues were the result of physical limitations or problems brought on by their illness.

Complexity of Motivating Factors

The results of this study demonstrate that some motivating factors differed among elders with each of the six mind frames, and, even in the cases where some similarities existed, a closer look showed that these factors were not the same. Family is an excellent example of this. Family was a motivator for both elders who were neither ready nor accepting of dying (Mind Frame 1) and for elders who were not ready but who had accepted their dying (Mind Frame 2). Yet how family motivated these elders' lack of readiness differed. Elders who had adopted Mind Frame 1 cited the importance of *providing* emotional and instrumental support to their family. Elders who had adopted Mind Frame 2 spoke of *receiving* emotional and instrumental support from their family. Thus, it is not enough for health care practitioners to know that family is an important influence on readiness to die. It is also important to understand just how family ties affect the terminally ill elder's readiness for and acceptance of their death.

Religious belief is another example of how a factor can appear to be the same across mind frames and yet can motivate elders to adopt different mind frames. Elders who were neither ready nor accepting of dying spoke of how God wanted them to fight to stay alive and did not want them just to accept their dying. God was important in a quite different way for some elders who explained their acceptance of death as based on their belief that time of death was God's decision. The religious belief that God decides time of death also served to motivate some elders who wished for death but who were not seriously considering hastening it. These differences raise the issue of whether the respondent's religious beliefs were of long standing and had led him or her to adopt the views towards death that had been described in the interviews, or whether the beliefs developed after the respondent's diagnosis in order to support the mind frame the respondent needed to be in at that time. Either way, the religious beliefs held by some respondents gave them support for their mind frame.

These are only two examples of the complexity of the motivating factors that needs to be taken into consideration when health care professionals are working with terminally ill elders. For example, strong family ties or religious beliefs cannot always be assumed to operate in the same manner. Instead, professionals need to uncover the specific nature of such ties or beliefs.

Palliative Care Program and Practice Implications

The overarching implication to emerge from this study is the need to develop palliative care programs from a holistic rather than a primarily medical perspective. The elders participating in this study provided quite a bit of evidence as to the importance of addressing not only their physical needs, but their spiritual, emotional, and social needs as well. Developing a program that meets these needs has several underlying implications.

Once elders have been told they have fewer than six months to live, the main goal of palliative care programs becomes ensuring that they receive a quality dying process. The term *quality dying process* is ambiguous and so necessitates defining. The qualitative information provided by the 96 terminally ill elders interviewed for this study serves as a step towards such a definition.

For elders participating in the current study, a quality dying process meant recognizing that each had his or her own psychosocial, spiritual, and physical needs, and that whether or not these needs were met had an impact on the mind frame that elders adopted towards dying. If palliative care programs were to adopt the definition of a quality dying process as holistic and individualistic, it would be important to develop instruments that ensure a comprehensive assessment of each elder's mind frame; the psychosocial, physical, and spiritual factors that led to its adoption; and the elder's level of satisfaction with it. If the elder is satisfied, then such programs can emphasize to their practitioners the importance of respecting the elder's wishes, even if the practitioner does not agree with them. However, if the elder is not happy with his or her current mind frame, then the elder and practitioner can address the factors that may allow for transitioning to another mind frame. It is crucial that palliative care programs acknowledge the fluidity of movement between mind frames (as evidenced by 15 of the 96 respondents who reported previous transitioning), such that elders' psychosocial, spiritual, and physical needs are continually assessed as they move through the dying process.

In an attempt to ensure that each terminally ill elder has a quality dying process, I suggest the following guidelines for palliative care programs. First, the design of these programs may best be guided by the input of clergy, nurses, physicians, and social workers so that all aspects of care are considered. Second, once programs have been established, it may be beneficial for staff to work as a team in order to ensure that each terminally ill elder has all of his or her needs met. Third, in order to develop effective care plans, it may be helpful to develop evaluation instruments that assess the spiritual, emotional, social, and physical needs of the elder, as well as his or her current mind frame towards dying and the elder's level of satisfaction with that mind frame.

It is important, however, to honor the elder's self-determination regarding his or her needs. This means that guidelines should be established that specify the need for practitioners to determine and honor what each elder feels are the most critical issues to be addressed. As was revealed in the current study, some terminally ill elders gave psychosocial issues higher priority than physical ones. Time is limited for these individuals, and it is important that elders be the ones to determine how their limited time is spent. Fourth, in the current study, sense of control served as a key motivating factor for not only considering a hastened death but also for developing a specific plan to carry it out. Although more research is necessary regarding the role sense of control plays in relation to a terminally ill elder's dying process, palliative care programs should include the assessment and fulfillment of control needs in their care plans. Finally, palliative care health professionals need to attend training sessions that allow them to explore their own values and beliefs regarding death. An increased self-awareness and comfort with dying and death could result in practitioners being more receptive to allowing terminally ill elders to express their fears and concerns honestly throughout the dying process.

Study Limitations and Research Implications

Although this study advanced knowledge on hastening death and had an unusually large sample size for a qualitative study, there were also limitations. First, the sampling technique used in this study was purposive, so the findings cannot be considered representative of the population of terminally ill elders. Second, the research design used for this study was cross-sectional and only captured the elders' mind frames at one point in time. I asked elders who were not currently considering a hastened death to recall whether they had ever considered hastening their death; in this way, I gained evidence regarding past mind frames. This evidence, however, was based on recall that could have been impacted by the elder's medication or current situation. I did not ask elders who were considering a hastened death about prior views regarding hastening death.

Therefore, I do not know whether they had been considering a hastened death since they were diagnosed as terminally ill or whether, at one time, they had not been considering a hastened death. The current evidence that terminally ill elders transition between mind frames is an important finding and one that would be best followed up by using a longitudinal research design.

Additional research on this topic using a random sample and a longitudinal research design may add support and clarification to the program and practice implications suggested by the current data. Qualitative studies focused on race/ethnicity, gender, social class differences, and sites of care are necessary in order to obtain information that will improve the care of terminally ill elders. In addition, future research on this topic should aim to develop a multidimensional assessment tool that not only captures elders' personal characteristics and their mind frames towards dying, but also assesses elders' spiritual, emotional, social, and physical needs.

References

Arias, E., Anderson, R., Hsiang-Ching, K., Murphy, S., & Kochanek, K. (2003, September 18). Deaths: Final data for 2001. *National Vital Statistics Report, 52* (3), 1–116.

Arnold, E. (2004). Factors that influence consideration of hastening death among people with life-threatening illnesses. *Health & Social Work, 29* (1), 17–26.

Back, A., Wallace, J., Starks, H., & Pearlman, R. (1996). Physician-assisted suicide and euthanasia in Washington state: Patient requests and physician responses. *Journal of the American Medical Association, 275,* 919–925.

Bernabei, R., Gambassi, G., Lapane, K., Landi, G., Gatsonis, C., Dunlop, R., et al. (1998). Management of pain in elderly patients with cancer. *Journal of the American Medical Association, 279,* 1877–1882.

Black, H., & Rubinstein, R. L. (2004). Themes of suffering in later life. *Journal of Gerontology: Social Sciences, 59B,* SI7–S24.

Breitbart, W., Rosenfeld, B., & Passik, S. (1996). Interest in physician assisted suicide among ambulatory HIV-infected patients. *American Journal of Psychiatry, 153,* 238–242.

Chin, A., Hedberg, K., Higginson, G., & Fleming, D. (1999). Legalized physician-assisted suicide in Oregon: The first year's experience. *New England Journal of Medicine, 340,* 577–583.

Chochinov, H., Hack, T., Hassard, T., Kristjanson, L., McClement, S., & Harlos, M. (2002). Dignity in the terminally ill: A cross-sectional, cohort study. *Lancet, 360,* 2026–2030.

Chochinov, H., Wilson, K., Enns, M., Mowchun, N., Lander, S., Levitt, M., et al. (1995). Desire for death in the terminally ill. *American Journal of Psychiatry, 152,* 1185–1191.

Cleeland, C., Gonin, R., Hatfield, A., Edmonson, J., Blum, R., Stewart, J., & Pandya, K. (1994). Pain and its treatment in outpatients with metastatic cancer. *New England Journal of Medicine, 330,* 592–596.

Emanuel, E., Fairclough, D., Daniels, E., & Clarridge, B. (1996). Euthanasia and physician-assisted suicide: Attitudes and experiences of oncology patients, oncologists, and the public. *Lancet, 347,* 1805–1810.

Emanuel, E., Fairclough, D., & Emanuel, L. (2000). Attitudes and desires related to euthanasia and physician-assisted suicide among terminally ill patients and their caregivers. *Journal of the American Medical Association, 284,* 2460–2468.

Ganzini, L., Harvath, T., Jackson, A., Goy, E., Miller, L., & Delorit, M. (2002). Experiences of Oregon nurses and social workers with hospice patients who requested assistance with suicide. *New England Journal of Medicine, 347,* 582–588.

Hetzel, L., & Smith, A. (2001). *The 65 years and over population: 2000* (Census 2000 Brief No. C2KBR/01-10). Washington, DC: U.S. Census Bureau.

Jacobson, J., Kasworm, E., Battin, M., Botkin, J., Francis, L., & Green, D. (1995). Decedents' reported preferences for physician-assisted death: A survey of informants listed on death certificates in Utah. *Journal of Clinical Ethics, 6* (2), 149–157.

Lavery, J., Boyle, J., Dickens, B., Maclean, H., & Singer, P. (2001). Origins of the desire for euthanasia and assisted suicide in people with HIV-l or AIDS: A qualitative study. *Lancet, 358,* 362–367.

Meier, E., Emmons, C., Wallenstein, S., Quill, T., Morrison, R., & Cassel, C. (1998). A national survey of physician-assisted suicide and euthanasia in the United States. *New England Journal of Medicine, 338,* 1193–1201.

Oregon Department of Human Services. (2000). *Oregon's death with dignity act: The second year's experience.* Portland: Oregon Health Division.

Oregon Department of Human Services. (2001). *Oregon's death with dignity act: Three years of legalized physician-assisted suicide.* Portland: Oregon Health Division.

Oregon Department of Human Services. (2002). *Fourth annual report on Oregon's death with dignity act.* Portland: Oregon Health Division.

Oregon Department of Human Services. (2003). *Fifth annual report on Oregon's death with dignity act.* Portland: Oregon Health Division.

Patton, M. (1990). *Qualitative evaluation and research methods* (2nd ed.). Newbury Park, CA: Sage.

Pessin, H., Rosenfeld, B., & Breitbart, W. (2002). Assessing psychological distress near the end of life. *American Behavioral Scientist, 46,* 357–372.

SUPPORT Investigators. (1997). Perceptions by family members of the dying: Experiences of older and seriously ill patients. *Annals of Internal Medicine, 126,* 97–106.

Volker, D. (2001). Oncology nurses' experiences with requests for assisted dying from terminally ill patients with cancer. *Oncology Nursing Forum, 28* (1), 39–49.

Address correspondence to TRACY A. SCHROEPFER, University of Wisconsin, Madison, School of Social Work, 1350 University Ave., Madison, WI 53706. E-mail: tschroepfer@wisc.edu.

Acknowledgments—Support for this article was provided by the John A Hartford Foundation Geriatric Social Work Doctoral Fellowship Program.

From *Journals of Gerontology,* vol. 61B, no. 3, 2006, pp. S129–S139. Copyright © 2006 by Gerontological Society of America. Reprinted by permission of the publisher.

UNIT 7

Living Environment in Later Life

Unit Selections

Key Points to Consider

- What are the advantages and disadvantages of keeping the seniors in their own homes by providing home health care services?

- What are the advantages old people who move into continuing care communities have?

- What are the advantages for seniors of living in a "Green House Home"?

- How was Beacon Hill turned into a place where older persons could live for their entire life?

- What home services are necessary to allow an older person to remain in their own home?

Student Website

www.mhhe.com/cls

Internet References

American Association of Homes and Services for the Aging
   http://www.aahsa.org
Center for Demographic Studies
   http://cds.duke.edu
Guide to Retirement Living Online
   http://www.retirement-living.com
The United States Department of Housing and Urban Development
   http://www.hud.gov

Unit 4 noted that old age is often a period of shrinking life space. This concept is crucial to an understanding of the living environments of older Americans. When older people retire, they may find that they travel less frequently and over shorter distances because they no longer work and most neighborhoods have stores, gas stations, and churches in close proximity. As the retirement years roll by, older people may feel less in control of their environments due to a decline in their hearing and vision as well as due to other health problems. As the aging process continues, the elderly are likely to restrict their mobility to the areas where they feel most secure. This usually means that an increasing amount of time is spent at home. Estimates show that individuals aged 65 and above spend 80 to 90 percent of their lives in their home environments. Of all the other age groups, only small children are as house- and neighborhood-bound.

The house, neighborhood, and community environments are, therefore, more crucial to the elderly than to any other adult age group. The interaction with others that they experience within their homes and neighborhoods can either be stimulating or foreboding, pleasant or threatening. Across the country, older Americans find themselves living in a variety of circumstances, ranging from desirable to undesirable.

Approximately 70 percent of the elderly live in a family setting, usually a husband-wife household; 20 percent live alone or with nonrelatives; and the remaining number live in institutions such as nursing homes. Although only about 5 percent of the elderly will be living in nursing homes at any one time, 25 percent of people aged 65 and above will spend some time in a nursing home setting. The longer one lives, the more likely he or she is to end up in a total-care institution. Because most older Americans would prefer to live independently in their own homes for as long as possible, their relocation—to other houses, apartments, or nursing homes—is often accompanied by a considerable amount of trauma and unrest. The fact that the aged tend to be less mobile and more neighborhood-bound than any other age group makes their living environment crucial to their sense of well-being.

Articles in this section focus on some of the alternatives available to the aged: from family care to assisted living to nursing homes. In "Oh, Lord, Don't Put Me in a Nursing Home," Barbara Basler points out how much less expensive it is for states to

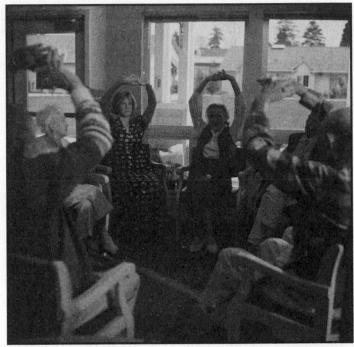
© Keith Brofsky/Getty Images

provide home care services that allow people to stay in their homes rather than moving them to a nursing home. In "Where to Live as We Age," Susan Fine points out the advantages to seniors who move into the "Green House Home" rather than the traditional nursing home. Christine Larson in "Finding a Good Home, Taking Care of Your Parents: A Guide to Making the Wisest Senior Living Choice" points out the different choices children of aging parents have as to where is the best place for Mom and Dad when their health prevents them from continuing to live independently. In "Declaration of Independents: Home Is Where You Want to Live Forever. Here's How," Barbara Basler tells how Beacon Hill in Boston turned itself from a residential neighborhood into a nonprofit association, which provides services to its residents on a 24-hour-a-day basis.

Oh, Lord, Don't Put Me in a Nursing Home

BARBARA BASLER

S hirley Miller, an 85-year-old widow, has lived on the 10th floor of an aging rent-subsidized apartment build-ing in Winter Park, Fla., for 21 years, close to her friends, church and doctors. Miller remains sharp and independent, but one health problem after another has left her unable to maintain her daily routine on her own.

So a year ago she applied for help with cleaning, meals and personal care from the state's Medicaid and elder care programs. Though she qualifies for help, she was put on a waiting list.

Today Miller weighs barely 100 pounds. She eats only when friends bring her food. She cries because she cannot clean her home or even bathe herself properly.

And she has yet to receive any help from the state.

"I'm afraid now I'll die before they get to me," she says, in a voice just above a whisper.

Programs that help older Americans like Miller live indepen-dently in their own homes—and out of nursing homes—have not been keeping pace with the needs of people age 85 and older, the fastest-growing age group. Across the nation more than 300,000 individuals are already on Medicaid waiting lists for home or neighborhood services.

Now, shocking budget deficits produced by the deepening recession are forcing state lawmakers to freeze or even cut these lifelines for older residents. At least 46 states plus the District of Columbia face shortfalls this year or next; and an estimated $350 billion in state deficits loom over the next 30 months, according to the Center on Budget and Policy Priorities (CBPP), a Washington think tank.

"Every program, every bill and every policy issue will be affected by the economy," William Pound, executive director of the National Conference of State Legislatures, wrote in a recent NCSL report on the budget outlook.

At least 22 states and the District of Columbia are cutting or proposing cuts to home and community services or are signifi-cantly increasing what low-income people must pay for them, according to the CBPP. In a recent national survey of state area offices on aging—which direct many such state programs—70 percent said they anticipate "severe" budget cuts.

Alabama, for instance, has ended homemaker services for more than 1,000 older adults. Rhode Island now charges

Call to Action

Protect Medicaid

Many states are considering Medicaid cuts that could swell the number of uninsured Americans and the num-ber of home and health care workers who lose jobs. AARP urges members to tell their state legislators not to cut health care for people who can't afford it. For contact information, go to http://capwiz.com/aarp/dbq/officials/ or check your phone book blue pages.

low-income older residents more for adult day care. And the Florida legislature, grappling with deficits of more than $2.8 billion for 2009, lopped almost $2 million from the state's Community Care for the Elderly program—which supplies home care, meals, adult day care and a host of other services—before Republican Gov. Charlie Crist vetoed the cut.

Such reductions around the nation could undo progress in shifting funding for long-term care away from nursing homes and into services that give people more choices for where to live. Some of these home services are fully funded by the states; others are part of Medicaid, the joint state and federal health care and long-term care program for low-income Americans. On average more than 21 percent of all state spending goes to Medicaid, which makes its programs a tempting target for bud-get cutters.

By law, state Medicaid programs are required to pay for nurs-ing home care for those who qualify for help with long-term care, and the majority of long-term care dollars go to these facil-ities. But the federal government also gives states the option to develop services that help people who qualify for long-term care to remain in their own homes—a choice nine of 10 older Ameri-cans prefer over nursing homes, according to AARP research. From 1995 to 2007, total Medicaid spending on such services more than doubled to 41 percent, according to the Kaiser Com-mission on Medicaid and the Uninsured. These programs now serve some 2.8 million Americans.

Reducing these services, experts say, is a false economy because it forces people into nursing homes, which cost the state more. Florida's Community Care for the Elderly, for example, spends about $5,000 a year to help one older person remain in her home; more extensive state Medicaid home services cost $8,000 per person, and the average cost of a Florida nursing home is $65,000.

"Home care, meals, help for Alzheimer's caregivers—all help the state save money by keeping people out of nursing homes, and that's a message we want to take to legislators," says Randy Hunt, CEO of the Senior Resource Alliance, an area office on aging in Orlando. Hunt knows that lawmakers now working on Florida's 2010 budget are staring at an estimated shortfall of $5 billion.

In the coming months, states will be looking for sources of new revenue—higher taxes on cigarettes, sales taxes on the Internet, increased traffic fines—and trying to find the least harmful cuts they can make. Reluctant to chop a whole program or service, lawmakers may freeze or cut fees to those who provide the services, including not only nursing homes and hospitals, but also agencies that supply home care workers and health aides. Such cuts, though, eventually tend to translate into problems of access and quality of care, says Nick Johnson, director of the state fiscal project for the CBPP.

Unfortunately, even the economic stimulus package assembled by Congress and President Obama—with its billions of dollars of state aid, including more than $87 billion for state aging and Medicaid programs—does not fully protect these home and community long-term care services. "The stimulus money will give states a baseline, so cuts may not have to be so drastic," says Donna Folkemer, group director for health at the NCSL. "But it probably won't allow new programs or even help them to hold on to all the current programs."

And standing still can be moving backward. Consider Florida. While its Community Care for the Elderly escaped cuts this year, for nine years it has gone without a budget increase while its target population of older residents has grown by 700,000, according to Jack McRay, advocacy manager at the AARP Florida state office in Tallahassee. Today, 50,000 older Floridians are on waiting lists for these kinds of home services, state experts say, and 2,272 people died last year while on lists.

Those numbers worry Shirley Miller, who, up until she was 80, earned extra money by working the night shift at the reception desk of her apartment building. "When you've been independent all your life, you don't want to ask for help," Miller says. "But I just can't keep up anymore. I need help."

Where to Live as We Age

SUSAN FINE

Christine Cleary, 91, puts down her crochet work as she happily describes her new residence in Cohoes, a suburb of Albany, N.Y. "It doesn't smell like a nursing home," she says appreciatively. "There's no disinfectant odor." Cleary also enjoys how much quieter it is than most nursing homes—no beeping machines and clattering carts.

People stay healthier and happier in friendly settings.

Cleary lives with 11 other elderly people in a Green House home, a comfortable residence that offers meals, support, and nursing care at a cost comparable to that of a private room at a large, impersonal home. Each person has his or her own room and bath around a sunny living area with a big dining table that can accommodate all of the residents. An open kitchen allows seniors to put in their two cents about meal preparation, and they have easy access to a garden and patio.

Residential eldercare is a big business today. Nearly 1.4 million seniors live in nursing homes in the United States. But in 18 towns and cities from Birmingham, Ala., to Winthrop, Wash., a new model of care is being tested. While these Green House homes may not soon replace the 16,000 nursing homes in the U.S., they're changing the way our nation cares for its oldest citizens.

Geriatrician Dr. Bill Thomas, created The Green House Project with the hope of revolutionizing eldercare. In 2001, he wandered into the Robert Wood Johnson Foundation wearing a sweatshirt and Birkenstocks and shared his vision. The foundation was so impressed by his ideas it agreed to support a pilot program. With the foundation's help, Dr. Thomas eventually partnered with NCB Capital Impact, a national nonprofit organization that offers assistance to underserved communities, to roll out a plan. Two years later, the first Green House homes were constructed in Tupelo, Miss.

The success of the Green House model lies in trading a typical nursing home's top-down organizational structure for a self-managed team of workers who share the tasks involved in caring for their residents, including housekeeping and cooking. Most important, Dr. Thomas says he wanted to create residences that avoided the loneliness and expense of at-home care and the coldness of an institution. "We only have two populations who live in institutions in our society: criminals and the residents of nursing homes," he says.

"When my mother was at home alone, I worried about her nourishment and loneliness," Leslie Kellam says, explaining why she moved her parent from Florida to the Cohoes Green House.

Kellam's mother, Natalie Siegel, 83, says, "Here, I feel safe. At home, my aide might move my wheelchair, and I'd forget that it wasn't next to me. I worried about falling."

Green House residences go to great lengths to be not just homelike but to be home. Diana Lloyd, director of nursing at Cohoes, doesn't permit the use of traditional hospital carts to deliver pills. "If we introduce one cart," she says, "there will soon be carts for laundry and for drinks, and we'll become an institution." But it wasn't practical to ask the nurses to go to the medicine chest for each patient's dosage. "First we tried a rolling knapsack," Lloyd says, "before we settled on a tea cart one might find in a family home."

A comfy residence could replace nursing homes.

Residents are called "elders," not "patients." Unlike in most nursing homes, residents can have pets, and instead of mandated mealtimes, they can choose when to eat. Simple changes like these appear to improve seniors' behavior and health. "Because it is quieter," one administrator explained, "the elders are less agitated." According to a recent University of Minnesota study, Green House residents were less depressed and were able to perform daily functions longer than people in regular nursing homes.

Doctors say they receive fewer urgent calls at night. Because the staff interact so closely with the same residents every day, they can tell when there's been a significant change in a person's condition and can explain symptoms in greater detail.

Darlene Shaughnessy's uncle has lived in a Green House home outside Detroit for the past six months. Before moving there, Daniel Shaughnessy, 81, lived alone, and neighbors checked in on him. Once they called Darlene after he hadn't answered the phone for a few days. She found her uncle curled in a ball in a corner of a room, having suffered a serious stroke. He weighed about 80 pounds.

Today, Shaughnessy has recovered from the stroke and weighs a healthy 180 pounds. "I like it here," he says of his Michigan Green House, where residents dance hip-hop in their wheelchairs and play Nintendo Wii games.

About 30% of traditional nursing homes are beginning to incorporate some aspects of the Green House model, like breaking themselves down into smaller "households." Preliminary research on Green House homes indicates that their approach may result in lower staff turnover and in residents' spending less time bedridden, with fewer complications.

"The No. 1 reason nursing home reform has lagged is that people don't believe the system can really be changed," Dr. Thomas says, "even though it costs a lot of money and doesn't generate a lot of well-being." But the good news is that if these models offer similar costs and happier residents, they could become the new way to live as we age.

Finding a Good Home

CHRISTINE LARSON

Soon after Jeanne Erdmann's father passed away in 1995, it became clear that her mother, then 85, would one day need a new home. Although her mom, Florence Greco, was still in relatively good health, "she didn't like living by herself anymore," says Erdmann, 53, a science writer who lives in Wentzville, Mo. So six years ago, Erdmann and her husband invited Greco, who lived in a nearby county, to move in. "She didn't like being here at first," says Erdmann. "We have a lot of farms around us and no neighbors that you can see from the house, so she felt isolated." Erdmann and her husband also had to adjust, curtailing their evening activities to keep Greco company at night. Although Erdmann gets a break now and then when one of her two sisters takes Greco for a while, "the day in and day out wears you down," Erdmann says, especially as her mother has gradually required more care over the years.

Still, Erdmann and her mother agree the arrangement suits them. "I'm very lucky," says Greco. "I took care of my mother until she passed away, and I took care of my husband until he passed away, and I have very nice daughters and they're taking care of me."

Erdmann is one of 19 million Americans caring for someone over age 75, typically a parent or a grandparent, who may or may not live with them. Often called "informal caregivers," these adult children or relatives provide 75 to 80 percent of all long-term care in the United States. Many, like Erdmann, struggle to find a living situation that gives parents both the assistance they need and the independence they desire. Historically, older adults have lived on their own, with their children, or in nursing homes. Today's seniors, however, face a rapidly expanding array of housing choices. New programs, services, and technology are helping people to stay in their homes longer. Federal and state lawmakers are shifting funds from nursing homes to home- and community-based health services. Even nursing homes and retirement communities are offering in-home services ranging from housekeeping to telemedicine. The wide assortment is encouraging new models of independent living, such as elder cohousing. Meanwhile, the number of assisted-living facilities has grown substantially in the past decade, as have continuing-care retirement communities, which bring independent living, assisted living, and nursing homes together on one campus. The changes are putting pressure on nursing homes to create smaller, warmer environments.

Still, the search for the right fit for a parent can be frustrating and time-consuming. Not all options are available in every community, and cost structures can be baffling. Here's a look at trends in housing alternatives:

Aging in place. Suzanne Stark, 80, has a pacemaker, a broken foot, and a 17-pound cat named Zenobia. When the cat had to be rushed to the vet recently, Stark called Beacon Hill Village, a nonprofit association that helps residents of the Boston neighborhood stay in their homes as they age. For a $35 fee, the association dispatched a helper who boxed the cat and drove Stark to the vet. "I have a daughter in Brookline who has two jobs and children who are 5 and 9," says Stark. "A big push for me was to not have her take total responsibility for me."

Forget the old joke about being nice to your kids because they pick out your nursing home. The vast majority of Americans, like Stark, grow old in their own communities. "People want to be where their family and friends are," says Elinor Ginzler, director of livable communities for AARP. Founded in 2001, Beacon Hill Village helps them do that. Open to neighborhood residents over age 50, membership costs $550 a year for individuals or $780 for households. Low- or moderate-income members like Stark, however, pay just $100 a year. Services include things like a weekly ride to the grocery store, nearby exercise classes, and access to a geriatric-care manager. And there's a concierge service of sorts: Need a plumber? A home-health nurse? Beacon Hill Village will set it up through screened providers at a 10 to 50 percent discount. "I would worry about living alone if I didn't have it," says Stark of her Village membership. Similar organizations are being developed in Denver; Washington, D.C.; Madison, Wis.; and elsewhere.

Other communities are creating a different version of the neighborhood-based retirement program. The state of New York is bringing social workers, health programs, and other aging services directly into some 50 "naturally occurring retirement communities," apartment complexes, housing projects, or neighborhoods where the population is growing older. These small programs have produced big results. For example, in Deepdale Garden Co-op, a Queens apartment complex where 60 percent of residents are over 60, city funds and philanthropic grants helped an onsite team—including a nurse and two social workers—reduce residents' risk of falling by addressing medical factors like low vision and hypertension, as well as

At Your Service

These websites offer tips and advice for adult children caring for aging parents:

www.eldercare.gov The federal Eldercare Locator can put caregivers in touch with local senior services.

www.familycaregiving101.org Two associations teamed up to help new caregivers learn the ins and outs of their roles.

www.longtermcare.gov This new federal website spells out senior living alternatives and the various payment options.

www.medicare.gov/nhcompare Compare nursing home quality data and find state inspection agencies at this federal website.

www.strengthforcaring.com Connect and chat with other caregivers at this site, sponsored by Johnson & Johnson.

installing grab bars and fixing cracked sidewalks. Communities in 20 states are launching similar programs.

In other areas, adult children are increasingly turning to an emerging class of professionals to help aging parents stay in their homes. Geriatric-care managers—typically for-profit social workers or nurses specializing in elder issues—can attend doctor's appointments with the patient, supervise medication, hire and oversee home health assistants, or find and evaluate assisted-living or nursing homes. Typical cost: $80 to $200 an hour (and rarely covered by insurance). The National Association of Professional Geriatric Care Managers (*www. caremanager.org*) can provide local referrals.

Joel Kazis, 53, of New York arranged for a Boston geriatric-care manager to work with his parents, who live in Boston. For example, she helped them find a geriatric-care physician and evaluate assisted-living facilities. When they opted for an apartment instead, she found a move coordinator, someone to cook and clean, and made sure grab bars were installed in the bathroom. She even found a geriatric-care manager to assist the couple when they spent a few months in Florida. His folks, Kazis says, "needed additional resources, and I needed someone familiar with those resources."

Even nursing home and assisted living companies are jumping on board. For example, the Sears Methodist Retirement System in Abilene, Texas, a nonprofit that runs 12 senior living facilities, is currently testing a high-tech service called Seniors Safe@Home. It uses sensors to monitor whether clients have gotten out of bed, used the bathroom, or visited the fridge. Automated systems dispense medications and monitor conditions like blood pressure and blood sugar levels. Data are screened by a call center and uploaded to a website that clients' children can access.

Boomerang parents. Forget kids who head straight from college to their old bedrooms. Out of 36 million people age 65 or older, about 13 percent live with their adult children or other

family members. But the older generation requires a lot more hand-holding. When Greco moved in with her daughter, she was generally in good health, except for severe arthritis and high blood pressure. Over the years, however, Erdmann has found herself doing more and more for her mother. She manages her mother's three medications, watching to make sure she takes each one. Always fearful of falls, she's never far away when her mother bathes. She drives Greco to doctor's appointments, fills out all her medical forms, and spends hours on the phone every month sorting out billing or insurance problems. Meanwhile, she says, her mother has started to suffer from short-term memory loss, and Erdmann has become less comfortable leaving her alone during the day.

Such gradual increases in care are one reason why many adult children don't think of themselves as caregivers. "They say, 'I'm just doing what any good daughter would do,'" says Gail Gibson Hunt, president and CEO of the National Alliance for Caregiving, a nonprofit coalition of caregiving organizations. As a result, she says, adult children don't think to look for help. That omission can have serious consequences for both the caregiver and the aging parents, since stress can harm caregiver health and lead to a lower quality of care.

One thing that can help ease the strain is proper training. The American Red Cross, hospitals, and nonprofit aging organizations offer courses for family caregivers that cover safety, nutrition, and legal and financial issues. Professional help can also be a godsend. Roughly 1.4 million people receive home-health services, sometimes paid for by Medicare, Medicaid, HMOs, or other insurance. Senior-living companies are also starting to offer home-based services. In Ohio, Kendal Corp., a Pennsylvania firm that owns 14 senior communities, has launched Kendal at Home, which, for an initial membership fee starting at $7,600, plus a monthly fee of $294, offers a lifetime guarantee to provide long-term care services.

States and federal lawmakers are recognizing the home trend. Vermont, for example, is already paying some family members $10 an hour to provide home care to Medicaid recipients who might otherwise be in nursing homes. Other states are following suit, and the federal Centers for Medicare and Medicaid Services has designated $1.75 billion in grants to encourage them. Most of these programs, however, are in the early stages and apply only to very low-income seniors.

Perhaps more immediately helpful for relieving the strain is respite care, someone to take over while caregivers take a deserved break. Some people arrange for a relative or paid caregiver to come. Others find assisted-living facilities that will take a family member for a short stay. In some communities, local Area Agencies on Aging pay for respite care.

Senior Cohousing

In 2002, a group of longtime friends in Davis, Calif., all in their 70s and 80s, sat down to talk about the future. Many had worked together at the University of California-Davis. Now, they faced a new challenge: "We wanted to spend our last years together and help each other as we aged," says John Jungerman, 84, a retired physics professor from UC-Davis.

The rapidly expanding array of housing choices is encouraging new models of independent living, such as cohousing.

Jungerman and his friends are getting their wish. After four years of negotiating for property, lobbying the city council for residential zoning, and coordinating with architects and builders, he and his wife, Nancy, were the first of 13 residents to move into Glacier Circle, the country's first elder cohousing community. Residents own their apartment or townhome (there are eight attached residences, all wheelchair accessible) and a portion of a separate common house that includes a kitchen, dining and living rooms, and a housekeeper's apartment. They also share chores and maintenance expenses. "We've been talking about sharing the cost of a nurse if several of us needed one," he says. Each home has its own kitchen, but residents share three meals a week—two of them whipped up by a professional cook—together in the common house. On Thursdays, it's potluck. In addition to spontaneous after-dinner socializing and movies, the residents meet every week to discuss new furniture for the common house, hiring a gardener, or business at hand. At least 20 other groups around the country are starting their own cohousing communities.

Like any group endeavor, cohousing presents daunting challenges. First, it's costly. Each family spent $350,000 to $450,000. Estate planning is tricky. All want heirs to be able to sell the property without changing the spirit of the community. And making group decisions can be difficult. "We definitely have more work on our hands than people who move into big retirement facilities," says Jungerman. "But it keeps our lives feeling meaningful."

Assisted living, continuing care. In 2003, Nina Liebman, 65, of New York City gave her 93-year-old father, Jules Roskin, a choice: move to an assisted-living facility or agree to a home health aide. The Albuquerque, N.M., resident suffered from congestive heart failure and Liebman felt it was no longer safe for him to live alone. He opted for a health aide, who gave him his medications and helped him with dressing and grooming, as well as shopping, cooking, and cleaning. But he resented the lack of privacy. Next he agreed to try assisted living. The decision turned out to be the right one, allowing Roskin to keep his fiercely guarded privacy until his death in 2004. "People came when he needed them," says Liebman. "Someone could help him, but then he could be by himself. That was very important to him."

An assisted-living residence charges a monthly fee—the national average is $2,968, according to MetLife—for room, board, and services such as laundry, transportation, housekeeping, and medication management. The fee goes up for higher levels of service, such as meals delivered to your apartment or dementia care.

Some assisted-living homes are part of continuing-care retirement communities. These promise to care for residents for the remainder of their lives; they move to the various facilities

as their needs demand. Unlike assisted-living facilities, most CCRCs don't simply charge rent and a service fee. Instead, seniors pay a hefty entrance fee, which can range from $70,000 to more than $1 million. In addition, there is a monthly fee that may or may not increase as the resident's level of care goes up. If this sounds like an insurance policy, there's a reason: Most CCRCs are actually considered a form of insurance and are overseen by state insurance regulators, as well as by state agencies that license assisted-living and nursing homes. Because of the complexity of fee structures, if you and your parent decide to go with assisted living or a CCRC, it's critical to understand what it will cost, what services are provided, and how those costs will change if your parent needs additional care.

The security of assisted living and CCRCs can bring adult children peace of mind, while older parents often like the idea of no home upkeep. "I'd maintained a home for 62 years, and I really didn't want the responsibility anymore," says Nellie Snook, 84, who moved into a CCRC in Chapel Hill, N.C., in 2004. But assisted living and CCRCs may not suit those who don't like crowds. And you must be in good health to join. Most CCRCs accept only new residents who can start off in independent living.

Nursing homes. After Kathleen Berthay's husband died four years ago, Berthay moved to a 140-bed nursing home in Tupelo, Miss. At the time, Berthay, who is blind, could reasonably have expected to live the rest of her days in a shared, hospital-style room eating meals delivered on a tray. Instead, as part of a "Green House" project launched by Mississippi Methodist Senior Services in Tupelo, Berthay, 81, moved out of the home in 2003 and into a house she shares with just nine other people. Berthay eats with her housemates at a common table in the dining room, sharing meals prepared by a certified nurses' aide who also cleans the house and helps Berthay and other residents with bathing, dressing, and other daily tasks. When doctors and physical therapists visit, they ring the doorbell.

The search for the right file for a parent can be frustrating. Not all options are available in every community.

"This is the best thing that ever happened to old people," Berthay says. The Green Houses—so named to connote growth and life—have yielded impressive results since they first opened in 2003. "The Green Houses are revolutionizing the model of care within nursing homes," says Rosalie Kane, a professor of public health at the University of Minnesota. Her research shows that compared with nursing home residents, people living in the Green Houses score better on measures of quality of life and show slower declines in their abilities to perform daily tasks.

Efforts are underway to launch Green House projects in every state. Traditional nursing homes are scrambling to keep up. Some are starting to offer private rooms, replacing dinner trays with dining room buffets, and training staff to be more autonomous. At a growing number of nursing homes run by Beverly

Living and Golden Living, hospital-style care is giving way to "neighborhoods," where large institutions are subdivided into groups of 12 to 24 residents, who take part in choosing music or planning activities and share family-style meals in small dining rooms. And the companies are aiming to have the same staff take care of the same residents all the time.

When considering nursing homes, look for these types of efforts to make care more homey and personal. "You don't have to trade in your ticket to quality of life to get a certain level of personal care and monitoring of healthcare," says Kane. That's a lesson that adult children are learning in their search for the best old-age care. "All the time I was helping my father, I was thinking, 'What if this were me? Would I want to be in a place like this?'" says Liebman. The answers that baby boomers arrive at will no doubt shape the future of aging as they demand better care for their parents and, eventually, for themselves.

Declaration of Independents

Home Is Where You Want to Live Forever. Here's How

BARBARA BASLER

Suzanne Stark, 79, lives in a book-lined apartment in central Boston's lovely Beacon Hill neighborhood. Independent and active, the author and freelance writer nevertheless acknowledges there are times when problems arise and she needs help. Like when her beloved cat Zenobia became suddenly, violently ill, and Stark couldn't get her into a carrier to take her to the veterinarian.

"I tried everything, and then I called Beacon Hill Village," she says. "I said, 'I know this is weird, but can you send someone to help me get this cat in the carrier?' And they did."

Beacon Hill Village is a revolutionary, all-encompassing concierge service created by residents who want to grow old in the homes they have lived in for years. Now, they can do that, confident that even as they age they can deal with almost any contingency, large or small, without relying on relatives or friends. To preserve their independence, they can turn to the village, as the nonprofit association is known, which helps its 320 members find virtually any service they need—from 24-hour nursing care to help with a wayward cat, often at a discounted fee.

Their innovation is so appealing that a national expert on aging at the Massachusetts Institute of Technology asserts it could well change the way Americans—and the rest of the world—grow old. "The assisted living and the die-with-a-golf-club-in-your-hand communities had better take notice," says Joseph Coughlin, director of the MIT AgeLab, a think tank on aging.

This fresh concept is already attracting attention far beyond the quaint cobblestone walkways of Beacon Hill. In the three years since it started, the village has received more than 200 inquiries—from places as diverse as Manhattan and Las Vegas.

The group's grassroots creators are now writing a how-to manual so others can replicate the village in their own neighborhoods. And MIT is working on a plan of the concept that could be used around the world.

"With Beacon Hill Village you have life, you don't have retirement," Coughlin says. The village not only links members to carefully vetted personal trainers, caterers, house cleaners, plumbers and computer advisers, it also offers them a number of free benefits such as weekly car service to the grocery. Other free benefits include monthly lectures by notable Bostonians, exercise classes and special health clinics—all activities that take place in neighborhood churches, schools and a community center.

The village hasn't yet had a request it couldn't help fill, says Judy Willett, the social worker hired to direct the association and its two other full-time employees. "We even had a member in the hospital call and ask us to find someone to pick up her betting slips at the track. And we did," she says.

"We wanted everything you'd find in a retirement community or assisted living—but we wanted these services in our own homes," explains Susan McWhinney-Morse, 72, the president of Beacon Hill Village, who was one of the 12 residents who helped create it. "We didn't want to leave the neighborhood we love."

Village founder and member J. Atwood "Woody" Ives, 69, says, "Even the places they call active retirement communities tend to be depressing. They're so artificial—everybody there is old." But, he says, by staying in his own neighborhood, "I see college students, couples, young families, old people. There is a great mix here, and I think that adds to the quality of life."

Any neighborhood resident age 50 or older can join the village. Its members include retirees in their 90s as well as working people in their 50s and 60s. "The younger ones join because they like the convenience of our services or they need help caring for a parent who lives with them," Willett says. "They want to support Beacon Hill Village, make sure it will be there as they age."

Membership costs $550 a year per person, $750 a year per couple and $100 a year for lower-income residents, who also get a $250 credit toward services. And the village has people who charge as little as $15 an hour for odd jobs.

The woman the village sent to help Suzanne Stark with Zenobia spent all afternoon with them—driving Stark and her cat to the vet, waiting, then driving them to the animal hospital and finally home. "That saved Zenobia's life," Stark says. The cost of the service: $35.

In many cases remaining at home and using the village's à la carte services is much cheaper than assisted living, Willett says. If, however, someone becomes ill enough to need 24-hour care or other expensive services, the total costs probably will equal those of a nursing home, "but with one big difference: You are in your own home."

Village employees not only provide information and referrals, they telephone members to check that each job was completed satisfactorily. Although members are entitled to highly personalized attention, the tiny staff—operating out of a one-room neighborhood office—has never been overwhelmed because only

How to Build Your Own Village

Huddle: Form a core group of about a dozen high-profile neighbors with diverse skills and backgrounds.

Count Your Chickens: Research your community—the number of residents over age 50, their average income, etc. Beacon Hill Village used census information to determine if there are enough people to support the venture.

Know Your Customers: Commission a survey to find out what services people want and what they will pay for them.

Line up Players: Contact key local businesses and health providers—from local hospitals and home care agencies to repair services—to gauge their interest in working with your group.

Do the Math: Draw up a business plan, estimating membership income and service costs. Beacon Hill Village used Harvard MBA alumni. Local universities or colleges may offer similar free consultation.

Pass the Hat: Raise seed money. 30 percent of your estimated budget. Much of Beacon Hill Village's start-up money came from contributions by neighborhood residents who believed in the idea.

Get a Chief: Hire a director who will be the face and voice of your enterprise as you continue to recruit members and service providers.

The leafy streets of Beacon Hill are lined with 19th-century townhouses where people such as Henry James and Louisa May Alcott once lived. Today's residents live in a dense mix of fine homes, imposing apartment buildings, condos and even subsidized housing for older people, but they still tend to be well heeled and well educated. Can their aging solution really be transplanted to other, very different communities?

Yes, says Coughlin, because innovations "always start at the top, rather than the middle or the bottom. Of all the ideas we've seen here at the AgeLab, this one has got a better chance of going mainstream than many others."

Establishing this city-bred idea in the suburbs and beyond may actually be easier "because the cost of living, the cost of services is much less expensive there than here," says Sue Bridge, 66, one of the founders who, with help from alumni volunteers from Harvard University's School of Business, wrote the village's business plan.

Coughlin points out that "some of the best-knit communities in America are not in the city but in the country, in rural agricultural areas where institutions of faith often organize services and contacts for people."

Transportation in the suburbs or exurban areas could be an issue, but he does not see it as an insurmountable problem. "You have to think creatively," he says. "Missoula, Montana, for example, uses its airport shuttles in the off-peak hours to ferry older residents where they want to go and to take families to visit relatives in nursing homes."

"What we need," Coughlin says, "are folks with the passion to work these things out." Those people may be in a neighborhood association or they may be entrepreneurs "who see an explosion of disposable income and a demand for services that needs to be met."

One of the biggest obstacles to this effort to change the way people age has been the residents themselves. Village research shows that of the 13,000 people in the Beacon Hill area, 14 percent are age 60 or older, and some of these people were the most resistant.

"We couldn't believe all of the people we approached about joining who told us, 'That's a great idea, but I'm not ready yet,' " says board member Ives. "These were people in their 80s and 90s. People just hate to admit they need any kind of help."

Instead, "too many deal with aging by cutting back on where they go and when, what they do, who they see," says Bridge. "Their lives become more and more constricted. When they join the village, suddenly life opens up again."

One resident who initially resisted the village is now a booster. "They treat me like a queen," says Dorothy Weinstein, 97, who recently signed up for a village trip to New Hampshire to see the fall leaves. "They've been a saving grace."

She uses the village grocery service and calls the office when she needs an escort to her clinic appointments. The village even has volunteers who accompany her on neighborhood walks.

A resident of Beacon Hill for 53 years, still living in the house where she and her late husband raised their sons, Weinstein wouldn't think of moving.

"Where would I be as content as I am here?" she asks. "I look out my window at the park. I see people passing. I talk to old neighbors I know. This is the way I want things."

about a third of the members call the village frequently. Another third use it now and then, while the remainder draw mainly on its social offerings—lectures, weekly lunches in a local restaurant and day trips to places like the Newport Jazz Festival.

"The social aspect is the secret sauce here," says MIT's Coughlin. "Just bringing services to your door doesn't ensure a good life. People, especially older people living alone, need to be engaged, they need reasons to go out, to be a part of a community. And the village works to give them that."

The core group of 12 residents laid the groundwork for the project with meticulous research, drawing up a business plan, vetting and recruiting a number of businesses and health providers, all of them eager to have a reliable stream of customers. Two key concerns joined their effort early and helped anchor it—Harvard Medical School's Massachusetts General Hospital and House-Works, a Boston home services company.

The gifted amateur organizers, however, were canny enough to realize they needed help. By donating their own money and raising contributions from others in the neighborhood who believed in the idea, they hired professionals to help market the village concept to residents. They also approached several foundations for money for the subsidized memberships.

The village still relies on foundations and support from board members and the community, but membership is growing by about eight new members a month.

"Membership fees pay for about 50 percent of our expenses, and within a year we think that will rise to 60 percent," Willett says.

UNIT 8

Social Policies, Programs, and Services for Older Americans

Unit Selections

Key Points to Consider

- What are some of the problems a society must consider in facing an increasing aging population?

- What are the different ways that the financial solvency of the Social Security program could be achieved without privatization?

- What are the advantages and disadvantages of privatization of the medical drug benefit program?

- What does William Greider propose as a new retirement program to replace all those that are now having financial difficulties or being terminated?

- What new medical care practices does Patricia Barry believe would improve medical practices and costs?

- Which country did Mike Edwards rank at the top in terms of government benefits provided to its older citizens?

Student Website
www.mhhe.com/cls

Internet References

Administration on Aging
http://www.aoa.dhhs.gov

American Federation for Aging Research
http://www.afar.org

American Geriatrics Society
http://www.americangeriatrics.org

Community Transportation Association of America
http://www.ctaa.org

Medicare Consumer Information from the Health Care Finance Association
http://cms.hhs.gov/default.asp?fromhcfadotgov=true

National Institutes of Health
http://www.nih.gov

The United States Senate: Special Committee on Aging
http://www.senate.gov/~aging

It is a political reality that older Americans will be able to obtain needed assistance from governmental programs only if they are perceived as politically powerful. Political involvement can range from holding and expressing political opinions, voting in elections, participating in voluntary associations to help elect a candidate or party, and holding political office.

Research indicates that older people are just as likely as any other age group to hold political opinions, are more likely than younger people to vote in an election, are about equally divided between Democrats and Republicans, and are more likely than young people to hold political office. Older people, however, have shown little inclination to vote as a bloc on issues affecting their welfare despite encouragement by senior activists, such as Maggie Kuhn and the leaders of the Gray Panthers, to do so.

Gerontologists have observed that a major factor contributing to the increased push for government services for the elderly has been the publicity about their plight generated by such groups as the National Council of Senior Citizens and the American Association of Retired Persons (AARP). The desire of adult children to shift the financial burden of aged parents from themselves onto the government has further contributed to the demand for services for the elderly. The resulting widespread support for such programs has almost guaranteed their passage in Congress.

Now, for the first time, there are groups emerging that oppose increases in spending for services for older Americans. Requesting generational equity, some politically active groups argue that the federal government is spending so much on older Americans that it is depriving younger age groups of needed services.

The articles in this section raise a number of problems and issues that result from an ever-larger number and percentage of the population living to age 65 and older. In "Dignified Retirement: Lessons from Abroad," the author discusses how the retirement age of people in different countries affects their economic stability and growth. In "Social Security's 70th Anniversary: Surviving 20 Years of Reform," the author reviews the success of the Social Security program and why he believes it will be financially solvent for well into the future. In "The Corporate Beneficiaries of the Medicare Drug Benefit," the author points out how privatization

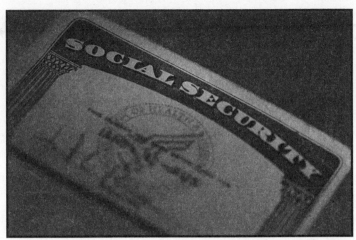

© Comstock/PunchStock

of the program imposed large costs on seniors, people with disabilities, the government, and health care providers.

Patricia Barry, in "Coverage for All," reviews Massachusetts and Vermont's universal health care coverage programs, and points out that these may well be the direction that health care coverage in the United States is headed in the near future. William Greider, in "Riding into the Sunset: The Geezer Threat," gives the economic problems of the current retirement funds and proposes a mandatory and universal saving system that he believes would be more durable than the current programs. In "The New Face of Health Care," the author discusses a number of new medical practices that would improve health care and lower costs. Mike Edwards, in "As Good as It Gets," shows the advantages that older persons living in the Netherlands have over other countries throughout the world in terms of the number and quality of retirement programs and government services they are provided. In "Population Aging, Entitlement Growth, and the Economy," the *AARP Public Policy Institute* observes what would have to be done with the current social service programs and federal taxation to keep the government deficit no worse in 2050 than it is today.

Dignified Retirement
Lessons from Abroad

Sylvester J. Schieber

There aren't many mysteries about the financial challenges posed by the aging of America's population. While little consensus exists on how to shore up Social Security, there is widespread understanding that the system will be in deficit within a decade of the first baby boomers' retirements, which start in 2008. The Medicare financing outlook is even bleaker; the federal health-insurance program for the elderly is already in the red even as a costly new prescription drug benefit is being implemented. Front-page stories about corporate pension plans that go belly up or are cut back, at the same time that retiree health-benefit programs are curtailed, add to the general anxiety.

But perhaps the biggest concern Americans should have about their retirement system is the sheer inertia that has prevented the nation from addressing its problems. For more than two decades, we have known about the demographic challenges facing Social Security. We knew before prescription drug benefits were added to Medicare coverage that the system was in trouble. It makes for a sad spectacle indeed that we enjoy the rare advantage of being able to see the future with clarity yet are unwilling to act.

Meanwhile, other countries have started to address some of the same challenges, and they have done so with greater inventiveness and determination than the United States has shown. The list of pioneers ranges from the familiar example of Chile to the less noted examples of Sweden, Germany, and Canada. All offer lessons from which America can learn.

By some measures, America's aging problem is relatively minor compared with what other developed countries face. For every retired person in America, there are currently about four working people. (Australia, Canada, and the United Kingdom have similar ratios.) In Japan, the ratio is closer to three workers per retired person; in Italy, it's down close to two, and Germany is not much better off than that.

The demographic future also looks at least as favorable for the United States as for any other developed country. The retirement burden on American workers is not expected to be any greater in 2030 than it already is today in Germany or Italy. By that year, Germany's burden is expected to be twice and Italy's 2.5 times America's. Italy will have only one active worker per retiree. Other developed countries, such as Switzerland and the Netherlands, will be in better positions than that but will still face bigger burdens than the United States.

Perhaps the most important lesson to be learned from abroad comes from countries that are less reliant on pensions to provide income security to older people. They do not rely as much on pensions for the simple reason that many older people in these countries are still working. Japan presents an especially interesting case. It has the most rapidly aging population in the developed world, but its retirement burden in 2030 is expected to be attenuated because older people in Japan tend to work later into life than their counterparts in most other developed countries. The average retirement age for Japanese men is nearly 67.

The undeniable fact is that many people, especially in the world's developed economies, are retiring at ages when they could still be highly productive. An astonishing 38 percent of Italians in the 50-to-54-year-old bracket are already out of the labor force, and hardly anyone in Italy between 60 and 64 still works. Granted, Italy is an extreme case; even in Sweden, workers are less likely to retire early. But the trend toward early retirement is widespread.

The most significant influence on when the majority of people leave work behind is the structure of the retirement system: An earlier "normal" retirement age or more generous benefits for early retirement lead, predictably, to more retirements. In Iceland, 81 percent of the population between the ages of 60 and 64 is still in the labor force, largely because of incentives in the retirement system that encourage people in that age bracket to continue working. Even in the United States, 47 percent are still economically active during those years. In Europe, the comparable numbers range from 22 percent in Germany to only 14.5 percent in France.

In Iceland, the average man works until age 67. In France, his counterpart retires at 59. Such variations help explain the range of costs associated with different retirement systems. In France, the average remaining life expectancy for a male at the typical retirement age is 20.5 years. It is 13.7 years in Iceland. All else being equal, a male retiree in France will cost about 60 percent more in retirement benefits than one in Iceland simply because of the longer duration of retirement.

Slowing Economic Growth

Pension payouts are not the only cost of retirement. By withdrawing their labor from the economy, retirees also slow economic growth, making it harder to underwrite retirement costs. If a country has a growing elderly population that does not contribute to national output and workers have an incentive to retire in their fifties, the particular method of financing retirement—pay-as-you-go, like Social Security, or fully funded retirement accounts—doesn't matter a great deal. There will, in any case, be trouble down the road.

Most government-run retirement systems around the world operate similarly to the U.S. Social Security system: Benefits paid to current retirees are financed on a pay-as-you-go basis, out of revenues from current workers. There's little or no "money in the bank." Beneath this level of general similarity, however, there are some significant differences in how public pension systems are structured, how large a role private pension plans play, and, most important for our purposes, how willing policymakers have been to make the hard choices needed to ensure the survival of these systems.

One little-appreciated difference between the American system and most others has to do with its basic architecture. Most other countries have two-tier publicly financed retirement systems. The United States has a single tier.

In most of those other countries, virtually every citizen is entitled to a basic first-tier benefit upon reaching retirement age. In some cases, this benefit comes in the form of a universal "demogrant"; in others, recipients face income or assets tests that may reduce the size of the benefit or, in some cases, eliminate it.

On top of this basic benefit, these countries provide a separate, second tier of retirement benefit that is proportional to a worker's preretirement earnings. The second-tier benefit usually accounts for the largest share of the total retirement pension.

What's important is that the first tier is explicitly funded by general tax revenues, not by earmarked employer and employee contributions. As a result, the first-tier basic benefit seems to voters less like "their" own money, less like something they are entitled to. And that makes it politically easier for policymakers to adjust this part of the retirement system.

In the United States, the whole Social Security benefit is based on earnings, but it includes elements of the first- and second-tier benefits provided in other countries. Low-wage workers receive larger benefits relative to their earnings than those with high earnings, an arrangement that hides the character of the implicit basic benefit in our system. Yet workers with higher levels of covered earnings receive larger absolute benefits, which links payouts to covered earnings levels, albeit indirectly. Virtually all benefits are financed through payroll tax contributions. The structure of the U.S. system has led people to believe that they have "paid for" their benefits even though the benefits are highly subsidized.

Such perceptions matter a great deal. In Canada, for example, legislators were able several years ago to impose a means test on the basic pension through the income tax system, reducing benefits for higher-income retirees. Australia, too, has cut back its basic benefit, though with a twist. All Australians are still entitled to a relatively generous basic benefit, set at roughly 25 percent of the average worker's earnings, but it is subject to a means test that reduces recipients' benefits as their earnings and assets increase. In the past, Australians nearing retirement age did everything they could to avoid losing out under the means test—going on shopping sprees, taking round-the-world voyages, or doing whatever else it took to jettison some of their wealth. As a result, Australia in the early 1990s implemented a mandatory retirement savings program designed literally to force workers to save so much that many would fail the asset and income tests.

There has been a lot more innovation around the world in the second tier of public pensions. These pay-as-you-go programs are usually financed by contributions from both employers and employees, and they have traditionally promised workers a future "defined benefit" linked to their earnings during their working years. Social Security is such a system. Americans of working age are reminded of this every year when they receive a statement in the mail from the Social Security Administration showing, based on their contributions so far, how big a Social Security check they can expect in retirement. Such defined-benefit programs are in the deepest trouble, and reforms are under way from Canada to Japan and Sweden.

Some countries have shifted their retirement programs to a more fully funded basis—meaning they are now putting "money in the bank" to pay for future benefits. In the late 1990s, for example, Canada raised the contribution levels of employers and employees and created a separate, non-government board to invest the the money in stocks and bonds, seeking higher returns. The United States has been reluctant to pursue similar policies because of political concerns over how the government might manage what could become the largest pool of investment capital in the world.

Defined-Contribution Places Burden on Individual

Traditional defined-benefit programs guarantee people a certain fixed payout in the future. But several countries have moved toward a bigger role for "defined-contribution" plans. In such systems, the ultimate payout is not fixed in advance but is determined by the level of return on the invested money. In some countries, employers select the defined-contribution plan provider. In others, individuals choose from a series of authorized private-fund managers. The investment risk in both cases is largely borne by the individual account holder, although some systems provide a guaranteed minimum return of some sort. The theory here is that at retirement, workers will simply receive benefits in accordance with what they have contributed.

Since the 1980s, a number of countries have even adopted defined-contribution plans as the primary element of their second tier. The example that has received the most attention is Chile, which radically reformed its pension system in 1981. In essence, the Chileans transformed their severely dysfunctional pay-as-you-go system into private individual retirement accounts. The accounts are mandatory, fully funded, fully vested, and portable. Workers must contribute 10 percent of their annual earnings to their retirement accounts and choose where to invest their savings from funds offered by highly regulated, specialized, private-fund management companies. Workers also must purchase term life insurance and disability insurance from their pension managers. All told, the package comes to about 13 percent of gross pay. At retirement, participants have a retirement nest egg whose size will vary depending on how the investments have performed.

Two main criticisms have been leveled against the Chilean system: The fund management companies have extracted very high fees, and large numbers of Chileans are not covered because they are self-employed or too poor, or for other reasons. However, the system has been reasonably successful, with many workers enjoying more secure retirement prospects than they did under the old system. A number of other Latin American countries have followed the Chilean example.

Roughly a decade after Chile acted, Australia embarked on an equally radical reform. Beginning in 1992, employers were obliged to contribute a share of workers' pay (now nine percent) to privately operated retirement funds. As a result, most workers will accumulate enough assets so that they will not qualify for Australia's meanstested first-tier basic pension until much later in their retirement (as they exhaust their savings) than under prior policy. Australian voters accepted this change because there would not be significant reductions in basic pensions for many years and because those affected would have a bigger pot of personal savings at retirement.

Sweden created supplemental private accounts without much fuss during the mid-1990s as part of a larger reform of its pension system; it now requires that workers contribute 2.5 percent of covered pay to individual accounts invested through government-approved investment managers. At the same time, Sweden made a revolutionary change in the traditional pay-as-you-go system that still provides the main pension benefit for Swedes. Under the new setup, workers continue to pay contributions to the system, and they amass retirement accounts—even though in reality their contributions are quickly paid out to current retirees. But as the change is phased in, workers' accounts will be treated as what they really are: virtual or "notional" accounts, with no assets backing them. The accounts are bookkeeping devices. As a result, there is no defined benefit. Benefits are not determined until a worker reaches age 61, when they will be set in a two-step process.

In the first stage, a basic benefit will be determined on the basis of the group's remaining life expectancy. As life expectancy increases in the future, monthly pensions will decrease to keep the total lifetime value of pensions relatively constant. In the second step, the benefit will also be adjusted so that each age group's expected lifetime benefits will be covered by what is anticipated in worker contributions during the course of its retirement period. This latter demographic adjustment will keep the system in balance as the number of retirees grows relative to workers. The result will almost certainly be a reduction in benefits, as well as much less strain on the Swedish economy.

The individual accounts Sweden mandated in the 1990s were not hugely controversial. Political leaders educated the public about the need for reform, and the accounts were part of a larger overhaul. The system's alterations were to be implemented in the future on a gradual basis. It is remarkable that attempts in the United States to shift toward such supplemental personal accounts in our Social Security system, most recently by the Bush administration, have proved so controversial, denounced as somehow being an abrogation of the "social" character of the U.S. system. The accounts that most American supporters have talked about range from 2 percent to 4 percent of earnings, not much different from the 2.5 percent Sweden has legislated.

Policymakers in Germany and Japan took a long, hard look at the Swedish example several years ago when they grappled with their own painful reforms. Neither was willing to move to Swedish-style notional accounts, but in both cases they adopted provisions for their defined-benefit systems that mimic the demographic adjustment the Swedes will use in determining future benefits. German and Japanese leaders took that route, most observers agree, in part because they thought it would be easier to get people to accept reforms if it were not so clear what the implications of the changes would be.

Americans are now experiencing—unwittingly, for the most part—the effects of just such a delayed reform undertaken in 1983, during Ronald Reagan's presidency. Congress raised the age at which Social Security benefits would be paid, but it deferred implementation until 2000. As a result of the reforms, people retiring this year will need to wait until eight months after their 65th birthday to stop working if they want to receive full benefits; people who are now 46 or younger will need to wait until their 67th birthday. There is a lesson in the fact that this delayed reform provoked virtually no protest in 1983 or when it began phasing in 17 years later.

Private versus Public Pensions

Private pensions are the other big element involved in thinking about how to pay for retirement. Such pensions loom larger in the retirement landscape of some countries, such as the United States, than others, but it seems clear that their role is likely to grow everywhere. As a rule, where public pensions are rich, private pensions tend to be spare, and where public plans are small, private pensions tend to be more substantial. In the past, it made little sense for a German employer to provide a generous pension, for example, since the country's public pension already allowed workers to retire at virtually the same standard of living they enjoyed while working.

But the remorseless logic of demographic change has led even the Germans to try to strike a new balance between public and private pensions. As part of a controversial package of public-pension tax increases and benefit cutbacks in 2000, the Social Democratic government of Chancellor Gerhard Schröder created tax incentives designed to encourage employers to establish voluntary supplemental retirement savings plans for workers and thus to take some of the pressure off the public system. Schröder's successor, Angela Merkel, recently declared that private pensions must be increased and that it will be necessary for Germany to push the normal retirement age up to 67.

Because Americans as a whole are not as dependent on the national pension, the United States enjoys some advantages in addressing the challenge of an aging society. Shoring up Social Security should be a much more manageable task than it has been in countries such as Germany and Sweden, where retirees are heavily dependent on public pensions. And mandating private pensions or savings programs, as many countries have already done, should not be as disruptive or expensive as it might be in countries where employers and workers do not already have a lot of experience with voluntary private plans. Requiring that all workers have supplemental accounts to boister the national pension, as Sweden has done, would seem to play to the generally successful American experience with 401(k) plans.

What remains an obstacle is the fear that such accounts will unduly expose workers to the risks of the stock and bond markets. There are risks in financial markets, and anyone who argues otherwise is misleading us about the choices we face. At the same time, many Americans have forgotten the painful 1977 Social Security reforms that reduced benefits for the "notch babies" (people born between 1917 and 1922) by as much as 20 percent relative to prior law. If U.S. workers aren't required to save some added amount of their pay in individual accounts, the Social Security benefit reductions that loom in the future probably will be far more widespread. If America doesn't address this problem soon, the eventual cutbacks will likely have to include some people on the verge of retirement, if not those already retired. Every path has risks, but the risks are greater in doing nothing until the onset of a crisis.

If the United States does not take to heart the lessons that some other countries have learned, it will be forced to repeat the unpleasant experiences of those that refused to act until there was no alternative. The Germans discovered that they had no choice but to reduce pension benefits, not just for future retirees but for existing ones. The Japanese learned that legislators confronted with such a crisis may come to blows on the floor of parliament. The future that looms before the United States is neither a blur nor a mystery. Its outlines can be seen with all the clarity of an actuarial table, and so can the choices.

Mr. Schieber is vice president of U.S. Benefits Consulting at Watson Wyatt & Company. From "Paying for It," by Sylvester J. Schieber, Wilson Quarterly, Spring 2006, pages 62–69.

Social Security's 70th Anniversary: Surviving 20 Years of Reform

L. RANDALL WRAY

Social Security turned 70 on August 14, [2005], although no national celebration marked the occasion.[1] Rather, our top policymakers in Washington continue to suggest that the system is "unsustainable." While our nation's most successful social program, and among its longest lived, has allowed generations of Americans to live with dignity in retirement, many think it is time to retire Social Security itself. They claim it is necessary to shift more responsibility to individuals and to scale back the promises made to the coming waves of retiring baby boomers.

Even the nonpartisan Social Security Administration has been enlisted in the effort to lower expectations, posting on its website the following caution to today's 26-year-old: "Unless changes are made, when you reach age 62 in 2041, benefits for all retirees could be cut by 26 percent and could continue to be reduced every year thereafter. If you lived to be 100 years old in 2079 (which will be more common by then), your scheduled benefits could be reduced by 32 percent from today's scheduled levels." Private accounts, lower benefits, and—perhaps—higher taxes are the prescribed remedy for "unfunded" trillions of commitments we have made to tomorrow's seniors. In this note, I provide a brief assessment of the curious transformation of America's most popular and efficient safety net into a program that is widely regarded as requiring thorough reform.

There is no question that Social Security has been under attack by well-organized and well-funded opponents for the past two decades. As my colleague Max Skidmore has documented, the enemies of the program have been there from the beginning, but they have had little success until recently (Skidmore 1999). Originally, the program was criticized on the basis that it was socialistic. However, the framers of the Social Security Act anticipated such claims and consequently formulated the program as if it were an insurance plan, with payroll taxes that could be counted as "contributions" and "benefit payments" that bore some relation to the contributions. Americans came to believe that they earned benefits because they "paid into" the program. And because the program was never means tested, it enjoyed wide support. Hence, rather than socialistic welfare, the program has been viewed as little different from a pension plan. For several decades, this misconception

effectively quashed criticism, so the program was expanded, rather than cut (Wray 2001).

However, beginning in the 1980s, the critics seized on an apparent weakness. Slower economic growth after 1970, lower birth rates, longer life spans, and especially the coming retirement of a wave of baby boomers all supposedly threatened the long-run financial viability of Social Security. The enemies of the program formulated a two-pronged attack. First, they began a campaign to convince younger people that because of shaky finances they would never collect benefits equal to what they paid into the program (Skidmore 1999). This became an increasingly easy sell for younger, high-income workers because the redistributive aspects of the program provide fairly low "money's worth" returns for the "pension" provided by Social Security. (Note that the debate mostly ignored all the "non-pension" aspects of the program, such as disability and survivors' benefits, which make it a good deal for just about all Americans.) Second, the Greenspan Commission was formed in 1983 to resolve the long-run financial problems with "reforms" that included large payroll tax increases and a gradual rise of the normal age of retirement (Papadimitriou and Wray 1999a). These changes reinforced the claim that Social Security was a bad deal for younger workers, who were already seeing take-home pay fall during a period in which labor was under attack by the Reagan administration.

After the Greenspan Commission had "solved" the financial problems, the Social Security Administration adopted increasingly pessimistic assumptions for its long-run forecasts—as documented by Skidmore (2001) and by actuary David Langer (2000). Not surprisingly, a "looming financial crisis" reappeared, and hysteria about reforming Social Security was revived. Taxes would have to be raised, benefits would have to be cut, and, more importantly, the return on Trust Fund assets would have to be increased. As the stock market performed well throughout most of the 1980s and then picked up the pace in the 1990s, the enemies saw a chance to privatize the program while playing the role of savior. At the same time, the "friends" of Social Security, mostly Democrats and Big Labor, also saw a chance to exploit popular fears. They would play along with the enemies, pretending there really was a financial problem, so that *they* could save Social Security and thereby win votes. Polls consistently show that voters trust Democrats more on Social Security; hence, given a choice between Republican schemes to "save" the program through privatization or Democratic plans to "save" it by placing the Trust Funds off limits, the voters would choose the Democrats.

I have been writing about Social Security since the late 1980s, and in 1990, I published a critique of *Can America Afford to Grow Old?* a book by Henry Aaron, Michael Bosworth, and Gary Burtless that argued that the only way to take care of baby boomers would be to immediately increase national saving (Wray 1990, 1990–91; Aaron et al. 1989; Aaron 1990–91). This could be done, according to the authors, by running budget surpluses, adding to national savings, and increasing the size of the Trust Fund. Hence, this book could be seen as a road map for the evolving Democratic party position during the Clinton years. However, I argued at the time that a larger Trust Fund could not in any way provide for future retirees, nor would it add to national savings. Rather, the Trust Fund represents a leakage that lowers aggregate demand; all else being equal, this lowers economic growth and thus makes it more difficult to take care of future retirees. Aaron wrote a response to my piece, arguing that he had thought that such "vulgar Keynesianism" was "blessedly extinct" (Aaron 1990–91). According to Aaron, running budget surpluses to add to the Trust Fund would indeed increase saving and lower interest rates, thus stimulating investment and economic growth, making it easier to take care of retirees.

As we now know, the Clinton budget did turn sharply toward surplus, and those surpluses were projected at the time to continue for at least a generation. A number of economists advocated "saving" this surplus for future retirees. As laid out in the plan by Aaron, et al., President Clinton proposed to take a portion of each year's surplus and add it to the Trust Fund (Wray 1999a, 1999b). Essentially, this would allow double counting of the surplus run by Social Security, since most of the budget surpluses accrued during the Clinton years were due to payroll taxes that far exceeded program benefits. During the 2000 presidential race, Al Gore used Social Security "lockboxes" as a primary campaign issue, confusing an internal bookkeeping operation (as Social Security's assets in the Trust Fund equal the Treasury's liabilities to Social Security, this is a case of the government owing itself) with availability of "finance" for the government as a whole. A wide variety of economists (including Aaron) embarrassed themselves by claiming that this was "good economics," going so far as to sign a petition in support of the plan (Wray 1999b).

I was told by economic advisors to top Democrats and big unions that they realized lockboxes were nonsense but believed it was politically pragmatic to endorse irregular accounting as a means to "save" the program. I responded that there was no need to run budget surpluses in order to credit Social Security's Trust Fund; the government can immediately credit the Trust Fund with trillions of dollars of assets, offset by the Treasury's commitment to make timely benefit payments when and as necessary (Wray 1999b). Most importantly, I worried about the long-term damage that would be done to the program by creating a false crisis and then resolving it with a preposterous gimmick. Of course, the Democrats' strategy did backfire: Gore lost the election, the Clinton budget surpluses brought down the economy and morphed into huge deficits "as far as the eye can see," and President Bush took on Social Security "reform" as a major goal of his administration. Ironically, the Republicans now quote President Clinton whenever Democrats try to deny that the program faces a crisis, leaving Dems in the untenable position of either admitting they were lying in the 1990s or that they are lying now (Wray 2005).

During the Clinton years I wrote a series of pieces critical of alternative plans to "save" Social Security, including those proposed by Democrats as well as those advanced by Republicans (Wray 1999a, 1999b; Papadimitriou and Wray 1999a, 1999b). After reading one of these critiques (Papadimitriou and Wray 1999b), Charles P. Blahous, policy director for Senator Judd Gregg (R-NH), engaged me in a series of e-mail exchanges. He accepted my critiques of the Clinton plan, but was bothered by my critique of the Gregg-Breaux proposal (which, briefly, included partial privatization, a government-subsidized savings plan, and a combination of benefit cuts and tax hikes; Blahous had apparently played some role in formulating the plan, and many of its features were included in later reform proposals). He also insisted that there really was a Social Security crisis and that the only feasible solution would be to privatize. He raised a number of issues that appeared at the time to be rather bizarre: that the crisis would begin as soon as tax revenue fell below benefit payments (that is, long before the Armageddon date cited by many economists as the year in which the Trust Fund is expected to be depleted); that faster economic growth would make the problem *worse;* that under current law, benefits would have to be cut by more than a quarter as soon as the Trust Fund was depleted; and that Social Security was a terrible deal for blacks and for women. More interestingly, when President Bush appointed his Reform Commission to study the problem, none other than Blahous was picked as executive director.[2] Blahous's hand could be seen all over the various reports issued by the Commission, with many of the same arguments that he had made previously in e-mails to me. The Commission claimed that Social Security was "broken" and required a "complete overhaul"; it bemoaned the bad deal cut for women and minorities; it engaged in a sleight of hand by comparing its "reforms" against "current law benefits" that were actually a quarter below those promised in the current benefit formula (none of the proposed reforms came close to providing the legislated benefits); it claimed that the present value of Social Security's shortfall was $3.2 trillion; and it proposed partial privatization and benefit cuts as the solution (Wray 2001).[3] What appeared then to be bizarre claims are now commonplace.

However, terrorism and security issues forced Social Security to the back burner during the first Bush term. After reelection, Bush felt he had a mandate to return to privatization of Social Security. At first, supporters of privatization claimed that it would resolve the "financial crisis"; eventually, the President admitted that the private accounts would worsen the program's finances (Wray 2005). Finally, he returned to the Commission's suggestion to drop wage indexing of future benefits (at least for all but the lowest-income workers) and hinted that he would consider elimination of the cap on wages subject to taxation (Wray 2005). If successful, these changes would substantially erode the support of middle- and upper-income earners, who would face huge cuts to benefits and higher taxes. Partial privatization would almost certainly lead to lower retirement payments for many lower-income workers (with management fees eating up the returns on their small accounts). Further, as many middle- and upper-income workers would opt for the privatization alternative, the amount of benefits received directly from Social Security by them would fall toward insignificance (Krugman 2005). Over the long haul, the nonprivatized portion of Social Security would be converted to a "welfare" program, important only to low-income people. This could be the last straw for what has long been America's most successful and popular government program.

The truth is that Social Security does not, and indeed *cannot,* face any financial crisis. It is a federal government program and as such cannot become insolvent. Social Security benefits are paid in the same way that the federal government makes expenditures for all of its other programs: by cutting a Treasury check or, increasingly, by directly crediting a bank account. Social Security is an unusual program only in that we pretend the payroll taxes "pay for" benefits; in reality, trying to maintain a balance between these flows is purely a politically inspired accounting procedure. Any federal government spending must be accounted for, but it cannot be *financially* constrained by specific or even general tax revenues. Further, the Trust Fund does not and cannot provide finance for Social Security. So long as the full faith and credit of the U.S. government stands behind the promised benefits, they can and will be paid, whether the Trust Fund has a positive or negative balance. Many proponents of the current system who understand this economic reality still want to accumulate a Trust Fund on the argument that it provides political protection. Perhaps the Trust Fund provided cover at one time, but it no longer serves even that purpose. It is precisely because there is a Trust Fund that the privatizers are making headway: if there were no Trust Fund, there would be nothing to privatize. Indeed, some of the privatizers see the trillion and a half dollars in the Trust Fund as a potential boost to flagging equity markets. Further, the eventual "exhaustion" of the Trust Fund plays a critical role in all of the schemes to increase returns on assets through privatization. Hence, the irregular accounting only hinders development of a clear understanding of the issues involved.

Social Security provides a substantial measure of security for aged persons, survivors, and disabled persons—and their dependents. It has never missed a payment, nor will it ever do so, as long as the full faith and credit of the U.S. government lies behind the program. Reform might be desired, and might even be necessary, but not because of any mythical looming financial crisis. Our nation is undergoing slow but important demographic changes that probably warrant informed discussion of the future shape of Social Security. While the baby boomers receive all the attention, other demographic and economic changes may be more important, including a greater proportion of female-headed households, higher immigration and the rising proportion of "minority" populations (already a majority in several states), and increasing economic inequality. Combined with the disappearance of employer-provided defined benefit pension plans and reduced employment security, these trends actually might strengthen the arguments for more generous and secure publicly provided safety nets—*not* for benefit cuts and privatization. However, none of these challenges rises to the level of a programmatic crisis; we will have years and even decades to make adjustments to Social Security should we decide they are necessary. In the meantime, happy 70th birthday, Social Security, with many happy returns.

Notes

1. Interestingly, the only reference to the anniversary available on the Social Security Administration's website is an *Orlando Sentinel* editorial by Jo Anne B. Barnhart, commissioner of Social Security, who notes that while the program has paid "approximately $8.4 trillion in benefits to nearly 200 million people," and while the benefits for "our parents, grandparents, and great-grandparents . . . are secure and will be paid . . . the same cannot be said for my teenage son and his friends" (Barnhart 2005).

2. Before that appointment, Blahous served as executive director of the business-sponsored Alliance for Worker Retirement Security from June 2000 through February 2001. He joined the National Economic Council on February 26, 2001, and now serves as special assistant to the president for economic policy.

3. See Diamond and Orszag (2002a) for a careful analysis of the Commission's reports. Blahous tried to defend the claims made for the various "reforms" in a memo characterized by *New York Times* columnist Paul Krugman as "hysterical. The number of non sequiturs and misrepresentations Mr. Blahous manages to squeeze into just a few pages may set a record" (Krugman 2002). See Blahous's response (2002) and Diamond and Orszag's rejoinder (2002b).

References

Aaron, Henry J. 1990–91. "Comment: Can the Social Security Trust Fund Contribute to Savings?" *Journal of Post Keynesian Economics* 13:2: 171.

Aaron, Henry J., Barry P. Bosworth, and Gary Burtless. 1989. *Can America Afford to Grow Old?* Washington, D.C.: Brookings Institution.

Barnhart, Jo Anne B. 2005. "Social Security Boss: Send Signal of Strength." *Orlando Sentinel,* August 11. www.ssa.gov/article081105.htm

Blahous, Charles P. 2002. "Problems with the Diamond/Orszag Paper on the Proposals of the President's Commission to Strengthen Social Security." June 18. Available from Peter A. Diamond, MIT, or Peter R. Orszag, Brookings Institution.

Diamond, Peter A., and Peter R. Orszag. 2002a. "An Assessment of the Proposals of the President's Commission to Strengthen Social Security." Washington, D.C.: The Brookings Institution. www.brookings.edu/views/papers/orszag/20020618.htm

———. 2002b. "A Response to the Executive Director of the President's Commission to Strengthen Social Security." Washington, D.C.: Center on Budget and Policy Priorities. www.cbpp.org/6-25-02socsec.pdf

Krugman, Paul. 2002. "Fear of All Sums." *New York Times,* June 21. www.pkarchive.org/column/062102.html

———. 2005. "A Gut Punch to the Middle." *New York Times,* May 2.

Langer, David. 2000. "Cooking Social Security's Deficit." *Christian Science Monitor,* January 4.

Papadimitriou, Dimitri B., and L. Randall Wray. 1999a. *Does Social Security Need Saving? Providing for Retirees throughout the Twenty-first Century.* Public Policy Brief No. 55. Annandale-on-Hudson, N.Y.: The Levy Economics Institute.

———. 1999b. "More Pain, No Gain: The Breaux Plan Slashes Social Security Benefits Unnecessarily." Policy Note 1999/8. Annandale-on-Hudson, N.Y.: The Levy Economics Institute.

Skidmore, Max J. 1999. *Social Security and Its Enemies: The Case for America's Most Efficient Insurance Program.* Boulder, Colorado: Westview Press.

———. 2001. "What Happened to the Social Security Surplus? An Examination of the Trustees' Projections." Paper presented at "The Social Security 'Crisis': Critical Analysis and Solutions" conference at the University of Missouri–Kansas City.

Wray, L. Randall. 1990. "A Review of *Can Americans Afford to Grow Old?: Paying for Social Security,* by Aaron, Bosworth, and Burtless." *Journal of Economic Issues* 24:4: 1175–1179.

———. 1990–91. "Can the Social Security Trust Fund Contribute to Savings?" *Journal of Post Keynesian Economics* 13:2: 155–170.

———. 1999a. "The Emperor Has No Clothes: President Clinton's Proposed Social Security Reform." Policy Note 1999/2. Annandale-on-Hudson, N.Y.: The Levy Economics Institute.

———. 1999b. "Surplus Mania: A Reality Check." Policy Note 1999/3. Annandale-on-Hudson, N.Y.: The Levy Economics Institute.

———. 2001. "Killing Social Security Softly with Faux Kindness: The Draft Report by the President's Commission on Social Security Reform." Policy Note 2001/6. Annandale-on-Hudson, N.Y.: The Levy Economics Institute.

———. 2005. "Manufacturing a Crisis: The Neocon Attack on Social Security." Policy Note 2005/2. Annandale-on-Hudson, N.Y.: The Levy Economics Institute.

Senior Scholar **L. RANDAL WRAY** is a professor at the University of Missouri–Kansas City and director of research at the Center for Full Employment and Price Stability.

The Corporate Beneficiaries of the Medicare Drug Benefit

Dean Baker

Millions of senior citizens and disabled people enrolled in Medicare Part D drug plans in 2006 discovered the "doughnut hole," the unusual $2,850 gap in coverage that was placed into the plan to save the U.S. federal government money.

The doughnut hole is peculiar because it goes directly against the general design of insurance. Usually, insurance policies are designed to protect holders against large losses. Policies typically have deductibles and/or co-pays with the assumption that most people can afford modest costs. After a certain level of costs, the share borne by the insurer typically increases—this is the bad event against which the policy holder is insuring themselves.

The Medicare drug benefit effectively takes the opposite approach. There is an initial deductible, and the basic formula provides for a 25 percent co-payment, but the benefits continue only until the beneficiary incurs $2,250 in drug expenses for the year. At that point, the beneficiary is directly and fully liable for the next $2,850 in annual expenditures, with no assistance provided through the benefit. Only if expenses exceed $5,100 for the year will the insurance again provide benefits, at that point paying 95 percent of additional expenses.

The size of this doughnut hole will grow in the future, since the basic benefit schedule is indexed to average per person drug spending, which is projected to grow at a rate of more than 8 percent annually. The expected size of the doughnut hole in 2007 is $3,078. By 2016, it is projected to grow to $6,100.

This peculiar design was adopted in order to limit the cost of the Medicare drug benefit. Starting in 2007, when most participants will be enrolled for the full year, the doughnut hole will transfer costs of about $20 billion to beneficiaries—these are costs beneficiaries will have to cover out of pocket, thanks to the doughnut hole.

There were other ways in which costs could have been contained. Most notably, the brand-name pharmaceutical industry successfully pressed Congress to prohibit Medicare from bargaining directly with the drug companies to lower prices. This passive acceptance of drug company monopoly prices may have added more than $40 billion to the annual cost of the program in its first years. Congress also stipulated that the program would be administered through private insurers rather than the existing Medicare program—a decision that the Congressional Budget Office (CBO, an independent Congressional research agency) estimates added nearly $5 billion a year to the program's expenses, and that imposed billions more in indirect costs on beneficiaries.

Pharma's Benefit

In adopting the Medicare drug benefit, Congress stipulated that Medicare could not directly negotiate price discounts with drug manufacturers, as is done by the Veterans Administration (VA) and the Healthcare systems in most other wealthy countries. As a result, prescription drugs cost far more under the Medicare drug benefit plan than is necessary. In the case of many drugs, the prices paid by insurers participating in the plan are more than twice as high as the prices paid by the VA.

Since the industry is already making a profit at the price for which it sells drugs to the VA, the higher price paid by the private insurers participating in the Medicare drug benefit is pure profit for the drug industry.

Comparing the Veterans Administration price for drugs with those available in the Medicare drug program shows the huge price differences between what Medicare is paying and what it might pay, if it negotiated as well as the VA. Multiplying this differential by the number of prescriptions in the Medicare plan reveals the excess profits earned by the industry for each drug— in just one year of the program. (In the accompanying table, the calculation of excess profits is based on the difference between a weighted average of the prices available through insurers participating in the Medicare drug benefit and the price at which the drug can be obtained through the Veterans Administration. The calculation is based on the assumption that 70 percent of the prescriptions for the top 20 drugs among seniors were used by seniors in the Medicare drug plan.)

For several of the drugs, the excess profits are substantial. The excess profits earned on Protonix, a heartburn medication, are just under $1 billion. The combined excess profits earned on the two dosages for Zocor, a cholesterol-lowering drug, are more than $1.6 billion. The combined excess profits for the two

PhRMA: Negotiating Drug Prices Will Eliminate Patient Choice

Much of the underlying data in Dean Baker's story comparing the costs of drugs under the Medicare prescription drug program with the costs negotiated by the Veterans Administration comes from the Boston-based Families USA. When Families USA released a June 2006 study with the data, the brand-name pharmaceutical industry lobby responded immediately.

"Families USA is attacking Medicare's prescription drug program despite overwhelming evidence that it is making a positive difference for seniors and the disabled," charged the Pharmaceutical Researchers and Manufacturers of America (PhRMA) in a statement.

"The truth is this program is providing better access to medicines for seniors and the disabled while costing taxpayers much less than anticipated. Just a few years ago, barely half of America's seniors had prescription drug coverage. Today more than 90 percent of them do."

PhRMA's key charge was that the VA system undermines patient choice, by restricting patients to drugs that appears on a formulary. The power to refuse to list drugs on the formulary, the industry group charged, is what gives the VA its negotiating power.

"Families USA wants the government to negotiate prices as a 'fix' for a Medicare program that is not broken. They ignore two crucial facts. First, the success of the Medicare drug program relies on private sector competition to contain medicine costs. Private plans are already achieving significant savings from pharmaceutical makers.

"Second, when governments set drug prices, patient choice vanishes. Allowing the federal government to negotiate drug prices would, according to experts, lead to restrictive formularies and keep patients from getting the medicines their doctors prescribe. While Medicare Part D plans in 2007 cover 4,300 prescription drugs on average, the VA plan includes only around 1,300 prescription medicines.

"Families USA ignores the lack of choice patients have under the VA program. In fact, of the 300 drugs Families USA examined in its report, only 65 percent are included in the VA formulary, compared to the 95 percent that are covered by the largest plan in the Federal Employee Health Benefit Program (FEHBP), which covers members of Congress. Additionally, of 132 brand drugs among the top 300 drugs, a mere 42 percent are covered by the VA formulary, compared to 95 percent covered by the FEHBP formulary."

Families USA responded in detail in a follow-up report. The assertion that the VA restricts patient access to drugs is misleading on three counts, the organization explained. First, access to drugs in the VA system is not limited to drugs on the VA formulary. Patients can get drugs off the formulary through a straightforward waiver process. Second, the VA negotiates low prices for all drugs, including those not on the formulary. Drugs not on the formulary are discounted almost as much as those that are. Third, "in some ways, the VA system actually gives broader access to prescription drugs than the formularies of Part D plans. Part D plans can require large copayments, impose quantity limits and restrict access through prior-authorization requirements and utilization review. The VA charges only a small copayment per prescription and rarely imposes restrictions on the use of co-formulary drugs."

"Claims that the VA formulary achieves cost savings by unduly restricting access are simply unfounded," concludes Families USA. "An overwhelming majority of VA physicians report that the formulary allows them to prescribe drugs that meet their patients' needs. Patients also believe their needs are being met: Access to drugs is an issue in less than one-half of one percent (.4 percent) of veterans' complaints about the VA health system."

"The VA pairs rational, cost-effective prescribing practices with the bargaining power of the government to achieve substantial cost savings. In contrast, Part D plans limit access without effectively controlling costs. A system of direct negotiation under Medicare would presumably differ in some ways from the VA in order to meet the particular needs of Medicare beneficiaries. But if Medicare were able to use its leveraging power to negotiate on behalf of its millions of beneficiaries, it would likely be able to obtain prices that are much more in line with those secured for the millions of Americans covered through the VA."

---

dosages of Lipitor, another cholesterol-lowering drug, come to $1.2 billion.

The excess profits on this small group of drugs is fairly sizable relative to the doughnut hole gap in coverage under the prescription drug plan. The excess profit earned on Protonix alone is almost 5 percent of the size of the doughnut hole. The excess profits on Lipitor are close to 6 percent of the size of the doughnut hole.

There are thousands of different types of drugs, dosages and delivery mechanisms, which in nearly all cases cost more than necessary under the Medicare drug plan, because Congress prohibited Medicare from directly negotiating drug prices with the pharmaceutical industry. If Medicare had been allowed to negotiate in the same way as the Veteran's Administration, the savings would have been enough to eliminate the doughnut hole gap in coverage, even using conservative assumptions.

The Congressional Budget Office has found that drug prices in other industrialized countries are 35 to 55 percent lower than in the United States. Those countries also do a better job than the United States at controlling drug price inflation. These countries use various mechanisms to control price, but they ultimately reflect the countries' bargaining power—drug companies are always free not to sell, if they don't like the price. Medicare would be a larger buyer than any one country, so it is reasonable to assume it could at least match, and likely undercut, the prices available in other countries.

Excess Profits from Top Prescription Drug Sales, in Millions of Dollars

Drug	Maker	Annual Prescriptions (in millions)	Excess Profits (in millions of dollars)
Zocor	Merck	11.2	$1,656.1
Lipitor	Pfizer	31.6	1,199.9
Protonix	Wyeth	16.4	990.4
Prevacid	AstraZeneca	22.2	603.1
Zoloft	Pfizer	27.0	585.2
Fosamax	Merck	17.9	543.9
Plavix	Bristol-Myer's	18.8	412.4
Norvasc	Pfizer	16.3	369.6
Nexium	AstraZeneca	22.9	358.5
Actonel	Proctor & Gamble	9.7	223.8
Celebrex	Pfizer	11.0	216.4
Aricept	Pfizer	4.3	143.9
Xalatan	Pfizer	6.9	130.2
Toprol XL	AstraZeneca	8.2	114.0
Other			12,852.4
Total			**$7,647.9**

Source: Center for Economic and Policy Research calculations from Families USA price data and RxList prescription data.

If Medicare as negotiator were to do only as well as the most-expensive industrialized country—reducing prices 35 percent and controlling inflation—it would, from 2006 to 2013, save $332 billion versus what CBO projects will be spent under the existing rules. If Medicare did as well as the least-expensive industrialized country—reducing prices 55 percent and controlling inflation—it would save $563 billion over the 2006–2013 period.

Instead of being allocated to eliminate the doughnut hole or for other public purposes, those monies are landing in pharmaceutical company coffers.

Aiding the HMO/Insurers

Big Pharma's subsidy is not the only corporate welfare component of the Medicare drug benefit. The decision to offer the benefit through private insurers instead of the existing Medicare system imposes two sets of additional costs.

The Congressional Budget Office projected in July 2004 that additional administrative costs due to the marketing expenses and profits of the private insurers would be approximately 10.7 percent of overall costs in the first year for which the program was in operation, for a total of $4.6 billion. These additional administrative costs exclude the inherent costs in running a large program, such as dispensing fees paid to pharmacies and other costs of processing claims. The additional administrative costs are incurred only because of the decision to use multiple private insurers: "expenses that drug plans would incur for marketing, member acquisition and member retention," according to CBO. The uncertainty around projecting costs into the future will also impose costs that a public insurer would not face. CBO "assumed that plans would incur costs as a result of having to bear financial risk—whether to offset the costs of purchasing

private reinsurance policies or to build up their own reserves in case their costs exceeded expectations."

CBO estimated that overall additional administrative cost would stay roughly the same over time, increasingly slightly to $4.9 billion by 2013.

From 2006 to 2013, according to CBO's estimates, the additional administrative cost from using multiple private insurers, instead of a single government payer, will total $38 billion.

The second set of expenses from having private insurers manage the plan involve the time spent by beneficiaries and healthcare providers in navigating the additional complexity of a system with multiple insurers. Quantifying this cost is difficult, but it is possible to calculate the general order of magnitude. A survey by the Medicare Payment Advisory Commission found that more than half of the people who had signed up for a Medicare Part D plan (the survey was conducted in February and March 2006) had spent more than eight hours examining their options.

Assigning the economy-wide average hourly compensation for workers as the value of this time implies that the cost of this selection averaged $240 for the beneficiaries who went through this process. More than 20 million people are enrolled in Medicare Part D. More than 11 million of them did not previously have prescription drug coverage from Medicare or Medicaid (though many had prescription drug coverage through other, private providers).

It is understandable that many seniors would have viewed this expenditure of time as a substantial and unnecessary burden. In principle, this will be a one-time expenditure of time, since most seniors will probably opt to remain with the plan they have chosen. However, it is possible that changes in their prescription drug usage or changes in the plan coverage may make their current plans less desirable. It may also be the case that some insurers may opt to leave the market. In such circumstances, beneficiaries will be forced to go through the process of selecting a plan again.

Time costs are also incurred by doctors and other healthcare providers in helping beneficiaries navigate the system. No reliable data exists yet to measure how much time the benefit is actually requiring from providers, but there is some anecdotal evidence suggesting that the cost is substantial.

Of course, even the simplest benefit would require some amount of time from doctors, as they would still be required to consider cost as a factor in choosing medicines. But this time would be far less if there were just a single set of prices and rules. Also, if Medicare had bargained drug prices down closer to their production costs, price differences would usually not be large. This would allow doctors to make their prescription decisions based primarily on their assessment of the best drug for their patients.

In addition to the demands on doctors' time, the complexity of the plan is also placing a large burden on pharmacists. They have had to learn the rules for the various plans that are part of the Medicare program. Pharmacists have also had to deal with slip-ups with the system, which have often left people without proper coverage. In these cases, pharmacists have frequently opted to still provide drugs to customers in the hope of getting payment later, rather than sending Medicare beneficiaries home without necessary medication. Such situations have involved large amounts of time, and exposed pharmacies to financial risk.

A Peculiar Program

The peculiar features of the Medicare Modernization Act have imposed large costs on seniors, people with disabilities, the government and healthcare providers. The rule that prohibits Medicare from negotiating price discounts directly with the pharmaceutical industry, has added hundreds of billions of dollars to the cost of the program over its first decade. In addition, the decision to only provide the benefit through private insurers substantially increased both the cost and complexity of the program.

These costs are not unavoidable expenses associated with a major program. They are the result of counterintuitive rules and designed-in complexity, all crafted to serve the interests of the program's big financial beneficiaries: Big Pharma, and the insurance plans.

DEAN BAKER is co-director of the Center for Economic and Policy Research, in Washington, D.C.

Coverage for All

**Two states have enacted universal health care plans.
Are they leaders or simply anomalies?**

PATRICIA BARRY

After years of mounting evidence that the U.S. health care system has become dysfunctional—with nearly 46 million uninsured, costs escalating and some of America's largest employers cutting back on benefits—something unexpected happened this spring: two states enacted laws intended to create near-universal health coverage for their residents, starting next year.

What riveted the attention of health policy experts was that both these measures, though very different, had strong bipartisan support. In both Massachusetts and Vermont, they were passed by Democratic-controlled legislatures and signed into law by Republican governors. Only two lawmakers in Massachusetts voted against that state's bill, with its landmark—and highly controversial—requirements that all residents purchase health insurance and most employers contribute or face penalties.

Across the nation, the "first reaction to Massachusetts was marveling at the political accomplishments—how they were able to craft a compromise between a Republican governor and two Democratic leaders with very different ideas," says Paul Ginsburg, president of Washington's Center for Studying Health System Change. "And that's going to inspire other states to try."

For over a decade, since the Clinton health reform proposals tanked, Washington, riven by opposing ideologies, has remained in near-paralysis over the rising tide of uninsured and underinsured Americans. The right wing promotes more private insurance options, mainly high-deductible health savings accounts. The left wing favors a national "single-payer" system, run by the federal government.

Most Americans, however, want universal health coverage—whether private or public or mixed—that they can afford, according to recent opinion polls. The bipartisan Citizens' Health Care Working Group set up by Congress reported last month that of 23,000 people contacted, "over 90 percent . . . believed it should be public policy that all Americans have affordable coverage." The group has called on Congress to guarantee such coverage by 2012.

So, will the Massachusetts and Vermont initiatives point the way for other states or even the nation? And, for consumers,

just how universal, affordable and dependable is the coverage they're planning?

Massachusetts

No state has ever attempted to require all residents to buy health coverage. Under the new law, people in Massachusetts who are uninsured must buy coverage by July 1, 2007, and all businesses with more than 10 employees that do not provide insurance must pay a "fair share" contribution of up to $295 per year to the state for each worker.

That concept of "shared responsibility" was a major political key to the law's passage, experts say. Companies that already provide health insurance welcomed the opportunity to level the competitive playing field with those that do not. Even so, Gov. Mitt Romney, in signing the law, vetoed the $295 assessment on employers—a veto the legislature overrode.

Individuals who do not comply will lose their personal tax exemption in 2007 and after that will face fines of 50 percent of the monthly cost of health insurance for each month without it. But there is a caveat. They will not be compelled to buy insurance if they can't find affordable coverage. The state has not yet defined what "affordable" will mean. And it does not intend to set levels of premiums, deductibles and copayments.

The state has become the first to adopt an idea promoted by the Heritage Foundation, a conservative Washington think tank. The law sets up a clearinghouse—called the Connector—intended to link uninsured individuals and companies having fewer than 50 employees to a choice of "affordable" health plans designed by private insurers and regulated by the state.

The Connector aims to offer these two groups the advantages that many people in large employer-sponsored groups now enjoy—deeper discounts, premiums paid out of pretax dollars and an opportunity to change plans every year.

And it offers them a further unique advantage. Their coverage will be portable. If they change full-time jobs, or are part-time or temporary employees working several jobs, their coverage remains in place.

This is a fundamentally different approach to solving the problem of the uninsured, says Edmund Haislmaier, a Heritage Foundation expert who helped formulate the Massachusetts law. "If you make the insurance stick to the people instead of to the job, you'd probably solve at least half this problem with no new money."

The law also offers subsidized coverage (no deductibles, premiums on a sliding scale) to residents with incomes up to 300 percent of the federal poverty level (about $29,000 for an individual, $40,000 for a couple, $60,000 for a family of four). And it aims to make health coverage more affordable for young adults.

The law has plenty of detractors from both ends of the political spectrum. AFL-CIO President John Sweeney called the mandate for people to have insurance an "unconscionable" step that will "bankrupt many middle-class families." Michael Tanner, director of health studies at the libertarian Cato Institute, said that it presages "a slow but steady spiral downward toward a government-run national health care system."

For Massachusetts residents, the devil will be in the details. Just how much people who are not eligible for subsidies will have to pay in premiums, deductibles and copays under the private plans provided through the Connector is not yet known, though early estimates place monthly premiums at about $300 for an individual and $600 for a couple.

Comprehensive employer-sponsored health policies for a family in Massachusetts currently run about $12,000 to $14,000 a year. How will insurers offer new options for less?

Some believe it can't be done. The choice could be between costly plans that offer good benefits and inexpensive plans that cut benefits or have very high deductibles, says David Himmelstein, M.D., associate professor of medicine at Harvard Medical School and co-founder of a physicians group that promotes a national single-payer health system. The law, he says, "will force you to purchase either something you can't afford or something you can afford but which will be nearly useless in the actual coverage it offers."

Supporters also acknowledge the challenges. "We're very aware of the issues around cost sharing," says John McDonough, executive director of MA HealthCare for All, a grassroots group that helped get the law passed. "It will take a huge amount of implementation by [all] stakeholders to make sure that this is done well and done right" over the next few months. But he adds: "They're fully committed to doing that."

Vermont

Unlike the "stick" of mandated coverage proposed by Massachusetts, Vermont's new law is more of a "carrot" that lawmakers hope will achieve the same goal—near-universal health care coverage in the state by 2010.

Vermont will provide a new voluntary, standardized plan—called Catamount Health—for uninsured residents. It will be offered by private insurers, and its benefits and charges will be similar to those in the average BlueCross BlueShield plan in Vermont. Unlike Massachusetts', the Vermont plan has defined costs. Enrollees will pay $10 for office visits; 20 percent

Highlights of the Massachusetts Law . . .

- All residents required to have health insurance by July 1, 2007.
- All employers required to offer insurance or contribute up to $295 a year for each uninsured employee.
- Fines for residents and businesses not complying—except individuals unable to find "affordable" policies, or businesses with 10 or fewer employees.
- The Connector links individuals and companies with under 50 employees to a choice of "affordable" private health plans paid for out of pretax dollars.
- Health insurance obtained through the Connector is portable when enrollee changes jobs.
- Subsidized premiums on a sliding scale for enrollees with incomes of up to 300 percent of the federal poverty level.

. . . and the Vermont Law

- Catamount Health plan for uninsured residents starts Oct. 1, 2007.
- Businesses with more than eight employees pay up to $365 a year for every uninsured employee.
- Plan offers portable coverage through private insurers and defined benefits and costs, including annual caps on out-of-pocket spending.
- Subsidized premiums on a sliding scale for enrollees with incomes of up to 300 percent of the federal poverty level.
- Incentives for enrollees with chronic conditions who participate in a disease management program; payments for doctors who promote preventive care and healthy living.

coinsurance for medical services; tiered copays of $10, $30 or $50 for prescription drugs; and a $250 annual deductible for an individual or $500 for a family for in-network services (double those amounts for out-of-network). Another big benefit: Out-of-pocket expenses will be capped at $800 a year for an individual and $1,600 for a family using in-network services (almost double for out-of-network).

Premiums have yet to be determined but are likely to be around $340 a month for an individual. People with incomes below 300 percent of the federal poverty level would be eligible for premium subsidies.

Plan supporters are confident it will attract uninsured Vermonters without the need for a mandate because its benefits are more comprehensive than the only other plans that many can now afford. "Most folks tell us they do not want to be in a high-deductible health saving account where they're paying maybe $5,000 out of pocket before they reach some kind of catastrophic benefit," says Greg Marchildon, state director for AARP Vermont, which helped drive the new legislation. "They basically describe it as paying to be uninsured."

Employers are not required to provide health insurance, but those with more than eight employees must help fund Catamount Health by paying a dollar a day for every uninsured worker.

The other centerpiece of the Vermont law is a landmark program offering special care with financial incentives—such as waived deductibles and free services and testing—to people with chronic illness.

Vermont is the first state to formally recognize that about 80 percent of health care dollars are consumed by people with chronic conditions (such as diabetes, high blood pressure, heart disease and obesity) and that many cannot afford the screening and services that prevent expensive complications.

In terms of holding down costs as well as improving general health, "the last thing you want for those patients is high copays, deductibles or anything that will deter them from ongoing routine medical management," says Kenneth Thorpe, chairman of the health policy department at Emory University in Atlanta and the main architect of the Vermont legislation.

"If this is done well—and experts in Vermont believe it will become the gold standard for how you manage chronic disease," AARP's Marchildon adds, "we think that over time we're going to save tens of millions of dollars."

Will Other States Copy?

Other states will be closely watching Massachusetts and Vermont over the next year to see if they can implement their laws or if they'll run into roadblocks.

Analysts point to a number of reasons why other states may not rush to replicate those laws in their entirety. Both states, for example, have far smaller uninsured populations than the national average, tight regulations on health insurers already in place and, above all, sufficient financing (mainly from federal dollars) to fund the programs for at least a few years.

"But individual components of the reforms—yes, I think you will see states replicating them," says Laura Tobler, a health policy analyst at the National Conference of State Legislatures. She cites as examples Massachusetts' compulsory insurance and its Connector program and Vermont's chronic care program.

Yet experts on each law say the whole state system must be changed to achieve universal coverage. Haislmaier of the Heritage Foundation says the unique approach in Massachusetts is "to reform the market, not the products, to create a single unified mechanism that gets rid of these distinctions between [insurance for] individuals and small groups and large groups."

In Vermont's case, says Emory's Thorpe, reform "can't just be about costs or the uninsured. You've got to convince people who [already] have health insurance that they are going to get more affordable and better-quality health care with less administrative hassle than they have today."

Financing also relies on an integrated system. As more residents get coverage, the funds the two states now use to pay the hospital bills of the uninsured will be shifted to subsidies that help more low-income enrollees get coverage.

Many experts say Massachusetts and Vermont set aside ideologies to forge a compromise, and that this could well spur a renewed debate on national health coverage in the 2008 election.

"The whole history of national health [reform] has been of people overreaching and getting nothing," says Ginsburg of the Center for Studying Health System Change. "A lot of people have interpreted the term 'universal' as meaning single-payer, and that's a source of confusion. To me, universal just means that everybody's covered, no matter what the mechanism."

Reprinted from *AARP Bulletin*, July/August 2006, pp. 8–10. Copyright © 2006 by American Association for Retired Persons (AARP). Reprinted by permission.

Riding into the Sunset
The Geezer Threat

WILLIAM GREIDER

In 1900 Americans on average lived for only 49 years and most working people died still on the job. For those who lived long enough, the average "retirement" age was 85. By 1935, when Social Security was enacted, life expectancy had risen to 61 years. Now it is 77 years—nearly a generation more—and still rising. Children born today have a fifty-fifty chance of living to 100. This inheritance from the last century—the great gift of longer life—surely represents one of the country's most meaningful accomplishments.

Yet the achievement has been transformed into a monumental problem by contemporary politics and narrow-minded accounting. "The nation faces a severe economic threat from the aging of its population combined with escalating health costs," a *Washington Post* editorial warned. Others put it more harshly. "Greedy geezers" are robbing from the young, bankrupting the government. Painful solutions must be taken to avoid financial ruin. Or so we are told.

A much happier conviction is expressed by Robert Fogel, a Nobel Prize-winning economist at the University of Chicago and a septuagenarian himself. America, he reminds us, is a very wealthy nation. The expanding longevity is not a financial burden but an enormous and underdeveloped asset. If US per capita income continues to grow at a rate of 1.5 percent a year, the country will have plenty of money to finance comfortable retirements and high-quality healthcare for all citizens, including those at the bottom of the wage ladder. When politicians talk about raising the Social Security retirement age to 70 in order to "save" the system, they are headed backward and against the tide of human aspirations. The average retirement age, Fogel observes, has been falling in recent decades by personal choice and is now around 63. Given proper financing arrangements, he expects the retirement age will eventually fall to as low as 55—allowing everyone to enjoy more leisure years and to explore the many dimensions of "spiritual development" or "self-realization," as John Dewey called it.

"What then is the virtue of increasing spending on retirement and health rather than goods?" Fogel asked in his latest book, *The Fourth Great Awakening and the Future of Egalitarianism* (2000). "It is the virtue of providing consumers in rich countries with what they want most." What people want is time—more time to enjoy life and learning, to focus on the virtuous aspects of

one's nature, to pursue social projects free of economic necessity, to engage their curiosity and self-knowledge or their political values. The great inequity in modern life, as Fogel provocatively puts it, is the "maldistribution of spiritual resources," that is, the economic insecurity that prevents people from exploring life's larger questions. Everyone could attain a fair share of liberating security, he asserts, if government undertook strategic interventions in their behalf.

Fogel's perspective is generally ignored by other economists, but sociologists and psychologists recognize his point in the changing behavior of retirees. The elderly are redefining leisure, finding "fun" in myriad activities that lend deeper meaning to their lives. An informal shadow university has grown up around the nation in which older people are both the students and the teachers. They do "volunteer vacationing" and "foster grandparenting." They rehab old houses for the needy, serve as self-appointed environmental watchdogs or act as ombudsmen for neglected groups like indigent children or nursing-home patients. They dig into political issues with an informed tenacity that often withers politicians. In civic engagement, they are becoming counselors, critics, caregivers and mentors equipped with special advantages—the time and freedom to act, the knowledge and understanding gained only from the experience of living.

When the "largest generation" reaches retirement a few years from now, the baby boomers will doubtless alter the contours of society again, perhaps more profoundly than in their youth. Theodore Roszak, the historian who chronicled *The Making of a Counter Culture* thirty-six years ago, thinks boomers taking up caregiving and mentoring roles will inspire another wave of humanistic social values (perhaps expressed more maturely this time around). "More than merely surviving we will find ourselves gifted with the wits, the political savvy and the sheer weight of numbers to become a major force for change," Roszak wrote in *America the Wise* (1998). "With us, history shifts its rhythm. It draws back from the frenzied pursuit of marketing novelties and technological turnover and assumes the measured pace of humane and sustainable values. We may live to see wisdom become a distinct possibility and compassion the reigning social ethic." The "retired," he predicts, will seek to become reintegrated with the working society and claim a larger role in its affairs. Some elderly may reclaim the ancient role of respected "elders" who keep alive society's deeper truths and remind succeeding generations of their obligations to the nation's longer term. None of these possibilities are likely to unfold, however, if the promise of economic security for retirement is eviscerated in the meantime.

Fogel's optimism sounds eccentric amid the gloom and doom of the Social Security debate and the more threatening deterioration under way in private pensions and personal savings. Fogel skips over the snarled facts of current politics. He thinks big-picture and long-term. He won the Nobel Prize by producing unorthodox economic history that traced the deeper shifts in demographics and living conditions across generations, even centuries. His thinking is especially provocative because the conclusions collide with both left and right assumptions. Fogel is a secular Democrat, yet he extols the conservative evangelical awakening as a valuable social force. He sounds alternately conservative and liberal on economic issues, yet he thinks government should engineer a vast redistribution of financial wealth, from top to bottom, to insure equitable pensions for all.

Fogel's solution is a new national pension system alongside Social Security—a universal "provident fund" that requires all workers to save a significant portion of their wage incomes every year to provide for their future. He proposes a savings rate of 14.7 percent (though taking Social Security benefits and taxes into account, a lower rate would suffice for a start). The contributions would be mandatory but set aside as true personal savings, not as a government tax. The accumulating nest eggs would belong to the individual workers and become a portable pension that goes with them if they change jobs, but the wealth would be invested for them through a broadly diversified pension fund. Employers would no longer be in charge (though they could still contribute to worker savings to attract employees). The government or independent private institutions would manage the money, investing conservatively in stocks, bonds and other income-generating assets while allowing workers only limited, generalized choices on their investment preferences.

Fogel's vision of expanding leisure and greater human fulfillment is actually receding at the moment. The time for big ideas is now.

The concept resembles the forced savings plans adopted in some Asian and Latin American countries, but Fogel's favorite prototype is American: TIAA-CREF, the pension system that exists for nearly all college professors (a nonprofit institution founded in 1917 by Andrew Carnegie). Another model could be the government's own Thrift Savings Plan, which manages savings wealth for federal employees. Lifelong healthcare, Fogel adds, could be guaranteed for all by setting aside another

9.8 percent from current incomes. "If you take the typical academic, we all have TIAA-CREF," he explains. "The universities require of us that we invest anywhere from 12.5 to 17.5 percent of our salaries in a pension fund—mandatory—but it's all in my name. I can leave it to whomever I want. It has entered my sense of well-being for many years. The fund has earned about 10 percent a year since the 1960s, so retirement is not a burden to the university."

Obviously, people with low or even moderate incomes could not afford such savings rates, and even diligent savings from their low wages would not be enough to pay for either retirement or healthcare. Fogel has a straightforward solution: Tax the affluent to pay for the needy. A tax rate of 2 or 3 percent, applied progressively to families in the top half of income distribution, could finance the "provident fund" for those who can't pay for themselves. "This is a problem, not of inadequate national resources, but of inequity," he observes.

Fogel's big thinking—a system of compulsory savings, with the federal government taking charge—sounds way too radical for this right-wing era, and probably even most Democrats would shy away from the concept. But keep Fogel's solution in mind as we examine the sorry condition of retirement security. The current political debate is not even focused on the right "crisis," much less on genuine solutions. It is not Social Security that's financially threatened but healthcare and the other two pillars of retirement security—employer-run pension plans and the private savings of families. Many millions of baby boomers realize as they approach the "golden years" that they can't afford to retire at all, much less retire early. They will keep working because they lack the wherewithal to stop. Retiring for them would mean a drastic fall in their standard of living. Fogel's vision of expanding leisure and greater human fulfillment is actually receding at the moment. The time for big ideas is now.

Grasshoppers and Ants

When George W. Bush launched Social Security reform with his promise of new personalized savings accounts for everyone, he did not seem to grasp that most Americans already have such accounts. During the past generation tax-exempt 401(k) and IRA accounts—the individualized "defined contribution" approach—became the principal pension plan for working people, displacing the traditional company pension provided by employers who assume the risks and promise a "defined benefit" to workers at retirement. The do-it-yourself version of pensions is a flop, as many Americans have painfully learned. When older employees look at their monthly balance statements, they are more likely to experience fear than Bush's romanticized thrill of individual risk-taking.

Picking stocks for themselves has left many employees, perhaps as many as 40–45 percent, without an adequate nest egg for retirement. When Bush explains further that he intends to divert trillions from Social Security to finance his "ownership society," it makes people even more nervous. Social Security pays very modest average benefits—roughly equivalent to the federal minimum wage—but it is the last safety net. For nearly half of the private-sector workforce, it is the only safety net.

The far more threatening problem is elsewhere—shrinking pensions, collapsed personal savings and soaring costs for health insurance.

The bleak reality is reflected in those 401(k) account balances. Of the 48 million families who hold one or more of the accounts, the median value of their savings is $27,000 (which means half of all families have less than $27,000). Among older workers on the brink of retiring (55 to 64 years old) who have personal accounts, the median value is $55,000. That's only enough to buy an annuity that would pay $398 a month, far short of middle-class living standards. What's strange and disturbing about their low accumulations is that these older workers have been investing during the best of times—the "super bull market" of soaring stock prices that lasted nearly twenty years. The Congressional Research Service summarized the sobering results: Median pension savings "would not by themselves provide an income in retirement that most people in the United States would find to be adequate."

This grand experiment was launched nearly twenty-five years ago by Ronald Reagan, but with very little public debate because the pension changes were obscured by more immediate controversies—Reagan's regressive tax cuts and massive budget deficits. His Treasury under secretary explained the reasoning: "The evidence of the past suggests that people do not behave like grasshoppers. They are much more like ants." For lots of reasons, most Americans turned out not to be like the proverbial ants, storing food for winter. People either misjudged their future need for savings or couldn't afford to put much aside or bet wrong in the stock market and got wiped out. But corporate managements turned out to be the true grasshoppers, living for the moment and ignoring the future. Companies took advantage of the 401(k) innovation to escape their traditional responsibility to employees. They dumped old defined-benefit pension plans and adopted the new version, which requires much smaller employer contributions and thereby reduces labor costs dramatically. Good for the bottom line, bad for the country's future.

"The whole thinking was: Let's relieve the employers of this burden and empower individuals," explains Karen Ferguson, longtime director of the Pension Rights Center in Washington. "The problem is, it has failed—and failed miserably—and no one wants to say that."

Pension protection is actually shrinking, despite the proliferation of 401(k) accounts and the alleged prosperity of the 1980s and '90s. In the private sector, fewer employees participate in pension plans of any kind now than twenty years ago, down from 51 percent to 46 percent (the defined-benefit company pensions that once covered 53 percent now protect only 34 percent). The value of pension wealth, meanwhile, fell by 17 percent for workers in the middle and below, mainly because their voluntary savings were weak or nonexistent, yet soared for those at the top—"an upsurge in pension wealth inequality," economist Edward Wolff of New York University observed.

In sum, pensions became less valuable. And fewer families have one. That helps explain why Bush's plan encountered popular resistance. In these circumstances, whacking Social

Security benefits or raising the retirement age does not sound like "reform." But neither political party has yet summoned the nerve to acknowledge the implications of the failed experiment or to propose serious solutions.

The most threatening problem is not Social Security; it is shrinking pensions, collapsed personal savings and soaring health costs.

The circumstances look even more ominous—the very opposite of Professor Fogel's sunny vision—because personal savings also collapsed during the long, slow-motion weakening of pensions. Given the stagnating wages for hourly workers and easier access to credit, families typically managed to stay afloat by working more jobs and by borrowing more. Saving for the future was not an available option for many. In 1982 personal savings peaked at $480 billion, then began an epic decline. Last year the national total in personal savings was only $103 billion—down nearly 80 percent from twenty-five years ago. As Eugene Steuerle of the Urban Institute points out, the federal government now spends more money on tax subsidies to encourage the individual forms of pension savings—$115 billion last year—than Americans actually save.

The one potential bright spot in this story might be real estate—the family wealth that accumulates gradually through home ownership and the rising market value of houses. Given the current housing boom and runaway prices in the hotter urban markets, many families might salvage retirement plans by selling their homes and moving to less expensive dwellings. The trouble is, families have been living off that wealth—borrowing, almost dollar for dollar, against the rising price of their homes through equity-credit lines or refinanced mortgages. From 1999 through 2003, the value of family homes rose by a spectacular $3.3 trillion, but families' actual equity in those properties changed little because mortgage borrowing rose nearly as fast.

Thus, people financed routine consumption by borrowing against their long-term assets—that's real grasshopper behavior. And the situation could turn very ugly if the housing bubble pops and home prices fall. People will find themselves stuck paying off a mountain of debt on homes that are suddenly worth less than the mortgages. They will not only need to keep working; they might also be filing for bankruptcy.

"Just as wealth and income are being redistributed to the wealthy, so is leisure."

—Economist Teresa Ghilarducci

How could this have happened in such a wealthy nation—especially during an era when stock prices were rising explosively? The basic explanations are familiar: rising inequality and reactionary economic policies, launched first by Reagan, then elaborated by Bush II and resisted only faintheartedly by Democrats. The corporate "social contract" was discarded; regressive tax-cutting rewarded capital and the well-to-do; numerous other measures fractured the broad middle class. The wages of hourly workers—80 percent of the private-sector workforce—have been essentially unchanged in terms of real purchasing power for three decades (no one in politics wants to talk about that, either). The political system continues to defer to the needs of corporations despite the torrent of financial scandals and extreme greed displayed by egomaniacal CEOs. All these factors contributed to the erosion of retirement security. Economist Teresa Ghilarducci, a pension authority at Notre Dame, remarks, "Just as wealth and income are being redistributed to the wealthy, so is leisure."

In fact, Ghilarducci argues, allowing the pension system to deteriorate serves a long-term interest of business: avoiding future labor shortages when the baby-boom generation moves into retirement. "All this retirement policy is really a labor policy," she asserts. "It's motivated by these experts who say, Hey, wait, we're going to need to do what we can to encourage people to work longer. A whole range of economists and elite opinion makers is talking about a labor shortage where, God forbid, wages would increase. That's what they're worried about—making sure there isn't a corporate profit squeeze, that skill shortages and upward wage pressures are checked."

This development is already lengthening working lives, she finds. The average retirement age, rather than gradually declining toward 55, as Fogel foresees, has turned around in the past few years and is slowly increasing. "I'm not against older people working if they want to," Ghilarducci says. "I'm against policies that force them back into the workforce because they've lost their pensions or their healthcare costs have gone up."

O ne need not question the sincerity of the right's ideological convictions to see that their policy initiatives are also designed to benefit important political patrons. With the transition to 401(k) accounts, corporate employers were major winners. Ghilarducci's examination of 700 companies over nearly two decades found that their annual pension contributions dropped by one third—from $2,140 to $1,404 per employee—as they shifted from defined-benefit pensions to the less expensive defined-contribution model. Not surprisingly, the traditional company pension began to disappear or shrink as large industrial companies hacked away at the uncompetitive costs. The number of younger workers with the traditional form of pension is much smaller and falling fast.

Wall Street banks and brokerages were big winners too, since they began competing for the millions of new "investors" with their individual stock accounts. This enormous influx of customers helped fuel the long stock-market boom and encouraged the exaggerated promises made by both corporations and financial firms. The overall economy was probably damaged too, because mutual funds competed for customers by going after rapid, short-term gains rather than focusing on the long-term

investments financed by patient capital. When the stock-market illusions burst in 2000, the meltdown evaporated lots of retirement accounts too, especially for those innocent risk-takers who had bet their savings on NASDAQ's high-flying tech stocks.

The most damning fact about the 401(k) experiment is that it has failed to fulfill the original purpose: boosting savings for ordinary Americans. Academic studies have confirmed that the personal accounts produced "very little net savings" or "statistically insignificant" gains. While every worker could participate in theory, the practical reality is that only the more affluent families could afford to take full advantage of the 401(k) tax break—sheltering their annual 401(k) contributions from income taxes. But typically they did so simply by moving money from other conventional savings accounts into the tax-exempt kind.

More affluent Americans thus reduced their income taxes, but their net savings did not actually increase. For two decades, the federal government has been heavily subsidizing "savings" by the people who needed no inducement because they were already saving. Think of it as welfare for the virtuously well-to-do. A rational government would phase out such a misconceived program. Bush is instead proposing to make the contradictions worse by adding still other tax-exempt savings vehicles designed to benefit the affluent.

The old system of defined-benefit pensions had many strengths by comparison, but it was never a solution to the national problem either. Even at their peak, the traditional corporate pensions left out half of the workforce. Larger companies, especially in unionized industrial sectors, provided strong benefits for their employees, responding to labor's bargaining demands and to attract well-qualified people. But the millions of very small firms, where more Americans work, almost never offered pensions. The burden either seemed too costly or too complicated to administer. Generally, their workers are the folks who depend solely on Social Security.

The corporate pensions are also not portable (a problem the individual accounts were supposed to solve). And pension law gives corporate managers ample latitude to game their pension funds to enhance the company's bottom line. Stories of elderly retirees stranded by their old employers are now commonplace: broken promises on healthcare and other benefits that go unpunished. Instead of accumulating larger surpluses during the good times, the corporations often did the opposite, leaving their pension funds severely underfunded for the bad times, when shortfalls couldn't be overcome. Employees have no representatives to speak for them in the decision-making. If a corporate pension fund goes belly up, its liabilities are dumped on the government's insurance agency, which is getting strapped itself.

A logical and achievable solution exists to correct this mess. Government should create a new hybrid pension that combines the best aspects of defined-benefit and defined-contribution versions—one that requires all workers to save for the future and no longer relies on the "good will" of employers. Given modern employment patterns, workers do need a portable pension that stays with them, job to job. But their voluntary savings are simply too small and erratic—too vulnerable to manipulation by financial brokers—to produce secure results in the stock-market casino. Either they get lured into wild gambles or they park their savings in mutual funds that gouge them with inflated fees and commissions while catering to the corporations that are the funds' largest customers (this conflict of interest between large and small customers is endemic to the US financial system; guess who loses). The employees' money will produce far more reliable accumulations if it is invested for them by professionals at a major independent pension fund that works only for them.

The fundamental truth (well understood among experts) is that individualized accounts can never match the investment returns of a large common fund, broadly diversified and soundly managed, because the pension fund is able to average its results over a very long time span, thirty years or more. A few wise guys might beat the casino odds, but the broad herd of small investors will always be captive to the random luck of bad timing and their own ignorance. The right wing's celebration of individual risk-taking in financial markets is like inviting sheep to the slaughter.

The super bull market is over. Its gorgeous returns will not return for many years, maybe many decades. But a very large, diversified pension fund—managed solely in the interests of its contributors—provides the vehicle for "shared luck." It can smooth out the ups and downs among all participants, young and old, lucky and unlucky. It can invest for long-term economic development rather than chase stock-market fads. Good returns for retirees, good results for the economy.

These are the very qualities Professor Fogel envisions. They describe trustworthy pension systems, like TIAA-CREF, which reliably serves many thousands of individual employees (teachers and professors) who are scattered across many different employers (schools and universities). The present reform debate is not thinking this way. Collective action is out of fashion, especially if the government is involved. Significant reform would require institution-building. The transition would pose many technical difficulties. "There are obstacles, but I don't think that's the problem," Ghilarducci says. "The obstacle is imagination."

Pro-Life Pension Reform

The Pension Rights Center just conducted a year-long "conversation on coverage" that pulled together experts from business and labor, the insurance industry, Wall Street finance, academia, AARP and other interested sectors. The workshop sessions produced a long list of worthy ideas for patching up the broken system, but that was the problem: The proposals basically involved incremental tinkering with the status quo, not universal, mandatory solutions. To get all these diverse interests to join the conversation, Karen Ferguson confides, the center had to stipulate that "mandatory" would not be discussed.

"The bottom line is that the companies always have the upper hand, even though they've gotten huge subsidies and tax benefits," she explains. "The system is voluntary, so companies can always opt out." Indeed, the politics of pension reform is usually a discussion about what new favors and concessions should be granted to employers to get them to do the "right thing" for their employees. This political logic led to the current failure. "Voluntary" is a loser, as the past twenty years amply demonstrated, because it gives companies controlling leverage over what is possible. And even well-intentioned executives will always have to choose between the company's self-interest and its employees (guess who usually loses). Only the government has the reach and power to design and oversee a pension system that truly serves all. During the past generation, most corporations discarded their obligations under the old social contract. It seems only fair they should forfeit political control too.

A universal savings system that covers everyone because it is mandatory could prove to be as durable (and popular) as Social Security.

Plausible plans in addition to Fogel's do exist that offer genuine solutions. A universal savings system that covers everyone because it is mandatory could prove to be as durable (and popular) as Social Security. It balances equity by subsidizing the savings of lower-income workers. It creates authentic individual ownership and incentives to save more for the future, consume less in the present. It operates free of Wall Street profiteers and under government supervision, adhering to well-established principles of sound investing. Employers could be discouraged from further abandoning their obligations by penalties in the tax code. Many other nations, large and small and far less wealthy, have created such systems. Americans would need to craft their own distinctive version.

One promising example, designed by economist Christian Weller for the Economic Policy Institute, proposes a modest savings rate of 3 percent of wages, but combined with the existing Social Security benefits, it would approach the level of retirement security envisioned by Fogel. The government would contribute substantial savings for low earners and also match additional contributions made by the workers or their employers. Weller estimates this would cost around $48 billion a year—less than half the federal tax subsidy now devoted to all pension plans. Weller's design is robustly equitable, scaled to help the bottom rungs most and top income earners least. Combined with Social Security, low earners (wages of $24,000 or less) would enjoy a pension that replaces 83 percent of their peak working wages. Average earners would get 60 percent replacement, high earners only 48 percent. This makes sense, because higher-income families have much greater opportunity to augment pensions with other sources of income and savings. The working poor do not.

Essentially, Weller has updated and expanded a mandatory savings plan that was proposed nearly twenty-five years ago—a last gasp from the Carter Administration. Reagan's election and laissez-faire politics snuffed the idea. While still modest in scale, Weller's design represents a meaningful start toward Fogel's larger vision of a 15 percent savings rate. Since the

Social Security tax now collects 12.6 percent of wages jointly from workers and employers, it is not plausible at this point to add another 15 percent to labor costs for pension savings. However, as the new pension system matures and public confidence is established, a gradual transition can be pursued that adds little by little to the personal savings rate, offset by equivalent reductions in the payroll tax for Social Security—thus yielding greater savings and lower taxes. Both government systems would continue in place, one as the fundamental safety net of social insurance, the other as the universal, expanding pillar for comfortable retirement.

Ghilarducci thinks much of the accumulating wealth could be stored and invested by large private pension funds, organized by unions or other groups for workers at multiple employers (much like TIAA-CREF's role for universities). A successful existing model is the unified pension systems for the building and construction trades. Co-managed by unions and companies, they encourage industry and labor to collaborate on joint training and other productivity-enhancing endeavors that can raise the quality of work and wages.

While most politicians don't dare embrace a "mandatory" solution—not yet, anyway—it is not self-evident that ordinary Americans would reject one, if properly educated about the alternatives. Most people are conflicted. They know they need to save more—retirement is a very meaningful investment for them—but it's very hard to accomplish, given the competing pressures. They like the concept of personal accounts but are also aware of their vulnerability as amateur investors. In her conversations with union presidents, Ghilarducci finds they are more in favor of an "add on" national pension than raising the payroll tax for Social Security. "You can sell workers if their name is on it," she concludes. "If you had a system that says you must contribute 3 percent of wages to your mandatory savings account, you would actually have two-thirds of the workers grateful that they are being forced to save. You wouldn't get that if they were forced to pay another 3 percent in taxes into Social Security."

The retirement question—choices of mandatory or voluntary, universal or incremental—embodies a classic dilemma often facing liberal politics. Do reformers pursue the larger, more provocative approach that invites greater resistance but would fundamentally solve the problem? Or do they opt for smaller, safer measures that have a better chance of adoption and will demonstrate good intentions, if not a genuine remedy for society? For several decades, it seems obvious, most Democrats have chosen the side of caution: thinking small, offering symbolic gestures, avoiding fights over fundamental solutions. One can see where this strategy has gotten the party. The gestures are no longer taken seriously, since they don't lead anywhere. The public no longer associates Democrats with big ideas or principled commitments to authentic reform. We await incautious politicians with the courage to pursue their unfashionable convictions.

The New Face of Health Care

PATRICIA BARRY

As the Obama administration and Congress rev up for the Herculean task of reforming the health care system, one major goal is spelled out in a phrase the president and others often use: "to improve the quality of American health care while lowering its cost." The idea seems a contradiction. How do we get more for less? Doesn't "better" always cost more?

Not in health, it seems. The United States spends about $8,000 per person a year on health care—more than twice as much as Western countries that have universal health coverage and better medical results. The money spent "does not appear to buy us outstanding health," Paul Ginsburg, president of the nonprofit Center for Studying Health System Change, told the Senate last year. "By almost any measure, ranging from infant mortality to preventable deaths, the United States does not measure up well against other developed nations."

How to reverse that damning report has pre-occupied health policy brains for years. But increasingly eyes have turned to a few medical centers around the country as possible models for national reform. These centers—among them the Mayo Clinic, the Cleveland Clinic and the Geisinger Health System in rural Pennsylvania—have developed systems that change the way care is delivered and paid for.

What they have is a new way of doing business that rewards doctors and hospitals for taking better care of patients—instead of paying them for the number of patients they see and the individual services they use, as the widespread fee-for-service system does. Results suggest that improving quality may actually be the best way of reducing costs.

"That's the key, in my opinion, to getting the clinicians [onboard]," says Len Nichols, director of health policy at the New America Foundation, a Washington think tank. "If it's just about cost, there's no way they'll buy into it. But if it's also about improving patient care, then you can motivate them, because that's why they went to med school."

So how do these incentives work? To find out, the *AARP Bulletin* visited the award-winning, nonprofit Geisinger Health System, which has 750 physicians serving 2.6 million patients across 43 counties in Pennsylvania. Its flagship medical center—which began as a 70-bed hospital in 1915—dominates the small town of Danville in the Susquehanna River Valley.

Geisinger has developed several strategies to integrate its operations into a system that offers better care at lower cost: a coordinated approach to primary care; hospital surgery that comes with a warranty; electronic health records; and engaging patients in their own care. Obama's proposals for health care reform also advance these principles.

Best practices pay off "Some researchers believe that health care costs could be reduced by a stunning 30 percent—or about $700 billion a year—without harming quality if we moved as a nation toward the proven and successful practices adopted by the lower-cost areas and hospitals."

—President Obama, in his budget proposal for 2009

Coordinated Primary Care

A model known as the "patient-centered medical home" helps patients manage the complexities of their care in one setting, typically a family practice or clinic. "It's focused on putting patients and their families at the center of care, instead of doing what's convenient for the provider," says Janet Tomcavage, a registered nurse and vice president of medical operations in Geisinger's own insurance plan.

A team of doctors, nurses, technicians and a case manager who coordinates all care constantly monitors patients' needs, especially those with chronic conditions like heart failure, diabetes and lung disease. The team also helps patients navigate transitions into and out of the hospital or nursing home and puts them in contact with community social services.

The system has features unheard of in regular primary care. High-risk patients, for example, can call their case manager's cellphone anytime. Those with incipient heart failure are given scales that electronically transmit their daily weight directly from home to the clinic. If there's a spike indicating retention of fluid, the team is alerted and can take quick action to prevent a hospital emergency. "We're seeing a 12 to 13 percent reduction in heart failure admissions," Tomcavage says, not all due to the scales, but they help.

At a Geisinger medical home in Bloomsburg, one team is headed by a doctor, Karl Luxardo, and Maureen Conner, a registered nurse who's the case manager. Both say the system introduces "another layer of care" that allows them to help patients avoid medical complications—by rigorous monitoring and training them to better manage their own conditions.

"Maureen is another set of eyes and ears for me," Luxardo says. "She's making phone calls and spending the extra time on patients' questions and concerns that I might not have been able to address during the visit or that the patient may have forgotten to ask."

Conner says getting patients involved in their own care is a cornerstone of the medical home concept. "It's a big process," she says. "You have to gain their trust and get a relationship going."

Joaquin Mathew of Millville, a 71-year-old former paratrooper, has lupus, rheumatoid arthritis and heart problems. He calls Conner "my guardian angel" and "my lifeline." He looks after himself carefully, "but as soon as I sense anything is wrong, I call Maureen." It's that availability between scheduled appointments, Mathew says, that he appreciates most. "I try not to bother them with insignificant items, but it's good to know they're there," he says. "The connection's always maintained." He adds, "I get the feeling I'm special."

But why does this system, which requires major investment, save money? One reason is that Geisinger has changed the financial incentives for primary care doctors who work for its insurance plan. They get back half of any savings they've achieved in their medical home practices—through, for example, fewer hospital admissions and unnecessary tests—as compared with conventional practices. But they get the money only if they've also met a checklist of quality measures for preventive care, chronic disease management and so on, says Ronald Paulus, M.D., Geisinger's chief technology and innovation officer. "If they've saved $100,000, and have achieved 100 percent of the quality goals, they'd earn $50,000. If they've achieved 25 percent, they'd earn one-fourth of that amount [$12,500]."

So, Paulus says, the primary care practice is rewarded for efficiency but without sacrificing quality. "We didn't want the doctors and nurses to skimp on care to save in the short run but not have the patient do the best in the long run."

The other half of the savings goes to the Geisinger health plan to pay for extra services offered in medical homes. The incentives have paid off, Paulus says. In a region where patients are older, poorer and sicker than the national average, "the health plan earned 2.5 times its investment back in the very first year."

Surgery with a Warranty

Nationally, Medicare patients who are admitted to the hospital have an 18 percent chance of returning within 30 days. Typically, the surgeon does another operation and sends in a second bill, which the insurer or Medicare pays without question (except in the case of some preventable medical errors).

"You'd never do that with your car," says Alfred S. Casale, M.D., director of cardiothoracic surgery at Geisinger. "If you brought your car in, told them to rebuild the transmission and a week later the reverse gear was slipping, you'd demand they fix it because you paid them good money to fix it the first time."

In 2006 Geisinger embarked on a bold gamble to improve the situation. Starting with elective coronary bypass surgery, Casale and others drew up a 40-point checklist of best surgical practices developed by the American College of Cardiology and the American Heart Association. Each point on the list has to be checked off before a procedure begins, or it's canceled. Then Geisinger offered insurers what is in effect a warranty: Pay a flat price for each operation, and any further treatment arising from complications that put the patient back in the hospital within 90 days is free.

This system has so far succeeded in lowering the readmission rate by 44 percent and raised net hospital revenue by 7.8 percent.

Electronic Health Records

A vast room filled with black consoles humming away is the hub of Geisinger's electronic record system in Danville. Paulus says it allows "every one of our 750 doctors, whether they're spread across 20,000 square miles or right down the hall from one another, to use the same health record with all the information about a patient available at the click of a mouse."

Many patients are sold on it, too. About 119,000 have so far signed up to access their own records through personal por-monitor their own progress, schedule appointments and e-mail their doctors—and can do so from anywhere.

Hariteeny Fritz, 79, a retired banker from Bloomsburg, recalls the time she was in Bar Harbor, Maine, and developed double vision. Taken to a clinic there, she told the staff to use her password so they could access her entire medical record online. "There was this kind of disbelief," she says. "But it saved them a good deal of time."

Patients don't see everything in their records that the doctor does. "One of the things we don't share is physician's notes," e-health manager Jodi Norman says. Lab test results are posted quickly, but must be released by the doctor first. Sensitive results, such as HIV tests or just bad news, are withheld so that the doctor can discuss them in person with the patient.

Patient Involvement

"Where costs can really come down is in more engaged patients doing more preventive care for themselves," says Paulus. But lifestyle changes—like losing weight—are a tall order for many.

Yet with help from the medical home staff, patients can learn the value of their own efforts—quite often with the subtle prod of seeing a cool graphic in their e-health record showing their progress.

In another innovation, patients facing hip and knee replacement surgery are offered a two-hour class in which the whole team—surgeon, anesthetist, pharmacist, physical therapist and social worker—demonstrate what's in store and how they can improve the outcome.

Registered nurse Linda McGrail, who organizes the classes, says patients who take them are often ready to leave the hospital earlier and are less likely to be readmitted. That's because individually tailored plans for coping after patients leave the hospital, and the exercises they've begun even before surgery, make them "more confident and better able to bounce back."

As Good as It Gets

What country takes the best care of its older citizens? The Netherlands rates tops in our exclusive survey of 16 nations. But no place is perfect.

MIKE EDWARDS

Every week, Anna Sophia Fischer greets a clutch of tourists in the medieval central square of Utrecht and, with a spring in her step, guides them on a stroll among 14th-century Dutch monasteries and houses. She knows every arch, garden, and alley and, at 75, goes about her daily business by bicycle, as do the swarms of people around her. "You have to go by bike if you live in town," she says. (Could this be one reason that the Dutch live longer than we do—an average 78.6 years, compared with 77.3 in the U.S.?) A retired physician, Fischer is living her dream. "I wanted to do something different," she says. "I'm not rich, but I can do the things I want to do."

Wim van Essen, 69, is a former teacher, tall, vigorous, an ardent hiker, a fanatical chess player—and a one-man pep squad for the Dutch way of retirement. "You see how we live," he says, inviting a guest into his brick home in the leafy city of Amersfoort. There's a fireplace in the living room, a wildflower garden out back. Extra bedrooms upstairs await visiting grandchildren. On a coffee table are photos of Van Essen trekking in the Austrian Alps with his wife, Lamberta Jacoba Maria, nicknamed Bep. (Every year, the two of them take a major trip, partly subsidized by the government.) The couple receive government and work pensions and various perks. All told, it's a wonderful life, based on what Van Essen calls "a beautiful pension," which, when everything is added up, comes to about $45,000 a year.

In a world that is rapidly aging, the Netherlands, perhaps more than any other country, has created a society in which people have the luxury of growing old well, according to a survey conducted by AARP *The Magazine*. We weighed 17 criteria (see the table "And the Winner is . . .") in selected industrialized nations that approximate as closely as possible the lifestyle of most AARP members. We focused on key quality-of-life issues such as health care, work, education, taxes, and social programs.

But if you're already thinking of packing your bags, stop right there. The purpose of this report is not to encourage American retirees to immigrate to the Netherlands or to some of the other top scorers in our study. Most nations aren't keen to share their pensions and health care benefits with noncitizens just off a plane. Rather, our goal is to shed light on what retirees enjoy elsewhere in the world as a reference point for our own country's policies.

In the Netherlands, all citizens receive the full old-age pension at 65 if they've lived in the country for a minimum of 50 years between ages 15 and 64. Unlike our Social Security, however, the pension doesn't require a work history. The full amount per month is nearly $1,000 for singles and nearly $1,400 for couples, married or not. The old-age pension is in addition to an occupational, or employer-provided, pension based on payments over the years by worker and employer. And every pensioner gets a "holiday allowance" of about $700, thoughtfully paid in May, just in time for spring.

Pension generosity is a major reason that, by international measurements, only 6.4 percent of the elderly fall in the bottom quarter of income distribution, as compared with the U.S. percentage of 20.7. Although the U.S. has a far larger per capita income than the Netherlands— $26,448 a year versus $17,080—it scores poorly in two other comparisons: First, all Dutch citizens have government insurance for medical conditions and nursing-home care; 45 million Americans have no health insurance at all. Second, prescription drugs are available to all Dutch citizens, with few if any copayments; Americans get drugs in many different ways and those without insurance pay top dollar. Even when Medicare drug coverage begins in 2006, most enrollees will still face substantial out-of-pocket costs.

And the Winner Is . . . The **Netherlands,** Which Scored Highest on Key Quality-of-Life Issues Important to Older People and Society in General.

On a scale of 1 to 5 FIVE IS TOPS	Netherlands	Australia	Sweden	Finland	Switzerland	Norway	Denmark	Japan	France	Canada	Ireland	Spain	United States	United Kingdom	Germany	Italy
Mandatory Retirement	1	5	1	1	1	1	1	1	1	1	1	1	5	1	1	1
Age-Discrimination Laws	5	5	4	5	1	1	1	1	3	5	5	5	5	1	1	3
Unemployment Rate	5	4	4	2	5	5	4	5	2	3	5	1	4	5	2	2
College Education	4	3	2	2	2	5	4	3	1	3	2	2	5	3	1	1
Per Capita Income	3	3	2	2	3	5	3	2	2	3	4	1	5	3	2	2
Total Tax Burden	3	5	1	2	5	2	1	5	2	4	5	4	5	3	4	2
Home Care	3	5	2	3	2	4	5	2	2	4	1	1	2	1	2	1
Retirement Age for Full Benefits	3	3	3	3	3	1	1	3	5	3	3	3	1	3	3	3
Public Pension Replacement Rate	4	1	4	3	3	2	3	2	4	1	1	5	2	1	1	4
Employers Pension Coverage	5	5	5	5	5	3	5	3	5	2	3	1	3	3	3	1
Economic Inequality	4	2	5	5	4	5	4	3	4	3	3	3	1	2	4	2
Economic Inequality for the Elderly	5	1	5	5	4	3	5	5	4	5	3	4	2	3	5	4
Public Spending on Social Programs	3	2	5	4	3	4	5	1	3	2	1	3	1	3	5	4
Total Health Costs	4	4	4	5	3	4	4	5	4	4	5	5	1	5	3	5
Universal Health Care	5	5	5	5	5	5	5	5	5	5	5	5	4	5	5	5
Universal Rx	5	5	5	5	5	5	5	5	5	4	5	5	3	5	5	5
Life Expectancy at Birth	2	4	4	2	4	3	1	5	3	3	1	3	1	2	2	3
TOTAL	64	62	61	59	58	58	57	56	55	55	53	52	50	49	49	48

Understanding the Chart . . .

Mandatory Retirement Australia and the United States are the only countries on the list above that prohibit companies from making their employees retire at a certain age.

Age-Discrimination Laws The EU expects to have laws by 2006, but experts are skeptical that all countries will make the deadline.

Unemployment Rate In 2003, the Netherlands averaged lowest (3.8%); Spain, the highest (11.3%). The U.S. had 6%.

College Education The U.S. and Norway both get an A on this one: 28% of adults age 25–64 have a college degree.

Per Capita Income Compared with the countries above, the U.S. has the highest average standard of living; Norway is next.

Total Tax Burden Sweden collects the most taxes (51.4% of GDP).

Home Care In Australia and Denmark, more than 20% of those 65 and over receive home help—from medical care to tidying up. (In the Netherlands, its 12.8%; in the U.S., less than 10%.)

Retirement Age for Full Benefits Most grant benefits at 65. France is lowest—at 60—with citizens strongly protesting change; Denmark is 67.

Public Pension Replacement Rate Spain's retirement benefit as a percentage of an average workers earnings is highest, at 88%. Spain also has a high tax burden and the lowest income.

Employers Pension Coverage About 50% of U.S. workers have pension coverage at work. In some countries—Finland and Australia—employer pensions are required by law.

Economic Inequality Using an international definition, this is the percent of those whose income is in the lower quarter.

Economic Inequality for the Elderly In the U.S., the elderly fare slightly better than the general population.

Public Spending on Social Programs Income-support programs, such as social security and welfare, vary widely. Scandinavian countries traditionally offer the most.

Total Health Costs Americans spend the most (14.6% of GDP); Finland and Ireland, the least (7.3%).

Universal Health Care The U.S. is odd man out: 45 million—41%—have no health insurance, though most seniors have Medicare.

Universal Rx Canada has limitations and some gaps at the provincial level; 88% have coverage. The U.S. scores lowest, but changes in Medicare represent progress for the elderly.

Life Expectancy at Birth In the U.S., babies born in 2004 can expect to live to 77.3; in the Netherlands, to 78.6. Japan is highest at 81.9.

For more details on these criteria, go to www.aarpmagazine.org

Finland
Model Home

Drop a few coins into a slot machine in a local casino in Finland and you contribute to the care and comfort of retirees. Legal gambling in Finland is the exclusive province of the Slot Machine Association, a government-controlled nonprofit that pumps more than $50 million a year into the welfare of the country's 65-plus population (800,000 out of a total of 5.2 million).

Slot machine profits, for example, helped build the four-story Saga Senior Center, a complex of 138 units in Helsinki with cheerful apartments that are emphatically uninstitutional and that allow older people to have their own space and their own life. "It's the classiest senior home in Finland," says Leif Sonkin, a housing expert. "It's really like a spa." Indeed. Sunshine pours through the glass roof of the atrium, nourishing a lush semitropical garden. The swimming pool is indoor-outdoor and heated in winter. In the basement are saunas, essentials of Finnish life, and a well-equipped gym. (Pay no attention to its thick steel doors; the government requires bomb shelters in all buildings, a holdover from Cold War days.)

"The Saga center isn't a place for rich people," says administrator Mariana Boneva. A small apartment rents for about $600 a month. Most retirees can afford that, but "if they need it to live here, people can get a government housing subsidy," she adds.

Saga is one of three residences owned by the nonprofit Ruissalo Foundation. Although municipalities are charged by law with caring for older people, nonprofits have taken a major role; they operate more than half of Finland's "service housing" homes for the elderly. This shared responsibility is an extension of the egalitarian streak that started permeating policy in the 1950s, when Finland, along with Sweden, Norway, and Denmark, embraced an unabashedly liberal form of tax-supported welfare.

Finland's taxes are formidable. "I cannot say we love taxes," says Erikki Vaatanen, who lives with her husband, Orvokki, in the Wilhelmiina House, a new senior center. "But we know that schools, hospitals, and highways would go down if we didn't pay." Still, Vaatanen recently faced a drawback. After waiting a year for surgery for an arthritic wrist, she applied again, only to be told: "Little lady, you must wait two years more." So she went to a private physican for treatment and paid herself.

—M.E.

The European attitude is, we're all in this together and sooner or later we're all going to become older and need some help. The U.S. attitude is, we're all rugged individualists and we're going to take care of ourselves, not others.

How do the Dutch do it? How do their euros stretch further than our dollars? The key factor is lower costs. Although medicine isn't completely socialized—physicians and pharmacists, for example, aren't state employees—the government regulates almost all health expenses. That helps explain why, in the view of Professor Gerard F. Anderson of the Johns Hopkins Bloomberg School of Public Health, "in the U.S. we pay a lot more than anybody else for pretty much the same stuff." In analyzing health systems in the Netherlands and other industrialized nations, Anderson found that drugs, hospitals, and physicians' services were from 30 to 50 percent more expensive in the U.S., "and their health status is as good or better than ours."

Another factor is attitude. A strong feeling of "social solidarity," as Anderson sees it, makes Europeans inclined to be generous to older people, more willing to support them. "Their attitude is, we're in this together and sooner or later we're going to become older and we'll need some help," he says. "The U.S. attitude is, we're all rugged individualists and we're going to take care of ourselves, not others."

The Netherlands demonstrates its attitude toward older citizens (2 million are over 65) by showering them with numerous friendly perks, in addition to the big-ticket items such as pensions and health care. One example: seven days of free travel a year on the efficient rail system. "I go as far as possible," says Joris Korst, a 65-year-old civil servant in Nieuwegein. That's never very far in the Netherlands, which is only a third the size of Pennsylvania, but the destinations can be exhilarating—like the windswept beaches that Korst strolls in the West Frisian Islands. Museums, movies, concerts, campgrounds, and holiday bungalows are discounted, too. All this and a country that's worldly, prosperous, tolerant, steeped in art, and graced by canals, windmills, and tulip fields. What's not to like?

Health Care

The Dutch are accustomed to paying minuscule copayments for expensive treatment.

Dutch health insurance took care of teacher Van Essen when he needed a heart pacemaker. "He never saw a bill," his wife, Bep, recalls. Neither did civil servant Korst, who remembers that there were no charges when his wife, Trees, had cancer surgery followed by 32 chemotherapy treatments. "The whole country paid," he says, referring to the state-regulated insurance. In the U.S., those 32 treatments alone could have cost $30,000 or more, depending on the type and number of drugs used. Medicare might cover 80 percent, but the patient still could owe thousands.

Compare Trees's experience with that of Harold Powers, 79, and his wife, Ozelle, 82, retired educators in Tennessee. Powers paid about $200 of the bill for his bypass

Sweden
Shrinking Benefits

In a suburb of Stockholm, care for Aina Karlsson, 85, arrives twice a day, seven days a week. In the morning a *vårdbiträde* (care assistant) helps her bathe and dress; in the evening she helps her get ready for bed. Once a month she cleans the apartment that Aina shares with her husband, Einar. And twice a week she takes Aina to a gymnasium for exercise.

Life expectancy in Sweden is 80.4, one of the highest in Europe. Good care could be one reason. Aina has been receiving *hemhjälp* (home help) assistance since she suffered a stroke four years ago. Cost to the Karlssons: $159 a month. "Not very much," says Einar, a retired union official. To the municipal government, which provides Aina's care, the real cost is about five times greater. And if the Karlssons couldn't afford even $159, the government would provide a subsidy. "That's why Swedish taxes are so high," Einar says cheerfully, noting that income taxes shrink his own pension of $4,400 a month by a third.

Sweden is democratic, capitalistic, high-tech, and industrialized, well known for Ikea and Volvo. It is also well known as a prime example of a welfare state. Social spending, which includes payments such as pensions and welfare, equals 28.5 percent of GDP. In the U.S. it's 16.4 percent.

The income tax rate tops out at a breathtaking 58.2 percent, and there's a 25 percent VAT tax on most purchases. "Of course, many people say taxes are too high," remarks Nils-Erik Hogstedt, a home-care manager. "But the complaint isn't against the elderly. The great majority favor the care." Adds Pernilla Berggren, the manager of a retirement home: "People in Sweden are used to the community doing everything. You grow up expecting society to help take care of Mom."

Tens of thousands use *hemhjälp,* which enables people to remain in their own homes. "Sometimes we visit just once a month to clean," says Chatrin Engbo, head of a Stockholm district care office. "But if needed, we may go several times a day and at night."

This sounds nice—but expensive. To contain costs, the government recently sanctioned sharp cuts in home care by the municipalities, a move that upset many. "Home care used to include visits just to sit and have coffee two or three times a week, or just to take someone for a walk," says Berggren. "We do the essentials, but we can't afford those social moments anymore.

Reductions are also in the pipeline for the pension system, but for now a worker on the job for 30 years is customarily rewarded with a pension that replaces about 60 percent of his pay. (In the U.S. the Social Security replacement rate ranges from about 30 to 60 percent.)

The government's worry about future solvency began in the 1990s. The percentage of 65-plussers, almost one in five of the 8.9 million Swedes, is one of Europe's highest. As with U.S. Social Security, pension payments made by active workers support retirees. With low birth rates and the increase of pensioners, experts estimate that by 2035 the system will be seriously out of balance, with about two workers supporting each older person. (By then, America will be in the same boat.)

Looking ahead, the parliament recently approved drastic, complicated revisions. Out the window went the defined-benefit pension—a set amount based on salary and years of service—replaced by a system based on contributions by worker and employer. The benefit will be indexed to wage growth, with a built-in expectancy that the rate will grow 1.6 percent annually. If wages don't grow that much, the benefit drops. The plan phases in fully in 2019, with the retirement of those born in 1954.

There's yet another new wrinkle: mandated private investments. Besides paying into the pension's main part (employee and employer contribute a total of 16 percent of the worker's wages), all workers are required to put an additional 2.5 percent into their choice of investments—an idea that has become popular among world pension experts. A voluntary form of this setup is favored by President George W. Bush.

Swedes were optimistic in 2000, when this change took effect, even though many were confused by the hundreds of funds, Swedish and foreign, competing for their kronor. The timing proved terrible. The return averaged 3.5 percent in 2001, and then *katastrof!* Or so said a civil servant who saw a thousand dollars vanish from her stock account as markets toppled worldwide. More than 2 million Swedes lost 30 to 40 percent of their mandated investments. (By July 2004, the average fund had recovered nearly 19 percent.)

One likely outcome of the radically revised system: to earn higher pension benefits more Swedes will work beyond the typical retirement age of 60. Says Barbro Westerholm, president of the Swedish Association of Senior Citizens: "I've recommended to my children that they plan to work until they are 70."

heart surgery because Medicare picked up 80 percent of the tab and his private Medigap insurance (which costs extra) paid most of the rest. But, in addition, he and Ozelle spend about $3,000 a year for medicines, and Medicare won't cover any of that until 2006. Van Essen, on the other hand, pays nothing for the medicine he takes to prevent migraines. In 2003, however, the Dutch health ministry proposed that everyone make a copayment of $1.75 for each prescription—but backed down when the people protested.

There is also a government limit on the amount a hospital may bill an insurance company for a pacemaker—Van

O Canada!

The pain in her back was terrible, recalls Diane Tupper, who lives in a Vancouver suburb. When she finally got a consultation with a neurosurgeon—after waiting eight months—he said he could fix her spine. Then he delivered the bad news: "Our surgery waiting time is a year and a half to two years."

If Tupper, a 63-year-old lawyer, could hold out, her surgery would be free under Canada's universal-care system. But if she hopped over the border to St. Joseph Hospital in Bellingham, Washington, she could be in the operating room in days. The cost would be about $47,000. "I'm not a well-off person," Tupper says, "but I felt I didn't have any choice." Tupper took out two lines of credit, borrowed $14,500 from a friend, and went to Bellingham.

To many Americans, Canada may look like health care's promised land. Care for all 32.5 million citizens is paid for from taxes. Drugs are typically 30 to 50 percent cheaper than in the U.S.—which is why more than a million statesiders now get prescriptions filled in Canada.

But recently, Canada's system has fallen behind, hobbled by budget cuts, regulations, and shortages of physicians, nurses, and sophisticated equipment such as MRI machines. A recent survey put the backlog of unperformed procedures at 876,584. The waiting time for a hip replacement in Tupper's province, British Columbia, is nearly a year, even longer for a knee replacement.

Filling that gap are U.S. border cities such as Buffalo, New York, and Great Falls, Montana. Minot, North Dakota, attracts people needing CT scans and MRIs, for which they'd wait months in Saskatchewan. Randy Schwan of Trinity Health in Minot says Canadians are amazed to find that "a doctor says we've got to get a test, and the same day someone wheels them down the hall for that test." At the globally famous Mayo Clinic in Rochester, Minnesota, Canadians are the largest foreign-patient constituency.

Some provinces cover care outside of Canada under special circumstances. To trim the waiting list of cancer patients needing radiation treatment, Ontario picked up the bill for 1,650 people who went to the U.S. in 2000 and 2001.

So, get to a Canadian hospital's emergency room after a heart attack and you'll be treated promptly—with no worry about cost. But the system, once the nation's pride, has become, as one official says, "functionally obsolete."

—M.E.

These kinds of controls are not always painless. Just this past year, the Dutch government hit a nerve when it decided to boost the $6-per-hour cost of home care by 250 percent. Half a million citizens, most of them beyond the age of 65, have been receiving subsidized home visits by health professionals or workers who clean and tidy up (like most developed countries, the Netherlands wants to help people maintain their independence and avoid going into nursing homes as long as possible). However, at the increased rate of about $15 an hour, despite government subsidies, home care is rapidly climbing out of sight for many low-income retirees. This increase takes effect, moreover, at an awkward time when the country has a nursing-home waiting list of some 50,000.

Still, all things considered, the Dutch like their health care. In a Harvard School of Public Health survey (taken before the increase in home-care costs), 70 percent said they were satisfied with the system. The same study rated the satisfaction level in the U.S. at 40 percent. And this even when the U.S. spends far more on health care than any other nation in the world—an average of $5,440 per person, with a large share of that going toward retirees.

Canada, by the way, doesn't score much better. Just 46 percent say they are satisfied. Although Canadians receive low-cost prescription drugs, thanks to government controls, health services are underfunded and waiting periods for treatment are long (see the sidebar "O Canada!").

Waiting. That seems to be the tradeoff. Someone who needs open-heart surgery in the Netherlands might have to sit around for 14 weeks before a time slot and hospital space become available. Hip surgery? You're maybe looking at an average wait of eight weeks. Like much of Europe and also Canada, the Netherlands is short of hospital beds and medical staff. Dutch officials say no one has to wait for emergency attention, and some patients are being sent to Germany and Belgium for faster treatment. Still, the delays underscore a major difference between Dutch and U.S. care. Says one not-so-happy Dutch resident: "I don't care what they say. If you need open-heart surgery here, you can die before you get it."

"In America we love responsiveness," says Anderson, the Johns Hopkins expert. "We're the best on responsiveness." But ready access to care, he adds, is one of the reasons Americans pay more than people do in other countries. Anderson is one of a number of health specialists and economists who have been pointing out the built-in inefficiencies of U.S. care. Some critics argue that the huge number of health-insurance providers—HMOs, PPOs, Medicare, Medicaid, and all the rest—consumes far more in overhead than would one or two providers and that their many forms and complicated

Essen's was $5,750, plus the expense of the procedure. In the U.S., a pacemaker can cost as much as a car—$15,000 to $20,000, just for the device. The whole procedure can zoom up to $50,000. In the Netherlands, government pressure on hospitals, doctors, and manufacturers helps to keep costs down.

rules drive up hospital administrative costs. Others point to the huge sums spent advertising and marketing drugs and hospitals.

In Sweden, with its low birth rate and increasing number of pensioners, experts estimate that by 2035 the system will be seriously out of balance, with only about two workers supporting each older person.

Taxes

The Dutch in particular pay quite a lot to take care of one another. The personal income tax rate in the Netherlands isn't Europe's highest, but it's well up there, with a top rate of 52 percent on any income over $60,000. (The top U.S. rate has been going down during the presidency of George W. Bush and now stands at 35 percent. A family of four with an income of about $60,000 would be in the 25 percent tax bracket.)

Almost half of Dutch taxes go to the universal pension fund, known as the AOW, which provides the basic pension that everyone receives at age 65. The AOW takes a salary bite of 17.9 percent. Most Dutch workers have an employer-provided pension based on payments by worker and employer—that's another salary bite of 6 or 7 percent.

Then comes a bigger bite: a 12.05 percent contribution to help pay for basic state health insurance, known as the AWBZ, which, like the basic pension, is universal. Besides paying for care for grave illnesses and a place in a nursing home (after a wait), it also covers part (but less now) of the cost of home care. Most workers also have government-regulated insurance with private or nonprofit companies for lesser medical expenses and medicines. Employers usually pay most of this cost; the worker's share is only about 1.7 percent of income.

On top of that formidable raft of outlays, there's also a stiff value-added tax (VAT tax) of 19 percent on most things you buy. There's a 12 percent tax on food. And a whopping tax of as much as 40 percent on new cars (plus roughly $6 for a gallon of gas). Yet costs like these haven't stopped Wilhelmina and Cornelius van der Hoop, both retired teachers, from driving all around Europe towing a trailer.

The couple has a combined pension of about $41,000 after all deductions. "We have no reason to complain," Wilhelmina says. "All those taxes help other people."

In fact, polls show that the majority of Dutch citizens don't object to the large salary deduction that sustains the AOW. "The general attitude in the Netherlands—if you ask the man in the street—is that people who have worked their entire lives should be protected from poverty," says pension expert Maarten Lindeboom, an economist at the Free University of Amsterdam.

Dutch citizens with higher-than-average incomes usually invest in a private pension plan or annuities. That's what retired physician-turned-tour guide Anna Sophia Fischer did years ago. These investments put her annual income in the $60,000 range, where the taxman ordinarily takes a large bite. But thanks to reductions granted to people over 65, her tax is only about 30 percent of her income. As a physician, Fischer was well acquainted with the fabled liberality of the health system. "If you want a sex-change operation, the government will pay for it," she says. "I do think that goes a bit too far." A recent innovation: marijuana available by prescription for pain.

A noticeable difference in most of Europe's treatment of older people is the absence of laws that forbid discrimination and age-based mandatory retirement. In the U.S., mandatory retirement has been illegal for most occupations since 1986. Says one Dutch pension expert: "Here it is automatic that at 65 the job is over." The European Union has mandated that its 25 member states introduce laws against age discrimination by 2006, but the word is that loopholes will permit mandatory retirement to continue. Laurie McCann, senior attorney with AARP Foundation Litigation, concludes that the EU is a long way from either "talking the talk" or "walking the walk" when it comes to eliminating age discrimination.

Today some 14 percent of Americans 65 and older—about 4.8 million people in all—are still on the job; that's one of the highest rates in the industrialized world. Most European workers retire at age 60 or so, taking advantage of pension generosity.

The need for a ban on mandatory retirement hasn't seemed all that urgent. Frits Velker, a foreman at a Dutch plumbing and sheet-metal company, was 59 when the company was sold. "I looked around and saw so many other people who had retired early," he says. So Velker did too. His company pension is about $27,000, and when he turns 65 he and wife Gerrie will receive about $14,000 a year from the AOW, the state pension fund. In general, a worker in the Netherlands can expect a total pension equaling about 70 percent of his salary if he worked for 40 years. Thanks to cost-of-living adjustments, former teacher Van Essen's pension is slightly higher—72 percent of his salary—even though his teaching career stopped after 38 years.

Such generous retirement benefits are under siege all across Europe (and Japan). Cutbacks and proposed cutbacks in care and pensions provoked angry strikes last year in France, Italy, Germany, and Austria. Even in Sweden, shining star of the Scandinavian welfare-state constellation, benefits have shrunk. With increasing concern, governments are facing challenging demographics: swelling ranks of longer-living older citizens and thinning ranks of workers able—and willing—to pay for benefits.

MIKE EDWARDS, a writer and editor for *National Geographic* magazine for 34 years, has received national awards for articles on Chernobyl and pollution in the former U.S.S.R. Also contributing to this article was **SOPHIE KORCZYK,** an economist and consultant based in Alexandria, Virginia.

Population Aging, Entitlement Growth, and the Economy

Demographic aging—the graying of the baby boomers, increasing longevity, and low fertility rates—is changing the age structure of the United States. Many experts say these changes will have an unsustainable impact on the federal budget by causing rapid growth in federal spending for health and retirement benefits for older Americans, especially for Social Security, Medicare, and Medicaid.

Demographic aging may also negatively affect the U.S. economy and American families. Low fertility rates will slow the growth in the labor force; fewer workers will be available to support an aging population. A slower-growing labor force will slow economic growth. If left unchecked, increased deficits and government debt will choke off investment and further stifle economic growth. The slowing of economic growth will mean stagnant wages and slower family income growth as well. Health costs, which have outstripped economic growth even in prosperous times, will continue to increase faster than family incomes.

Can we afford our aging society? Is our fiscal future as bleak as many experts claim? In this report, John Gist takes a long-term perspective on these questions, examining the historical experience with "entitlements" and projecting out to the middle of this century. Looking backward, entitlement spending has actually been remarkably stable as a percentage of gross domestic product (GDP) for the past two decades, with one exception—health care. By 2016, Social Security will still consume about the same share of the economy as it did when Ronald Reagan was first elected president. Eventually, Social Security's costs will rise by two percent of GDP, but after 2030, when the last boomer has retired, Social Security will resume a gradual and manageable growth path. Other nonhealth entitlements will remain a smaller share of GDP than they were 40 years ago.

It is in health care only where entitlement growth presents serious future challenges. Rapid growth in health care costs is really nothing new, however. Overall health care costs, including Medicare and Medicaid, have risen faster than the economy for decades and are projected to do so indefinitely, with Medicare overtaking Social Security as the largest federal program within 20 years. However, contrary to much conventional wisdom, population aging is not the chief cause of this growth. An aging population accounts for only about one-sixth of Medicare's growth since 1970.

Our long-term budgetary challenge is to maintain the integrity of the social insurance programs that provide health and income security for current and future retirees without sustaining economic ruin. Our ability to achieve that goal will depend chiefly on two factors: the growth rate of health care costs and the willingness of the populace to be taxed. A starting point for avoiding a future "train wreck" would be to maintain the same level of spending restraint in our health programs that we have already achieved in the past decade *and* refrain from enacting any additional tax cuts, allowing revenues to rise automatically. This would hold the primary deficit (revenues minus noninterest spending) to a level in 2050 no larger than it is today. Because debt would still be rising in this scenario, additional policy solutions would be needed. Reforms to the health care system, making Social Security solvent, introducing greater budget discipline, getting people to work longer and save more would allow us to provide economic and health security while achieving fiscal stability and sustaining long-term economic growth.

For full report, see *AARP Public Policy Institute Paper* #2007–01.
In Brief prepared by John Gist, January 2007.

Test-Your-Knowledge Form

We encourage you to photocopy and use this page as a tool to assess how the articles in *Annual Editions* expand on the information in your textbook. By reflecting on the articles you will gain enhanced text information. You can also access this useful form on a product's book support website at *http://www.mhhe.com/cls*.

NAME:

DATE:

TITLE AND NUMBER OF ARTICLE:

BRIEFLY STATE THE MAIN IDEA OF THIS ARTICLE:

LIST THREE IMPORTANT FACTS THAT THE AUTHOR USES TO SUPPORT THE MAIN IDEA:

WHAT INFORMATION OR IDEAS DISCUSSED IN THIS ARTICLE ARE ALSO DISCUSSED IN YOUR TEXTBOOK OR OTHER READINGS THAT YOU HAVE DONE? LIST THE TEXTBOOK CHAPTERS AND PAGE NUMBERS:

LIST ANY EXAMPLES OF BIAS OR FAULTY REASONING THAT YOU FOUND IN THE ARTICLE:

LIST ANY NEW TERMS/CONCEPTS THAT WERE DISCUSSED IN THE ARTICLE, AND WRITE A SHORT DEFINITION:

We Want Your Advice

ANNUAL EDITIONS revisions depend on two major opinion sources: one is our Advisory Board, listed in the front of this volume, which works with us in scanning the thousands of articles published in the public press each year; the other is you—the person actually using the book. Please help us and the users of the next edition by completing the prepaid article rating form on this page and returning it to us. Thank you for your help!

ANNUAL EDITIONS: Aging 10/11

ARTICLE RATING FORM

Here is an opportunity for you to have direct input into the next revision of this volume.
We would like you to rate each of the articles listed below, using the following scale:

1. **Excellent: should definitely be retained**
2. **Above average: should probably be retained**
3. **Below average: should probably be deleted**
4. **Poor: should definitely be deleted**

Your ratings will play a vital part in the next revision.
Please mail this prepaid form to us as soon as possible.
Thanks for your help!

RATING	ARTICLE	RATING	ARTICLE
	1. Elderly Americans		21. Keep Pace with Older Workers
	2. You Can Stop "Normal" Aging		22. Color Me Confident
	3. Living Longer: Diet and Exercise		23. Work/Retirement Choices and Lifestyle Patterns of Older Americans
	4. Secrets to Longevity		
	5. Will You Live to Be 100?		24. Development of Hospice and Palliative Care in the United States
	6. Faulty Fountains of Youth		
	7. Failure to Thrive: Interventions to Improve Quality of Life in the Older Adult		25. The Grieving Process
			26. End-of-Life Preferences: A Theory-Driven Inventory
	8. Overweight and Mortality among Baby Boomers— Now We're Getting Personal		27. Mind Frames towards Dying and Factors Motivating Their Adoption by Terminally Ill Elders
	9. Lifetime Achievements		
	10. We Can Control How We Age		28. Oh, Lord, Don't Put Me in a Nursing Home
	11. Society Fears the Aging Process		29. Where to Live as We Age
	12. A Healthy Mind, a Longer Life		30. Finding a Good Home
	13. Research: Oldest Americans Happiest		31. Declaration of Independents: Home Is Where You Want to Live Forever. Here's How
	14. The Under-Reported Impact of Age Discrimination and Its Threat to Business Vitality		
			32. Dignified Retirement: Lessons from Abroad
	15. Alzheimer's—The Case for Prevention		33. Social Security's 70th Anniversary: Surviving 20 Years of Reform
	16. Brain Cancer: Could Adult Stem Cells Be the Cause—and the Cure?		
			34. The Corporate Beneficiaries of the Medicare Drug Benefit
	17. Trust and Betrayal in the Golden Years		
	18. The Extent and Frequency of Abuse in the Lives of Older Women and Their Relationship with Health Outcomes		35. Coverage for All
			36. Riding into the Sunset: The Geezer Threat
			37. The New Face of Health Care
	19. Retire Right		38. As Good as It Gets
	20. Money for Life		39. Population Aging, Entitlement Growth, and the Economy

ABOUT YOU

Name

Date

Are you a teacher? ❑ A student? ❑
Your school's name

Department

Address   City   State   Zip

School telephone #

YOUR COMMENTS ARE IMPORTANT TO US!

Please fill in the following information:
For which course did you use this book?

Did you use a text with this ANNUAL EDITION? ❑ yes ❑ no
What was the title of the text?

What are your general reactions to the Annual Editions concept?

Have you read any pertinent articles recently that you think should be included in the next edition? Explain.

Are there any articles that you feel should be replaced in the next edition? Why?

Are there any World Wide Websites that you feel should be included in the next edition? Please annotate.

May we contact you for editorial input? ❑ yes ❑ no
May we quote your comments? ❑ yes ❑ no